Herbal Treatment of Children

For Elsevier Butterworth-Heinemann

Commissioning Editor: Susan Young
Development Editor: Catherine Jackson
Project Manager: Andrew Palfreyman
Designer: George Ajayi

Herbal Treatment of Children

Western and Ayurvedic Perspectives

Anne McIntyre FNIMH

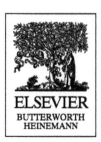

ELSEVIER
BUTTERWORTH
HEINEMANN

EDINBURGH LONDON NEW YORK OXFORD PHILADELPHIA ST LOUIS SYDNEY TORONTO 2005

ELSEVIER
BUTTERWORTH
HEINEMANN

First published 2005

ISBN 0 7506 5174 1

British Library Cataloguing in Publication Data
A catalogue record for this book is available from the British Library

Library of Congress Cataloging in Publication Data
A catalog record for this book is available from the Library of Congress

Notice

Medical knowledge and best practice in this field are constantly changing. As new research and experience broaden our knowledge, changes in practice, treatment and drug therapy may become necessary or appropriate. Readers are advised to check the most current information provided (i) on procedures featured or (ii) by the manufacturer of each product to be administered, to verify the recommended dose or formula, the method and duration of administration, and contraindications. It is the responsibility of the practitioner, relying on their own experience and knowledge of the patient, to make diagnoses, to determine dosages and the best treatment for each individual patient, and to take all appropriate safety precautions. To the fullest extent of the law, neither the publisher nor the editors assumes any liability for any injury and/or damage.

The Publisher

Working together to grow
libraries in developing countries

www.elsevier.com | www.bookaid.org | www.sabre.org

 ELSEVIER   BOOK AID International   Sabre Foundation

ELSEVIER your source for books, journals and multimedia in the health sciences

www.elsevierhealth.com

The Publisher's policy is to use **paper manufactured from sustainable forests**

Printed and bound by CPI Group (UK) Ltd, Croydon, CR0 4YY

Transferred to digital print 2013

Contents

Introduction

At the age of 16 I was given a book that, unknown to me then, was to have far-reaching effects in my life. The book was called *The Wisdom of India* (Yutang Lin 1966) and it included Hymns from the Rigveda, the Upanishads, The Bhagavad Gita and The Dhammapada as well as other ancient Indian texts. Its writings inspired me and resonated in a way that my Christian upbringing and regular church attendance had never done. I was delighted when I found a Buddhist meditation class locally and befriended the teacher who taught me much about the Buddhist way over the next couple of years while I was doing my A levels. When the pressure was on to find a suitable course at university I applied to study Eastern religion and Sanskrit and as soon as I could, after finishing my exams, I took a year out and set off to India to discover the source of such great wisdom.

Several years later, while living in a cottage on a small island off the East coast of England, growing my own food and harvesting as much from the wild as I could, I began to learn about the wild herbs that were growing around me. I realized that the earth provides the raw ingredients for our health and well-being and that, amazingly, herbs have the ability to keep us in balance on all levels of our existence – body, mind, emotions and spirit – if we could only understand their gifts to us to their fullest extent. I resolved to find a place to study herbal medicine and even managed to persuade my local education authority to give me a grant to study, which was a first in the UK.

Once in practice as a medical herbalist I continued to study, constantly searching for more pointers towards understanding the human organism and the keys to health and harmony, so that I could better serve my patients as well as my family and myself. Over the next few years I studied homoeopathy, aromatherapy, therapeutic massage and counselling. Around 1989 I heard about an eminent doctor from India, Dr Vasant Lad, coming to the UK to give a course on Ayurvedic medicine and applied immediately. Within a very short time I realized that here was the answer I was looking for to bridge that gap between my love of Eastern philosophy and my practice as a medical herbalist. Ayurveda is a body of knowledge and wisdom incorporating a complex system of medicine as well as guidelines for a way of living, the aim of which was not only freedom from suffering in mind and body but enlightenment itself.

Since then I have continued to study Ayurveda and slowly to incorporate its wisdom into my practice and now into my writing. Its effect has been a gradual transformation of my life as well as my herbal practice, that has evolved over the last 12–14 years, which is reflected here in my approach to the treatment of children. For the sake of clarity and understanding for readers, I have tried to keep the Western and Ayurvedic approach separate in treatment advice given in each chapter, although in practice my approach is more integrated.

The writing of this book is motivated by the growing interest in herbal medicine amongst mainstream and complementary healthcare practitioners. By some this interest has even been described as an enormous need for information in a climate of holism, health education and health promotion rather than illness and bio medicine. The intention of this book is to provide a practical guide for health professionals to inform them and to highlight the contribution of herbal medicines to the field of paediatric care. This book could facilitate the practitioners' inclusion of some herbs within their scope of practice, but for herbs to be used effectively they are always best prescribed to aid the homoeostatic mechanisms of the mind–body while addressing the underlying problems that give rise to ill health, including diet and lifestyle. There is no point for example, giving laxatives to a child with constipation who continues to eat a diet high in refined carbohydrates and deficient in fruit and vegetables.

Healthcare professionals often refer patients to a medical herbalist because of lack of knowledge of appropriate herbs for children and lack of confidence when giving advice about herbs. They may still want to refer on even once better informed, relying on the herbalists' greater knowledge and experience of herbs, but there could be a greater and more meaningful symbiosis between herbalist and mainstream healthcare professionals, each gaining from the other's specialist knowledge and skills. Healthcare professionals dealing with members of the public who would like to use herbal medicine, need to be aware of the indications and contraindications of herbs, even if they are not using them themselves, as part of their clients' health choice option. While many GPs, nurses and health visitors may have little knowledge of herbal treatments and have no interest in using them, they realize that many of their patients are already doing so. They may even have a medical herbalist amongst their practitioners working alongside them at their surgery where patients can consult the herbalist on the NHS. One advantage of orthodox healthcare practitioners being at least familiar with appropriate plant medicines for children is that it enables better conversation between practitioners and parents regarding the best treatment available for their child in a language that those keen to use complementary medicine will find meaningful.

There is an enormous wealth of wisdom and knowledge that has developed over thousands of years concerning health and disease that is still used by billions of people all over the world, which we are able to draw on in the prevention and effective treatment of children today. The world of complementary medicine may well contain much of this wisdom and at least can provide invaluable choice of therapies that can be used alongside allopathic medicine in primary health care. The availability of therapies including homoeopathy, acupuncture, massage, aromatherapy, nutritional medicine, and herbal medicine, provides choice when considering optimal health for children and families. As the name suggests, complementary medicine can be used to complement and support conventional medicine in both the prevention and treatment of disease and it fulfils a great need. Generally speaking, the children that I see in my practice are those with chronic problems for which orthodox medicine has not enough to offer or has not been successful in resolving in the long term. Asthma, eczema and other skin conditions, hay fever, sleep problems, behavioural problems, bowel disorders and a range of stress-related conditions are some that I frequently encounter.

As far as both Western and Ayurvedic herbal medicine is concerned, they have their roots in history that extend back thousands of years and in folk medicine, but their modern practice is being increasingly vindicated by research and scientific evidence that supports its traditional use. The popularity of herbal medicine over the past 20 years has been instrumental in motivating much of this research. In the first few years we have seen herbs being hailed as miracle remedies and panaceas, and because they were "natural" apparently they were devoid of the side effects of allopathic medicines that the public were beginning to voice their complaints about. The rebound effect then followed and alarms concerning the safety of herbs have been raised by one article after another about the dangers of many plant medicines. With insufficient real evidence the public and professionals alike are susceptible to media hype but with an increase in real information they will hopefully realize that the answer lies somewhere in between. Anyone using herbs or treating patients who take herbs, needs to be aware of their possible risks as well as their benefits, and to take advantage of up-to-date information increasingly available and to draw on the knowledge of professional herbalists when applicable. Today's medical herbalists have the best of both worlds, a blend of old and new, with their practice based on a thorough knowledge of the traditional uses of plant medicines as well as their biochemistry and pharmacology which is constantly updated. They can advise patients and professionals alike about the safe and effective use of herbal medicines and steer them through the quagmire of questions regarding dosage, interactions and contraindications, so that the confidence in herbal medicine that it deserves is ascertained.

The format of the book follows a systems approach including the main systems affected by "common" childhood illness, and has purposely omitted the cardiovascular, endocrine and reproductive systems because of the more complex and serious nature of problems affecting these systems. The age limit on childhood problems I have taken as adolescence. The health problems covered in the text are those that I have commonly encountered in my practice of nearly 25 years as a medical herbalist and those that I consider to be applicable to treatment using herbs. I have endeavoured to describe both the Western and Ayurvedic approach in most cases, including the herbs I use in my practice as well as in traditional practice in India. The text includes guidelines for treatment of infectious diseases that may not be common, due to widespread immunization. This does not necessarily mean that I am taking an anti-immunization stance, it is purely for the reason that parents *do* have choice on these matters and these infections do still exist and hence may require treatment.

To the orthodox eye, the herbal and Ayurvedic philosophy and approach to treatment of illness may follow some rather unorthodox/unconventional lines and it may well be said that there is little scientific justification for, for example, the use of mild diuretic and laxative herbs to clear the body of "accumulated toxins". Suffice to say that several ancient and respected systems of medicine, such as the Chinese, Tibetan and Ayurvedic systems, that have survived almost intact for at least 5000 years until the present day, providing the framework for the health care of literally millions of people, have such ideas central to their philosophy. For this reason the modern herbalist cannot overlook their consideration and their lack of inclusion in a book such as this would be a sad omission. It would mean that the use of herbs suggested was symptomatic rather than holistic and this would negate much of the rationale for considering the use of herbs here in the first place.

As Dr Andrew Dunford said in answer to the question "What is herbal medicine?" – "Phytotherapy can be defined as the study and application of the therapeutic effects of plant materials within an holistic context." (Eldin and Dunford 1999). The point is not simply to use herbs as drugs but in the wider context of holism, as well as in preventative health and health promotion.

Obviously the decisions regarding health care for children are largely made by parents, but the way forward in primary health care of children may well lie in these decisions being made in conjunction with informed knowledge of healthcare professionals, doctors, nurses and health visitors. An integrated approach to health care that considers a variety of treatment possibilities and is able to draw on what works best in each individual case is naturally preferable. This may be a herbal remedy or antibiotics, or both, supported by optimum nutrition and certain dietary modifications. It is fast becoming clear that complementary therapies and allopathic medicine *can* support one another and make for an integrated health service which not only can provide the best treatment for each child, but also minimize unnecessary spending of precious funds.

References

Eldin S, Dunford A 1999 Herbal Medicine in Primary Care. Butterworth-Heinemann, Oxford

Lin Yutang (ed) 1966 The Wisdom of India. Jaico Publishing House, Bombay

Chapter 1

Understanding herbs

PHILOSOPHICAL CONSIDERATIONS BEHIND HERBAL PRACTICE

We owe much to the scientific world and modern technology that has identified specific properties and interactions of botanical constituents, but at the same time we need to remember that this research for the most part vindicates the ancient use of such plants that goes back thousands of years. For professional herbalists, plant pharmacology is a modern development that augments their skill and knowledge, which is based on the accumulated knowledge and practice of countless generations. It is not the total foundation on which they base their practice, perhaps rather their ability to justify it to the world of science. In the "whole plant–whole person interactions" detailed knowledge of the effects of single constituents does not account for the multifactorial complexities involved (Hoffman). Interestingly it is not predominantly the world of science that has promoted the use of herbal remedies. The lead has come from the general public who have championed herbal medicine in their search for effective treatment of common and chronic ailments, and therapies that address the underlying causes of disease rather than simply treating the symptoms.

A "HOLISTIC" APPROACH

Not only are we rediscovering valuable herbal medicines but also the ancient medical systems that incorporate them, which have much to offer us, and provided a framework in which these herbs were prescribed. Basic to these traditions, East and West, is an understanding that health is derived from a balance of natural forces in the body and that symptoms and disease come from a disturbance of this balance. According to their philosophy, the body has a natural ability to regulate and heal itself, homoeostatic mechanisms that manifest themselves in the amazing feats that the body performs constantly as it protects, heals and regulates itself. This is known as the Vital Force, Prana or Qi. We maintain a steady state in temperature, blood sugar level, fluid levels, blood chemistry, heart and respiration rates despite the constant variables that could otherwise disturb our equilibrium. When poor diet, pollution, stress, overwork and other factors combine with inherited or constitutional predisposition to overcome our powers of adaptation and ill health results, the task of the practitioner is to enhance homoeostasis through the use of herbs and foods.

We have also been re-evaluating what is actually meant by health. Do we mean simply absence of symptoms that may well define health from an orthodox medical point of view, or can we really embrace the WHO definition: "The condition of perfect bodily, spiritual and social well-being and not solely the absence of disease and injury."? According to traditional medical philosophy, health depends on the harmony of body, mind and spirit and any symptom that arises needs to be seen in the context of the patient as a whole, their lives inner and outer. Bearing this in mind, ideally herbs need to be prescribed not only to redress specific physical imbalances, but also to attend to the deeper causes of imbalance. In practice the emphasis is on health and well-being rather than disease.

The aim of the professional herbalist is treatment that enables a patient to return to health with an understanding of the factors in their life that predisposed them to ill health in the first place. Health education is an integrated aspect of modern herbal practice. The result is that the patient benefits from the exchange not only with relief of symptoms but also better overall health and knowledge that will serve them as prevention for the future. Each patient is evaluated as an individual, the current symptoms exhibited are seen in relation to the complete medical history, past and present symptoms, and also to the patient's life as a whole. Only then can the correct strategy for treatment be developed. To illustrate, a child who presents with chronic sinusitis may not find a lasting and effective cure by simply taking antibiotics. Examination of past medical history may show that the child has a history of atopic eczema and asthma, recent development of hayfever in spring and early summer, and a long-term allergy to cats. Questioning about diet may reveal that the child was not breastfed, has chronically sluggish bowels, a high intake of milk products, white bread and sugary foods and drinks, and is not very keen on eating fruit and vegetables. Clearly there needs to be a considerable amount of dietary counselling for the family, as well as remedies that address the underlying problems of immunity combined with decongestant and antimicrobial herbs. In this instance one particular herb springs instantly to mind and that is chamomile; an excellent antimicrobial herb, with astringent and decongestant properties. Not only that but it is an outstanding remedy for atopic conditions as it soothes the histamine-mediated response.

THE HERBALIST'S TOOLS

The therapeutic tools of the herbalists are of course the roots, stems, barks, resins, leaves, flowers, fruits and seeds of plants. Today it is important that herbalists obtain their remedies from a sustainable source of herbs, for several valued herbs are becoming increasingly rare and even under threat of extinction. By definition a herb is any plant that has a therapeutic action in the body and naturally this includes most of the fruit and vegetable kingdom. Raspberries are full of vitamins and minerals. In addition to their nutritional value and delicious taste they have been used for thousands of years for throat and chest problems and the whole plant is well known for a variety of applications during pregnancy and childbirth (McIntyre 1994). Garlic and onions are excellent health-promoting and medicinal foods. They contain sulphur, germanium and selenium and are well known for their ability to enhance the immune system, reduce serum cholesterol levels, and as antioxidants to prevent free radical damage and prevent degenerative disease and cancer (Kuhn and Winston 2001).

From a "scientific" point of view, many herbal medicines are considered to be experimental. However, it is important not to forget that herbal medicines have stood the test of time, having been used and tested for thousands of years before the introduction of modern sophisticated drugs, and the human race has managed to survive! Many familiar and potent medicines of the 21st century were developed from herbs. Over the last hundred years or so scientists have isolated and then synthesized the active principles of these plants for use in pharmaceutical preparations. Cinchona bark, for example is the source of quinine, the anti-malaria drug; periwinkle is the source of vincristine, the anti-tumour drug, and the opium poppy is the source of morphine and codeine. Atropine, aspirin,

digoxin and ephedrine are all plant-derived drugs of unquestionable value. Long before the discovery of modern antibiotics, echinacea was one of the most commonly prescribed remedies for infections. It is clear this was well founded as echinacea has the ability to stimulate the production and activity of leucocytes and phagocytosis, to increase macrophage activity, T-cell activity and production of interferon (Kuhn and Winston 2001).

WHOLE PLANT MEDICINES

While science has tended to regard medicinal plants as a source of active ingredients, herbalists have preferred to stick to the use of whole-plant medicines and there are a variety of reasons for this. As plants were examined under the microscope and active ingredients identified, single constituents were isolated to replace whole-plant medicines. Then, as many of these were able to be synthesized in the laboratory, herbs that had been revered for centuries as powerful healers began to be considered old-fashioned and almost obsolete. The belief of pharmacologists was that if a man-made product was similar to one derived from the plant world it would be assimilated similarly by the body, and that it was superior to a plant medicine due to the fact that it was not subject to the relatively random laws of nature. Its active ingredients were quantifiable and therefore the dosage more reliable. However, this isolation and synthesis of potent active ingredients can have its drawbacks as it is likely to increase the risk of toxicity and side effects. The modern herbalist still advocates the use of the whole plant as a gentler and safer form of treatment.

There are many types of substance found in medicinal plants, all of which work synergistically together and probably have an equally important role to play therapeutically. The primary healing agents are the active constituents which seized the imagination of the early chemists and which have developed into modern drugs. Then there are other apparently secondary and less-significant agents, whose actual value should not be overlooked. These play an essential role in determining how effective the primary healing agents will be, by rendering the body more or less receptive to their powers. Some of these synergistic substances will make the active constituents more easily assimilated and readily available in the body, while others will buffer the action of other potent plant chemicals, thus preventing any possible side effects. It is the natural combination of both types of substances that determines the healing power and safety of the herbal medicines.

QUESTIONS OF SAFETY AND TOXICITY

Of most concern among orthodox healthcare practitioners, particularly to those unfamiliar with herbs, is the question of their possible toxicity, especially when it comes to prescribing herbs to children. Interestingly, parents and children are increasingly turning to herbal medicine and other forms of complementary medicines for their health needs, for both treatment of existing conditions and preventative health care. The main reasons for doing so are fear of unwanted side effects of orthodox drugs, along with more consultation time to address causes rather than symptoms. I can safely say that during 20 years of practice, I have rarely witnessed an adverse reaction in a child to a herbal medicine I have prescribed. Those rare cases that have occurred have consisted of mild rashes or slightly loose stools. Having said this, it is clear that herbs contain a huge variety of chemical components that, although generally safe, carry the potential of causing allergic reactions and idiosyncratic hypersensitive responses in the same way that foods do. Most of these can be avoided by familiarizing oneself with the chemistry of the herbal medicines that one is prescribing and giving herbs that are appropriate to a specific patient (having taken a detailed case history) in correct doses.

It is of course impossible to predict whether a child is going to react adversely or allergically to a herb, but there are certain herbs that are more likely to produce an allergic reaction, such as those from the aster family. (For more on plant chemistry and their reactions see Dr James Duke's Web page on the internet www.ars-grin.gov/duke. Dr James Duke was a former chief of the Medicinal Plant Resources Laboratory of the United States Department of Agriculture, who spent many years researching plants. He wrote 20 or more books and served as a consultant for the American National Institutes of Health on herbal remedies for the treatment of cancer and AIDS).

There are certain children who are more likely to develop sensitivities than others, particularly those that already have a history of food or chemical sensitivity or intolerance. It may well be that this arises due to problems in the gut, including imbalances in the intestinal flora, intestinal dysbiosis and chronic intestinal infections (Tillotson et al 2001) and certainly these patients may well benefit from dietary advice and herbal remedies.

On the question of safety, the risk of adulteration is one that obviously needs addressing. Adverse effects have indeed occurred on occasions due to adulteration with toxic herbs as well as mislabelling. In obtaining herbs it is essential that sources are reliable, preferably organic, as adverse reactions to pesticides and preservatives are difficult to quantify and may be confused with reactions to the plant itself. Indian herbs are considered more of a safety issue than European herbs, although the use of pesticides in Eastern Europe has also attracted negative attention. There are however reputable suppliers of Ayurvedic herbs as they increase in popularity and use, and their sources can be traced from organic growing conditions in India to their presence in dried form and formulae in British warehouses.

The question of drug interactions is a relatively new line of enquiry, since herbs and allopathic medicines have only been used in combination on a widespread basis for the last 30 years or so. It is now common for many patients to be taking prescription drugs from the doctor as well as herbs and nutritional supplements, either prescribed by a professional or purchased over the counter, and it is not easy to predict the outcome of such combinations. (For more information see Dr Duke's website www.ars-grin.gov/duke and books such as *Handbook of Herbs & Natural Supplements* by Linda Skidmore-Roth published by Mosby or Tieraona LowDog's book published by Proline Botanicals called *Safety, Toxicity, Drug Interaction & Contraindications of Botanicals* or *Botanical Medicines. The Desk Reference for Major Herbal Supplements* by Dennis J McKenna, Kenneth Jones, Kerry Hughes by Haworth Press).

I have prescribed herbs in my practice over many years to patients taking allopathic medicines and have encountered very few problems. Certainly it is possible that herbs can increase or decrease the bioavailability of drugs and nutrients and this is particularly important to know when patients are taking critical doses of powerful medicines such as cardiac medication or blood-thinning agents or prior to surgery. Herbs that contain a high proportion of mucilage or fibre, such as psyllium seeds, may inhibit absorption. Digestive herbs such as cayenne pepper and black pepper, that enhance digestion and absorption, can increase absorption of medicines, while herbs that act on the enzyme systems in the liver may alter the body's metabolism and thus blood levels of certain drugs. Several herbs have the ability to lower blood sugar levels and so need to be taken with care by insulin-dependent diabetics, as doses may need to be monitored. Grapefruit juice for example contains a substance known as "Bergamottin" which inactivates cytochrome P450-3A4, an enzyme which is responsible for metabolizing as much as 60% of all drugs including antihistamines, so it has a great potential for increasing the effect of many prescription drugs, which may certainly pose dangers (Tillotson et al 2001). Some herbs should be completely avoided by children as they are potentially harmful to the liver and their immature systems are obviously more susceptible to potential toxins than a mature adult body. Those with a high alkaloid content should be completely avoided.

The following herbs are contraindicated in children: *Aconitum* spp., *Adonis vernalis*, *Aristolochia* spp., *Arnica latifolia*, *Atropa belladonna*, *Bryonia* spp., *Buxus sempervirens*, *Catharanthus roseus*, *Convallaria majalis*, *Digitalis purpurea*, *Dryopteris filix-mas*, *Euonymus atropurpureus*, *Gelsemium* spp., *Hyoscyamus niger*, *Ipomoea purga*, *Mandragora officinarum*, *Phytolacca americana*, *Pilocarpus* spp., *Podophyllum* spp., *Pulsatilla* spp., *Rauwolfia serpentina*, *Tanacetum vulgare*, *Teucrium chamaedrys*, *Urginia maritima*, *Veratrum* spp., *Viscum flavescens*.

As far as research into herbal medicine is concerned, clearly there is a need for assurance that herbs are effective and safe, but whether this is possible from objective, quantifiable and reproducible data is so far not entirely clear. The study of the pharmacology of herbs can rationalize to some degree their effectiveness and their historical and current use by herbalists. It is also necessary in assessment of possible herb–drug interactions. Isolating single ingredients and testing them in laboratories on genetically bred animals however, may or may not be a reliable guide. It is questionable whether it is applicable or indeed useful in ascertaining the safety or efficacy of a herb to be prescribed professionally to a specific human individual with knowledge, expertise, correct dosage and in a "holistic" environment. Moreover much research is focused on identification of active components, which may not be valid when it comes to a consideration of whole-plant medicines as advocated by herbal practitioners. Also, to quote David Hoffman in his *Therapeutic Herbalism*, "using laboratory animals to demonstrate something already well known by practitioners is anathema to the herbalist's work of affirming life, an insane distortion of the search for knowledge and the desire for health."

Clinical trials may be a better way of evaluating herbal treatment but are also hard to quantify realistically. Their success relies on therapeutic outcomes being easy to discern, which is not always possible. They may not give due consideration to the complexity of human beings, and factors influencing their subjective and objective experience while taking the herbs in question. In addition, they still do not address the problem of evaluating herbs given after consultation with a professional herbalist that includes an evaluation of individual or constitutional needs and the role of diet and lifestyle, which can augment or detract from results. Nor does it address the huge question, regarding placebo, of the impact of the patient–practitioner relationship. Having said this, a brief glance of the main constituents of herbs is relevant, if only to fill in a little of the intricate jigsaw that is the world of medicinal plants.

THE CHEMISTRY OF PLANTS

As well as a variety of minerals, vitamins and trace elements, medicinal plants contain an array of substances known to have specific therapeutic actions in the body. Some of the most commonly occurring substances are as follows:

Volatile oils

Volatile oils are composed of a wide variety of chemical compounds and the different combinations of these in plants give us the variation in their aromas and therapeutic effects. Up to 60 different chemical constituents have been identified in some oils such as tea tree (*Melaleuca alternifolia*) oil, well known for its antiseptic properties. All volatile oils in fact are antiseptic, and enhance the function of the immune system in warding off bacterial, viral or fungal infection. Many oils have anti-inflammatory and antispasmodic properties, particularly those that contain sesquiterpenes such as azulene. Those in German chamomile (*Chamomilla recutita*) for example, are particularly applicable for the relief of inflamed and irritated conditions of the digestive tract, while those in dill (*Anethum graveolens*) relax spasm and colicky pain in the digestive system. Some oils have an expectorant action such as in thyme (*Thymus vulgon's*) and hyssop (*Hyssopus off.*), aiding the clearing of phlegm from the chest, while others are diuretic, useful in relief of fluid retention and urinary infections. While they exert their beneficial effects on the physical body, they also reach the brain and nervous system, meaning that aromatherapy has a wide range of mento-emotional applications. Since the time of the ancient Egyptians we have made use of the therapeutic properties of volatile oils. The art of employing the aromas of these oils, aromatherapy, also has a long tradition in the Far East.

Volatile oils can be taken into the body to exert these beneficial influences in a variety of different ways. They can be taken as culinary herbs in foods and drinks. When diluted in a carrier oil such as sesame oil, the oil can be rubbed on to the skin or inhaled through the nose. When inhaled olfactory receptor cells are stimulated and carry nerve impulses to the brain, especially the limbic system, thereby potentially affecting instinctual responses, emotions and memory. As the oils are inhaled molecules are also taken via the lungs to the bloodstream and the systemic circulation. Their actions are felt throughout the digestive tract, the urinary tract and the respiratory system, as well as affecting sweat, salivary, vaginal and lacrimal secretions. It is probable that the oils are passed in some amount through the breast milk. Fennel, dill and chamomile tea have been drunk for centuries by lactating women to soothe babies' colic and help induce sleep.

When oils are absorbed via the skin through massage or baths, they stimulate nerve endings in the skin, and messages are relayed to underlying tissues, muscles, blood and lymphatic vessels, and also via the nervous system to the pituitary gland, thereby having the ability to regulate the action of other endocrine glands, including the adrenals. These effects make aromatherapy of enormous benefit in treating hormonal problems and relieving stress and enhancing relaxation. Rose oil, for example, has a particular affinity for women. It has been used to alleviate tension and anxiety and symptoms related to the reproductive system, such as menstrual problems, PMS, emotional problems concerning sexuality and post-natal depression. Chamomile oil is excellent for fractious children (and mothers!) at the end of the day, relieving tension and irritability and encouraging deep and relaxing sleep for both.

Volatile oils can be absorbed into the body in as little as 30 minutes but their therapeutic effect can last for many hours. Once in the bloodstream, volatile oils are dispersed throughout the body, influencing the various tissues or systems according to the specific properties of the oils. Once they have exerted their beneficial action here, they are excreted from the body via the skin, the lungs and the urine.

Phenolic glycosides

These are a group of phenol compounds, which share antiseptic and anti-inflammatory actions when ingested and an irritant action when applied topically. They include arbutin in *Arctostaphylos uva ursi*, salicin, related to salicylic acid, the forerunner of aspirin, found in herbs including meadowsweet (*Filipendula ulmaria*), willow (*Salix* spp.) and wintergreen (*Gaultheria procumbens*). Thyme (*Thymus vulgaris*) is rich in antiseptic phenols and is frequently an important component of herbal cough remedies. Polyphenols have antioxidant and anti-inflammatory actions which contribute to their anticancer activity. Green tea leaves, for example, contain polyphenols.

Tannins

The main therapeutic action of tannins is astringent, brought about by their ability to bind albumin, a protein in the skin and mucous membranes, to form a tight, insoluble protective layer, which is resistant to disease. On the skin or in the mucosa of the mouth, the respiratory, digestive, urinary, and reproductive systems, tannins can separate bacteria that threaten to invade the body from their source of nutrition, thus improving resistance to infection. Tannins also have a healing action, protecting these areas from irritation while at the same time reducing inflammation.

Tannins occur widely in nature and are the main therapeutic constituents in herbs like witch hazel (*Hamamelis virginiana*), shepherd's purse (*Capsella bursa pastoris*), tormentil (*Potentilla erecta*) and oak bark (*Quercus robur*). Such herbs make useful mouthwashes for infected and bleeding gums, gargles for sore throats, remedies for catarrh, and inflammation of the gastrointestinal tract such as diarrhoea. They can be used externally as compresses to heal abrasions and cuts, and to treat burns and scalds. They can also be incorporated into lotions to bathe haemorrhoids and inflammatory skin conditions. Some herbs rich in tannins such as thyme have antioxidant properties.

Coumarins

This is a group of substances with fairly divergent actions. Those in melilot (*Melilotus officinalis*) have anticoagulant properties, similar to diocoumarol, derived from improperly cured sweet clover, which is a component of warfarin (Tillotson et al 2001). Bergapten in celery seed (*Apium graviolens*) is photo-reactive and can cause skin rashes and khellen found in visnaga (*Ammi visnaga*) is a powerful smooth muscle relaxant (Chevallier 1996). Other herbs containing coumarins have antimicrobial actions.

Bitters

There is a wide variety of compounds with a bitter taste that is found in medicinal plants and these have certain therapeutic actions in common. Bitters are characteristics of plant chemicals including monoterpenes and sesquiterpenes, iridoids and alkaloids. Bitter herbs exert their action mainly in the digestive tract, where they promote the secretions by the salivary glands and digestive organs including the liver, thus enhancing appetite, digestion and absorption.

By enhancing the function of the digestive system and improving digestion and absorption of nutrients, bitter-tasting herbs can have a nourishing and strengthening effect. They are prescribed for loss of appetite, gastritis, heartburn, poor digestion and to aid convalescence after illness.

Many bitter herbs have other actions, some are relaxant or sedative, some have protective effects on the liver, others are anti-inflammatory, or exert a beneficial action on the immune system, acting as natural antibiotics and antineoplastics.

Well known "bitter tonics" include dandelion, chicory, dock root and gentian. Their therapeutic action begins in the mouth, so for good effect they need to be tasted. This experience need not be as abhorrent to our taste buds as we might suppose. Chamomile and rosemary are important bitter remedies that even children manage to stomach!

Alkaloids

A diverse group of chemicals, these potent substances have in common the fact that they contain a nitrogen-bearing molecule and are pharmacologically very potent.

Many of the more toxic plants contain alkaloids, such as atropine in belladonna (*Atropa belladonna*) and morphine from the opium poppy (*Papaver somniferum*), the first alkaloid to be isolated in 1806 (Tillotson et al 2001). Caffeine, ephedrine, quinine, strychnine, nicotine and codeine are all alkaloids with diverse actions ranging from stimulants, bronchodilators, antimicrobials and anti-inflammatories, to narcotics and painkillers.

Mucilage

Mucilage is composed of polysaccharides, large sugar molecules that have the ability to draw water to them. When added to water it swells up to form a viscous, gel-like fluid. When taken orally mucilage forms a coating on the mucous membranes of the digestive tract and acts to protect them from irritation and inflammation.

Mucilage-containing herbs such as slippery elm (*Ulmus fulva*) are generally prescribed for their soothing properties, which also extend to the respiratory and genito-urinary systems. They are often used as laxatives as they loosen the bowel contents by absorbing water into the bowel and bulking out the stool; psyllium seeds (*Plantago ovata*) are a good example. One or two teaspoons of seeds left to soak in a cup of cold water for 30 minutes can be taken morning and night to relieve constipation.

Flavonoids

Flavonoids or flavonoid glycosides occur widely in nature and impart a yellow/orange colour to herbs such as cowslips and fruits like oranges and tomatoes. They tend to have a sweet or bitter taste. Many flavonoids have a diuretic action like those in buchu (*Barosma betulina*) and parsley (*Petroselinum crispum*). Some, like those in liquorice (*Glycyrrhiza glabra*), are anti-inflammatory and antispasmodic, while others have antiviral and antimicrobial properties (Tillotson et al 2001). Some are well known as bioflavonoids such as those that occur in vitamin C-rich fruits like blackcurrants and citrus fruits and which act synergistically with ascorbic acid to enhance the body's ability to metabolize it. These bioflavonoids, such as rutin in buckwheat (*Fagopyrum esculentum*) and those occurring in red and black grapes, elderberries, hawthorn berries and blueberries, are potent antioxidants, neutralizing free radicals and strengthening and healing peripheral blood vessel walls. They are used to treat a variety of vascular problems such as bruising and nose bleeds.

Saponins

Saponins are glycosides that form a soap-like lather when they are mixed with water. Soapwort (*Saponaria officinalis*), which contains a high proportion of saponins, was used in the past to manufacture soap. Other features shared by the many plants containing saponins are a bitter taste and haemolytic activity (Hoffman). On mucous membranes and blood vessel walls, saponins lower surface tension and have the ability to emulsify oils. Because they are able to dissolve red blood cells even when used in small amounts, they should never be injected directly into the bloodstream. Taken orally however they are hardly absorbed at all through an intact intestine but instead help to promote digestion and absorption of many other substances such as calcium and silicon.

Saponins often have beneficial action on the walls of veins and arteries, they decrease blood coagulation, blood sugar and cholesterol levels (Tillotson et al 2001). Those in horse chestnut (*Aesculus hippocastanum*), exert a beneficial effect on blood vessel walls, reducing fragility and oedema by making the vein wall less permeable. Some saponins have a diuretic action, such as those in horsetail (*Equisetum arvense*) and asparagus (*Asparagus off.*). Others have an expectorant effect, such as in cow-slips (*Primula veris*) and mullein (*Verbascum thapsus*), and several have hepatoprotective and immunomodulating effects including *Panax ginseng* and liquorice (Hoffman).

There are two main types of saponins, triterpenoid and steroidal. Steroidal saponins are similar in structure to human hormones secreted by the testes, ovaries and adrenal glands, and can resemble cholesterol, cortisone, oestrogen, progesterone and vitamin D. Triterpenoid saponins have the ability to regulate steroidal hormonal activity in the body and counter the effect of stress. Some have an action on the adrenal glands that mimic the activity of adrenocorticotropic hormone (ACTH). They are also reputed to enhance arterial circulation and improve the utilization of oxygen (Tillotson et al 2001).

Remedies containing these hormone-regulating properties are generally known as adaptogens, the most famous of which is ginseng (*Panax ginseng*). Others include liquorice, false unicorn root (*Chamaelirium luteum*), squaw vine (*Michella repens*), wild yam (*Dioscorea villosa*) and fenugreek (*Trigonella foenum-graecum*). Some of these such as wild yam and liquorice also act as anti-inflammatories.

Anthraquinones

These glycosides have a yellow colour that has often been used for producing commercial dyes. When taken internally they irritate and thereby stimulate the wall of the large intestine, increasing the force of muscular contraction and producing a laxative effect within approximately 10 hours of ingestion.

Anthraquinones are found in herbs like senna (*Cassia senna*), dock (*Rumex* spp.), cascara (*Rhamnus purshiana*), and Chinese rhubarb (*Rheum palmatum*) and can sometimes cause griping in the bowel. For this reason they are best combined with herbs such as ginger (*Zingiberis off.*) or fennel (*Foeniculum vulgare*) which reduce spasm and griping in the bowel. They should never be used over a long period of time as they can reduce the normal bowel reflexes and cause habituation.

Cyanogenic glycosides

Herbs containing cyanogenic glycosides have relaxant effects on smooth muscle and sedative effects on the nervous system. They are based on cyanide, a potent toxin, but when they occur in minute amounts in herbs such as elder (*Sambucus nigra*), mustard and wild cherry (*Prunus serotina*) they help to soothe the cough reflex and are useful for dry irritating coughs that disturb children's sleep.

Gums and resins

These are present in certain plants and act as protective chemicals, to be released when the plant is damaged. Some gums such as that found in Guggulu (*Commiphora mukul*) have the ability to enhance the liver's metabolism of cholesterol by promoting the uptake of LDL cholesterol from the blood (Tillotson et al 2001). The common marigold (*Calendula off.*) is high in resins with antimicrobial and anti-inflammatory effects.

THE HERBAL PHARMACY

PRESCRIBING HERBS TO CHILDREN

There are many ways that herbs can be administered to children to affect them beneficially. As long as they interact with the body chemistry in one way or another, they will exert their influence. The most obvious way that herbs can be taken is in daily diet. Salads with basil, coriander leaves, rocket and parsley, vinaigrette with garlic, fish with dill or sorrel, new potatoes with fresh mint, casseroles with bay leaves, biscuits and curries with ginger and pizza with oregano are often unknowingly our daily medicine. As the foods are absorbed from the digestive tract, the therapeutic constituents of the herbs enter the bloodstream and then circulate round the body. Most of the common culinary herbs contain a high proportion of volatile oils with antimicrobial properties and these would have been vital for health as well as enhancing culinary skills in the days before refrigeration.

The skin is highly absorbent and represents a large surface area. One simple way to administer herbs is to apply them in one way or another to the skin, where tiny capillaries under the surface will take the herbal constituents into the bloodstream. Dilute essential oils can be massaged, tincture-based rubbing lotions can be applied, as can ointments and creams, compresses and poultices. In addition, fresh herbs can be used, like dock leaves to soothe a nettle sting, yarrow leaves, marigold or lavender flowers to staunch bleeding from minor cuts and abrasions and relieve a minor burn.

The conjunctiva of the eye will also absorb herbal extracts. An eyebright (*Euphrasia off.*) or a chamomile eyebath or a marigold compress will relieve sore and inflamed eyes.

The nose and the nerve endings lying in it can provide another therapeutic pathway that is utilized by aromatherapists. By inhalation the messages from the herbs are carried to the brain and are also taken into the lungs where they are absorbed with oxygen into the bloodstream and circulated throughout the body.

Preparations for internal use

Infusions

Infusions are prepared using the soft parts of plants, leaves, stems and flowers. Take 1 oz/25 g of dried herb per pint (600 ml) of water or a teaspoon of herb per cupful of water. Double the amount of herbs if they are being used fresh. Place the herbs in a warmed pot and pour over boiling water. Cover immediately to prevent volatile oils escaping into the atmosphere. Leave to infuse for 10–15 minutes and then strain. The herbs can then be given immediately or stored in the fridge for up to 2 days. Some herbs need to be prepared as cold infusions as their therapeutic components may be destroyed by high temperatures. These include herbs that have a high proportion of mucilage like marshmallow (*Althea off.*) and comfrey (*Symphytum off.*) leaf. They are prepared in the same way but with cold water and left to infuse for 10–12 hours.

Infusions can be given three to six times a day depending on whether the ailment being treated is chronic or acute. Teas can be sipped, up to half a cupful (100 ml) at a time. Contrary to expectation many herbs are found by our pampered palates and especially those of children who are accustomed to sweet tasting foods and medicines, to taste strange, often even unpleasant. Although the bitters in some herbs need to be tasted to be effective, the bitter taste is generally not something we relish. However it is possible to combine several herbs together in an infusion so that aromatic, pleasant-tasting herbs such as peppermint, fennel, lemon balm, and lavender can disguise less-palatable herbs while not reducing their effect. Liquorice and aniseed also make excellent herbs for flavouring. Infusions can also be sweetened with honey if necessary.

Infusions are generally given warm to hot, particularly in the treatment of fevers, colds and catarrh. They are given lukewarm to cold for problems associated with the kidneys and urinary tract, such as kidney infections, cystitis and bed wetting.

Herbal teabags are sold in all high-street health-food shops and supermarkets and normally comprise the more aromatic, pleasant-tasting herbs like limeflower (*Tilia europaea*), fennel (*Foeniculum vulgare*) and peppermint.

Decoctions

The hard woody parts of plants have tough cell walls that require greater heat to break them down before they will release their constituents into the water. Bark, seeds, roots, rhizomes and nuts all need to be prepared as decoctions. To make their constituents more accessible to the water, break the herb up into small pieces with a pestle and mortar or smash with a hammer if the parts are very hard.

Use the same proportion of herbs to water as when preparing an infusion, just add a little more water to make up for losses during boiling. Place herbs in a stainless steel or enamel saucepan and cover them with water. Bring to the boil, cover and simmer for 10–15 minutes. Strain and drink in the same doses as an infusion. (See dosage, p. 14.)

Syrups

Syrups are an easy way to give herbs to children as they like their sweetness. They can be added to other preparations to mask their more unpleasant tastes. Pour 1 pint (600 ml) of boiling water over 2½ lb (1.25 kg) of soft brown sugar and stir over a gentle heat until all the sugar has dissolved and the solution comes to the boil. Either add tinctures in the ratio of one part tincture to three parts syrup and this will keep indefinitely or, alternatively, you can use an infusion or decoction in the following way: mix ¾ lb (325 g) sugar into 1 pint (600 ml) of the liquid and heat until the sugar has dissolved. This should be kept in a cool place, preferably the fridge. A dessert-spoonful can be given to children three or four times a day.

Honey can be used to persuade children to take herbs. Fresh, chopped or dried, powdered herbs can be infused in runny honey and given on the spoon.

Tinctures

Tinctures are concentrated extracts of herbs that use a mixture of water and alcohol or glycerol to extract the constituents of the plants and also to act as a preservative. According to herbal pharmacopoeias, there is a correct ratio of water and alcohol to plant matter for each herb depending on the constituents that require extraction. This can range from a herb:liquid ratio of 1:2 to 1:10. The alcohol ratio of the liquid can range from 25% alcohol for simple glycosides and tannins, to 90% for resins and gums such as those in myrrh (*Commiphora molmol*).

The herb can be used either fresh or dried, either finely chopped or powdered. Place the herb in a large jar and pour the alcohol and water mixture over it. Using dried herbs, the most frequently used ratio is one part of herbs per five parts of liquid. Fresh herbs are generally used in a ratio of one part herb to two parts liquid.

To illustrate:

To make 1 litre (1¾ pints) of chamomile tincture, take 200 g (7 oz) of dried flowers and pour over 1 litre (1¾ pints) of fluid. Chamomile requires a 45% alcohol solution and brandy or vodka would be perfectly adequate.

Place an airtight lid on the jar and leave to macerate away from direct sunlight for not less than 2 weeks, shaking the jar well about once a day. Then press the mixture through a press (such as that used for wine making) to extract as much of the fluid as possible, discard the herb, transfer the tincture to a dark bottle for storage and keep in a cool place.

Tinctures can also be prepared using neat cider vinegar, as the acetic acid acts as a solvent and preservative. Raspberry vinegar, for example, is a traditional remedy for coughs and sore throats. Glycerol can also be used. Glycerol-based tinctures have a sweet syrup-like taste which makes them a good medium for children's medicines. Pour equal parts of water and glycerol over the herbs in the same proportion of herb to liquid as for alcohol tinctures. Eighty per cent glycerol is required for more watery fresh herbs such as marshmallow (*Althea off.*) and coltsfoot (*Tussilago farfara*) to prevent deterioration. Peppermint, lemon balm, lavender, rose, basil, elderflowers and catmint (*Nepeta cataria*) are well suited to this method.

Because they are concentrated, only small amounts of tincture need to be given at regular intervals through the day. The dose will vary from five drops for babies to 10–20 drops for toddlers, $\frac{1}{2}$ tsp for children between 6 and 12 and up to a teaspoon for children over 12, taken in a little warm water, fruit juice or herbal tea, 3–6 times daily depending on whether the condition is chronic or acute. Tinctures can also be added to bath water, mixed with water to make compresses, mouthwashes or gargles, or stirred into a base to make ointments or creams. Tinctures require more preparation time but they have several advantages. They are easy to store, do not deteriorate in cold or damp conditions, take up relatively little storage space and keep almost indefinitely, although they are best taken within 2 years.

Tablets and capsules

Many herbs are available from herbal suppliers in tablet or capsule form. This is certainly a convenient way to administer herbs but it bypasses the taste buds on the tongue and this may reduce the therapeutic effects in some cases. However, only standard preparations will be available commercially, so should you require a specific combination of herbs to be given to a patient, these can be made up in vegetable gelatin capsules. Capsules can be filled with mixtures of the appropriate herbs using a capsule maker. There are two main sizes of capsule used by medical herbalists, size 0 which holds 0.35 g of powder and 00 which holds about 0.5 g. One or two of the size 0 capsules can be given three times daily and one of the size 00 three times daily.

Suppositories

The advantage of using suppositories inserted into the rectum is that the herbal remedy can be absorbed directly into the bloodstream through the mucosa of the rectum. This not only enables both local and systemic problems to be treated quickly and simply, but it also obviates the laborious process of giving herbs by mouth to travel the distance of the alimentary canal before being absorbed. It also overrides the risk of the child refusing to take the herbs by mouth because of their unpleasant taste.

Preparations for external use

Most herbal constituents are absorbed readily through the skin and the following preparations are designed to enhance this pathway into the body.

Herbal baths

A very pleasant and simple way to give herbs to babies and children is in a fragrant hot bath. There are various ways to add herbs to bath water. Dilute essential oils (one drop of essential oil per 5 ml teaspoon of base oil such as sesame oil) can be added. A muslin bag with fresh or dried aromatic herbs can be hung under the hot tap, or a pint (600 ml) of strong herbal infusion (double the standard dose described above) added to the water. The child can soak in the warm bath for 10–20 minutes.

When herbs are used in this way, the essential oils from the plants are taken in via the pores of the skin, which are opened up by the warmth of the water. The oils are also carried in the steam, which is simultaneously inhaled via nose and mouth into the lungs and from there into the bloodstream. From the nose, messages are carried from the oils via nerve pathways to the brain. Herbal medicines are in this way assimilated quickly and directly, bypassing the lengthy process of digestion necessary when herbs are taken by mouth. They are particularly useful for relaxing and soothing the nervous system and for easing mental and emotional strain. Lavender, basil, rose and chamomile are not only fragrant but also effective remedies for calming tension and anxiety and helping to promote sleep. Chamomile is well worth using for fractious children, particularly when they are unwell, for not only does it possess antimicrobial properties but it also helps induce sleep, nature's best way to ward off infection and enable self-healing. Rosemary baths while also relaxing, have a stimulating edge as they enhance blood flow to the head and enable greater alertness and concentration.

Hand and foot baths

Mustard foot baths were used by our mothers and grandmothers for all afflictions of cold and damp climates, from colds and flu to poor circulation and arthritis. The ancient tradition of hand and foot baths was made popular by the famous French herbalist, Maurice Messegue, who has written several books on herbal therapy based simply on this form of treatment. He recommends foot baths for 8 minutes in the evening and hand baths for 8 minutes in the morning. The hands and feet are, according to Messegue, highly sensitive areas of the skin, rich in nerve endings and despite some thickening of the skin from use, the constituents pass easily from the skin into the body. Hand and foot baths are excellent ways of treating babies and children who are required to keep still for only half the time recommended for adults, i.e. 4 minutes morning and evening.

Ointments and creams

Ointments and creams can be applied for treatment of skin problems and also for less superficial problems such as inflamed joints and headaches.

Any herb, fresh or dried, can be included in an ointment following this simple recipe:

> Macerate as much herb as possible in $\frac{3}{4}$ pint (450 ml) of olive oil and 2 oz (50 g) of beeswax for a few hours over a low heat in a bain-marie (double saucepan). After this time the constituents will have been taken up by the oil and the mixture can then be pressed through a muslin bag and the herb discarded. When the oil is still warm it can be poured into ointment jars where it will quickly solidify.

Creams can be made up easily by stirring tinctures, decoctions or a few drops of essential oil into a cream base such as aqueous cream. Two or three drops of chamomile oil (*chamomilla recutita*) mixed into 2 oz (50 g) of cream works well on many types of eczema.

Compresses

A clean cloth or flannel can be soaked in any of the following: a hot or cold infusion or a decoction; a dilute tincture; or water with a few drops of diluted essential oil. It should be wrung out and applied to the affected part. Compresses can be applied to help relieve symptoms such as headaches, abdominal colic, backache, boils, and painful joints. The treatment needs to be repeated several times for good effect.

Poultices

These are similar to compresses but involve using the herb itself rather than an extract of the herb. Place the herb, fresh or dried, between two pieces of gauze. If you use fresh leaves, stems or roots, they need to be bruised before being applied. If the herbs are dry, add a little hot water to powdered or finely chopped herbs to make a paste. Use a light cotton bandage to bind the gauze poultice to the affected part and keep it warm with a hot water bottle.

Liniments

A rubbing oil or liniment consists of extracts of herbs in an oil or alcohol base or a mixture of both. They are used in massage to relax or stimulate muscles and ligaments or to soothe away pain from inflammation or injury. They are intended to be absorbed by the skin to reach the affected part and so they often contain stimulating essential oil such as ginger or black pepper and are therefore not suitable for use on delicate baby skins, but can be used in older children.

Oils

Essential oils can be used with care for children and babies. They can be diluted in a base oil such as sesame oil (one drop of oil per 5 ml of base oil) for massage and in the bath. They can be used in burners (well way from children's reach) to permeate the atmosphere or in inhalations for a variety of symptoms such as colds, catarrh, coughs, insomnia and anxiety.

While essential oils are extracted by steam distillation from aromatic plants, infused oils can be prepared easily in the home. Finely chopped herbs can be placed in a jar with a tight-fitting lid, covered with oil such as olive or sesame oil, placed on a sunny windowsill and left to macerate for about 2 weeks. The oil will gradually take up the constituents of the plant as can be observed by macerating St John's Wort in oil. In a matter of minutes the oil will turn a deep red colour. (This is a very useful remedy for healing cuts and sores, and when massaged over the affected part can relieve painful nerve conditions such as trigeminal neuralgia and shingles.) After 2 weeks the oil can be filtered off and the remainder of the oil squeezed through a muslin bag. It should be stored in an airtight dark bottle to retain its therapeutic value for maximum length of time.

AYURVEDIC MEDICINES

Many of the Ayurvedic herbs recommended in the book are in traditional formulae and despite their unfamiliarity, the vast majority of them are available in this country from specialist herbal suppliers. The same formulae are mentioned in the book in different forms including powder (*churna*), tablets (*guti*), medicated ghee and herbal wines (*arishta/asavas*) as the medium the herb is given in can, to some extent, change or enhance the action of the herbs.

Gugguls are pills made with the purified resin of guggul (*Commiphora mukul*), a relative of myrrh. Guggul is purified by boiling it with various herbal decoctions such as Triphala and straining out the purified resin. A variety of different herbal powders or extracts are added to the purified guggul resin, often with ghee. They are mainly used for treating problems associated with toxicity, arthritis, nervous system disorders, skin problems, high cholesterol and triglycerides and obesity.

There are two types of herbal wines, *asavas* and *arishtas*. They are herbal fermentations made in a similar way to grape wine in large wooden vats and are considered easier on the digestion than other herbal preparations. Many contain spices that not only improve their taste but also their assimilation. They are particularly good for treatment of *Vata* problems. Asavas are made with fresh herbal juices and arishtas are made with decoctions of herbs, i.e. they have been boiled first. Dhataki (*Woodfordia fructicosa/floribunda*) flowers are added and they are left to self-ferment.

Herbal jellies/jams prepared with raw sugar, i.e. jaggery or with honey, are considered excellent tonics. The sugar acts as a preservative, improves the taste of the preparation and enhances their tonic properties.

Tailas-medicated oils are a speciality of Ayurveda. They are combinations of many tonic herbs and sometimes analgesic herbs, prepared mainly with sesame oil. They are used in massage and oleation therapy for external nourishment and are considered not as supplements to treatment but as a treatment in themselves.

Powders have the shortest shelf life and generally should be kept in dark containers, for no more than 6–9 months. Because herbs tend to deteriorate rapidly in the heat and humidity of India, powders are often made into tablets to extend their shelf life, or combined with pastes, ghee, and herbal extracts.

Medicated ghee will last for 6 months or longer if kept refrigerated. Tablets will keep for longer although they should be stored similarly away from direct sunlight. Herbal wines and jellies like chyawan prash will keep for up to 3 years (Frawley 2000).

Herbs are also given in different vehicles (*anupanas*), which vary according to the *doshic* balance of the patient they are given to. They help to carry the remedy to a certain part or tissue in the body, hence their name. Vehicles include warm or cool water, milk, ghee, honey and decoctions. The same formula can be given to balance different *doshas* but in a specific vehicle and often in combination with other formulae.

GUIDELINES FOR PRESCRIBING

The ways of prescribing herbal medicines vary considerably according to the condition being treated, the herbs employed, the age and build of the child, the constitution of the child, even the time of year. The dosage, the herbs chosen for administration, the type of preparation, the timing of administration and the duration of treatment all need to be evaluated.

Chronic conditions generally require mild herbal remedies which can safely be given, generally three times daily, over months at a time if necessary, while acute conditions may require stronger herbs given up to every 2 hours over a shorter period.

To illustrate, dandelion root has mild laxative properties which can be given to regulate digestion and elimination over a period, while senna root or castor oil have stronger laxative action for acute constipation or to clear heat quickly during a fever.

Some conditions, particularly fevers, colds, catarrh and problems associated with cold, require herbs to be given in hot preparations. Others such as urinary problems are better suited to cool preparations. Skin problems may improve more rapidly through administration of herbal teas as opposed to tinctures, while tinctures may be preferable when more concentrated medicines are required, such as the treatment of a virulent infection.

The herbs chosen may also dictate to some extent their method of administration. When giving teas, the aerial parts of a plant are prepared as infusions while roots, barks and seeds are better suited to decoctions.

The length of time herbs need to be given and the dosage will vary widely according to the nature of the condition as well as the age and constitution of the child. A predominantly *Kapha*-type child, well built with heavy bones and a comparatively sluggish metabolism, will generally require herbs to be given in larger doses and over a longer period of time than a small-framed, lightweight predominantly *Vata*-type child with a more sensitive body and faster metabolism.

There are two rules that are employed by some practitioners:

- Young's method: child's dosage = adult dose (generally 5 ml) × age divided by the age +12.
- Cowling's method: child's dosage = adult dose × age divided by 24.

Alternatively dosage can be calculated according to weight: child's dosage = adult dose × child's weight divided by 150 lb.

Generally remedies for *Vata* problems are given before a meal, for *Pitta* problems are given with a meal and for *Kapha* problems are given after a meal.

References

Chevallier A 1996 The Encyclopedia of Medicinal Plants. Dorling Kindersley, London, p. 59

Frawley D 2000 Ayurvedic Healing. Lotus Press, Wisconsin, pp. 361–362

Hoffman D Therapeutic Herbalism. Self published. 1997. California, USA

Kuhn MA and Winston D 2001 Herbal Therapy & Supplements. Lippincott, Philadelphia

McIntyre A 1994 The Complete Woman's Herbal. Gaia Books Limited, London

Tillotson AK, Tillotson NH, Abel R Jr 2001 The One Earth Herbal Sourcebook. Kensington Publishing Corps, New York

Chapter **2**

Monographs of Western herbs commonly used in the treatment of children

CHAPTER CONTENTS

Achillea millefolium : Yarrow

Family: Compositae
Part used: aerial parts
Taste/*Rasa*: bitter/*tikta*, pungent/*katu*, astringent/*kashaya*
Post digestive/*Vipak*: pungent/*katu*
Potency/*Virya*: cooling/*sheeta*
Dosha: PK- Vo

Constituents

Over 120 compounds have been found including volatile oil, sterols, bitters, tannins, salicylic acid, coumarins.

Actions

Diaphoretic, astringent, alterative, digestive, bitter tonic, styptic, antimicrobial, decongestant, anti-inflammatory, antispasmodic, analgesic, expectorant, haemostatic.

Indications

Colds, catarrh, fevers, diarrhoea, inflammation of the bowel, IBS, varicose veins, eruptive infections, wounds and ulcers, piles, heavy menstrual bleeding, first aid.

Introduction

Yarrow has been valued as a medicine since at least the times of the ancient Greeks and Romans. The name *Achillea* comes from the legend of Achilles who healed his companion's battle wounds with yarrow. The plant was still used as a first-aid dressing in World War I. Today *yarrow*'s main use is as an astringent internally and externally. It makes an excellent remedy for wounds. The volatile oils are anti-inflammatory and antiseptic (Candan et al 2003), the tannins are astringent and stem bleeding, the resins are also astringent and antiseptic while the silica promotes tissue repair.

Internal uses

Digestive system

Yarrow is an excellent herb for the digestive tract, stimulating the appetite, enhancing digestion and absorption. It helps relieve wind, colic and indigestion and other problems associated with poor digestion. The astringent tannins protect the gut from irritation and infection, so *yarrow* can be used in the treatment of diarrhoea, and inflammatory problems such as gastritis and colitis.

Circulatory system

A hot infusion stimulates diaphoresis and promotes perspiration. It has been used to reduce fevers as well as lower blood pressure and relieve problems such as poor circulation and varicose veins.

Immune system

The volatile oils in *yarrow* have been shown to have anti-inflammatory and antioxidant effects, which can be useful in the treatment of arthritis and childhood problems such as tonsillitis and conjunctivitis. By stimulating blood flow to the skin *yarrow* can help to bring out the rash in eruptive childhood infections such as measles and chickenpox.

Temperature

It reduces fevers and clears toxins, heat and congestion by aiding elimination via the skin and the kidneys through its diuretic effect.

External uses

Yarrow is still used as a healing remedy. With its antiseptic, anti-inflammatory and astringent actions and silica to promote tissue repair, it will speed healing of cuts and wounds, ulcers, burns and can be applied to varicose veins, haemorrhoids and skin conditions like eczema. An infusion makes a good vaginal douche, an eyebath, and a skin lotion for varicose veins and haemorrhoids.

Other uses

Yarrow's astringent effect is felt throughout the body, staunching bleeding from the nose, the digestive system and the uterus.

Precautions

None known.

Drug interactions

None known.

Research

- Candan F, Unlu M, Tebe B, et al 2003 Antioxidant and antimicrobial activity of the essential oil and methanol extracts of *Achillea* millefolium subsp. *millefolium* Afan. (Asteraceae). J Ethnopharmacol Aug; 87(2–3): 215–220

Allium sativum : Garlic

Family: Liliaceae
Part used: bulb
Taste/*Rasa*: all tastes except sour/*amla*
Post digestive/*Vipak*: pungent/*katu*
Potency/*Virya*: heating/*ushna*
***Dosha*:** VK- P+

Constituents

A variety of sulphur-containing compounds including allicin, alliein, lipids, antaocyanins, quercetin, kaempferol, glycosides, scordinins, tellurium compounds, essential amino acids, volatile oil, mucilage, germanium, glucokinins, vitamins.

Actions

Stimulant, carminative, expectorant, alterative, immunostimulant, antimicrobial, anthelmintic, lowers cholesterol, hypotensive, antitumour, rejuvenative, circulatory stimulant, digestive.

Indications

Colds, flu, chest infections, gastrointestinal tract infections, cystitis, worms, high cholesterol, hypertension, lowered resistance, thrush, catarrh, sinusitis.

Introduction

The humble *garlic* bulb, maligned for its powerful and lingering odour, is a wonderful medicine and has been valued as such for thousands of years. The ancient Egyptians used it for its energy-giving properties around 1500 BC and the Greeks and Romans, including Dioscorides and Galen, considered it a panacea and elixir of youth. Ayurvedic doctors in the 1st century AD in India prescribed *garlic* for heart disease, and for warding off infections. As recognized centuries ago, it is an effective antibacterial, antifungal, antiviral and antiparasitic remedy (Ankri and Mirelman 1999, Weber 1992). In an age of increasing drug resistance in bacteria, *garlic* may be of great value (Tsao and Yin 2001).

Garlic exerts its antimicrobial effects throughout the body. When absorbed from the digestive tract it circulates in the bloodstream and is excreted via the lungs, bowels, skin and urinary system, all of which are disinfected in the process. Recent research indicates that allicin is permeable through phospholipid membranes, which may account for its wide-ranging activity (Miron et al 2000).

Internal uses

Digestive system

Garlic has a beneficial effect on the digestion, stimulating secretion of digestive enzymes and bile, enhancing the movement of food through the gut and promoting absorption and assimilation of food. With its antimicrobial action it combats infection and aids the elimination of pathogenic bacteria in the gastrointestinal tract helping to restore the normal bacterial population of the gut after infection or orthodox antibiotics via the probiotic effects of fructo-oligosaccharides (Chow 2002). *Garlic* may also be of benefit in type 2 diabetes. It is an effective remedy for worms when taken on an empty stomach.

Circulatory system

In confirmation of the ancients' use of *garlic* for heart disease and high blood pressure, extensive research into the heart and circulation has indicated that *garlic* can significantly lower cholesterol, triglycerides, and low-density lipoproteins in the blood, although there is still controversy regarding its efficacy and correct dosage. However the German Commission E has approved *garlic* for the treatment of hyperlipoproteinemia in conjunction with other dietary measures and to prevent age-related atherosclerosis (Blumenthal et al 1994). It appears that *garlic* may interfere with cholesterol biosynthesis in the liver through a variety of mechanisms. The antithrombotic effects of *garlic* have also been extensively studied as have its hypotensive properties. *Garlic* has a vasodilatory action, increasing the flow of blood to the tissues and to the periphery of the body. This not only reduces blood pressure, but also increases the circulation, relieving cramps and circulatory disorders, such as Raynaud's disease.

Respiratory system

Garlic's antimicrobial properties can be put to good use in the treatment of sore throats, colds, flu and bronchial infections. Like other pungent remedies, *garlic* acts as a decongestant, helping to clear catarrh, and augmenting its antiseptic action in the respiratory tract. Its expectorant properties are helpful in coughs and may help to alleviate bronchial asthma, sinusitis, chronic catarrh, hayfever and rhinitis.

Immune system

Several in vitro studies indicate activity against viruses, including influenza B and herpes simplex type 1. In one study several viruses showed sensitivity at the highest concentration of *garlic* extract, including *vesicular stomatitis virus (VSV)*, *herpes simplex* 1 and 2, *para influenza type* 3 (Para-3), human rhinovirus and vaccinia virus. It was also shown that these viruses were inactivated by allicin. Of all the *garlic* preparations tested it was the products containing most allicin and other thiosulphinates which showed the highest antiviral activity. These products included crude garlic extract and powder and some but not all of the garlic tablets and capsules tested. Steam-distilled and oil-based products that did not contain thiosulphinates had no effect on the viruses (Weber 1992). Recent research has shown that *garlic* acts as a powerful antioxidant (Banerjee et al 2003) and its sulphur compounds have antitumour activities (Thomson and Ali 2003), while it is also said to protect the body against the effects of pollution and nicotine. Thus *garlic* may well help to slow down the ageing process, verifying our ancestors' use of *garlic* as a rejuvenative tonic and "elixir of youth".

Temperature

By causing sweating it helps resolve fevers.

External uses

Externally, *garlic* can be crushed and macerated in oil or made into an ointment to treat cuts and wounds, inflamed joints, gout and rheumatism, sprains, unbroken chilblains, athlete's foot, ringworm, stings, bites and warts. The effectiveness of garlic against the major pathogens involved in otitis media suggests it may be useful in management of this disorder (Klein 1999). An oil infusion can be used as eardrops to relieve ear infections and earache, and rubbed into the chest for chest infections and coughs. *Garlic* vinegar can be used for disinfecting and dressing ulcers and septic wounds. *Garlic* can also be used for oral and vaginal thrush when used locally. Trials have indicated success using allicin in treating thrush in newborn infants (Zhang 1992).

Precautions

Garlic is contraindicated in some sources in large doses during pregnancy. Large doses of raw garlic (possibly in excess of four cloves a day) may cause heartburn, flatulence and gastrointestinal upset. Raw *garlic* applied to the skin can cause contact dermatitis. Due to its reduction of platelet aggravation it may cause postoperative bleeding (Smith and Boon 1999). Except for small doses of cooked *garlic*, therapeutic doses of *garlic* should be discontinued 7–10 days before surgery due to antiplatelet activity. Gastrointestinal upset can occur in sensitive individuals.

Drug interactions

Anticoagulant/antiplatelet agent. Practitioners should be watchful of patients on warfarin who consume generous amounts of *garlic*. Antihypertensive medications.

Research

- Ankri S, Mirelman D 1999 Antimicrobial properties of allicin from garlic. Microbes Infect 1(2): 125–129
- Banerjee SK, Mukherjee PK, Maulik SK 2003 Garlic as an antioxidant: the good, the bad and the ugly. Phytother Res 17(2): 97–106
- Blumenthal M, Brusse WR, Goldberg A, et al 1994 The complete German Commission E Monographs. Austin Texas: American Botanical Council
- Chow J 2002 Probiotics and prebiotics: A brief overview. J Ren Nutr 12(2): 76–86

- Klein JO 1999 Management of acute otitis media in an era of increasing antibiotic resistance. Int J Pediatr Otorhinolaryngol 49(Suppl 1): S15–17
- Miron T, Rabinkov A, Mirelman D, et al 2000 The mode of action of allicin: its ready permeability through phospholipid membranes may contribute to its biological activity. Biochim Biophys Acta 1463(1): 20–30
- Smith M, Boon H 1999 The Botanical Pharmacy. Quarry Health Books. Ontario, Canada, p. 140
- Thomson M, Ali M 2003 Garlic: a review of its potential use as an anti-cancer agent. Curr Cancer Drug Targets 3(1): 67–81
- Tsao S, Yin M 2001 In vitro activity of garlic oil and four diallyl sulphides against antibiotic-resistant *Pseudomonas aeruginosa* and *Klebsiella pneumoniae*. J Antimicrob Chemother 47(5): 665–670
- Weber ND 1992 In vitro virucidal effects of *Allium sativum* (garlic) extract and compounds. Planta Med 58(5): 417–423
- Zhang RS 1992 A clinical study on allicin in the prevention of thrush in newborn infants. Zhongguo Zhong Xi Yi Jie He Za Zhi 12(1): 28–29

Anethum graveolens : Dill

Family: Umbelliferae
Part used: leaves, seeds
Taste/Rasa: pungent/*katu*, bitter/*tikta*
Post digestive/Vipak: pungent/*katu*
Potency/Virya: cooling/*sheeta*
Dosha: PK- Vo

Constituents

Volatile oil: including limonene, carvone; flavonoids: including daempfenol and vincenin, coumarins, magnesium, iron, calcium, potassium, vitamin C.

Actions

Carminative, alterative, expectorant, diuretic, anti-spasmodic, galactagogue, vermifuge, analgesic, relaxant, digestive, sedative.

Indications

Colic, wind, sleeping problems, coughs, asthma, urinary problems.

Introduction

The tranquillizing properties of *dill* have been known since the days of the ancient Greeks and Romans. Its name is said to come from the Saxon word dilla, to lull, due to the plant's ability to relax babies and children into a restful sleep. The volatile oil in *dill* seeds and leaves relaxes smooth muscle throughout the body.

Internal uses

Digestive system

Dill has a stimulating effect on digestion, enhancing appetite and digestion. As an antispasmodic and carminative *dill* releases tension and spasm in the digestive tract relieving colic and wind, indigestion and nausea and constipation as well as diarrhoea. It is an important ingredient in the famous Gripe water, used by generations of mothers to relieve babies' colic. In India *dill* is used as a vermifuge.

Nervous system

Dill has been used traditionally to help alleviate tiredness from disturbed nights and to strengthen the brain. The leaves were often cooked with fish to add flavour and to stimulate the brain. The relaxant properties of *dill* also help treat insomnia, and are good for stress-related digestive disorders, such as wind, colic and constipation.

Respiratory system

In the respiratory system *dill* acts as an anti-spasmodic and expectorant and has been used as an ingredient in medicines for coughs and asthma.

Reproductive system

In the reproductive system the antispasmodic effects can relieve painful periods and through its emmenagogic properties to regulate menstruation. In the East *dill* is given to women prior to childbirth to ease the birth. It increases milk in breastfeeding women.

Urinary system

Dill has diuretic effects.

Immune system

Research has confirmed the antibacterial (Singh et al 2002) and anticandidal (Jirovetz et al 2003) properties of *dill* and also that *dill* may have an ability to inhibit cancer formation. Various components of *dill* weed oil, including anethofuran, carvone and limonene have been researched and results look promising (Foster 1997).

External uses

Dill's analgesic and anti-inflammatory properties can help relieve pain and swelling. The essential oil is a useful ingredient of massage oils and liniments for abdominal pain, colic, arthritis and earache.

Drug interactions

None known.

Research

- Foster S 1997 Herbal Rennaisance. Gibb Smith, Utah, p. 82
- Jirovetz L, Buchbauer G, Stoyanova AS, Georgiev EV, Damianova ST 2003 Composition, quality control, and antimicrobial activity of the essential oil of long-time stored dill (*Anethum graveolens* L.) seeds from Bulgaria. J Agric Food Chem 51(13): 3854–3857
- Singh G, Kapoor IP, Pandey SK, Singh UK, Singh RK 2002 Studies on essential oils: part 10; antibacterial activity of volatile oils of some spices. Phytother Res 16(7): 680–682

Arctium lappa : Burdock

Family: Compositae
Part used: roots, seeds, leaves
Taste/*Rasa*: bitter, astringent, pungent; the root is also sweet
Post digestive/*Vipak*: pungent/*katu*
Potency/*Virya*: cooling/*sheeta*
Dosha: PK- V+ (in excess)

Constituents

Roots: up to 50% inulin, mucilage, pectin, poly-acetylenes, volatile acids, sterols, tannin, bitters, aldehydes, flavonoid glycosides (quercetin and kaempferol, asparagin, polyphenolic acid.
Seeds: 15–30% fixed oils, bitter glycoside (arctiin), flavonoids, chlorogenic acid.
Leaves: terpenoids, including arctiopicrin, sterols and triterpenols, mucilage, essential oil, tannin, inulin.

Actions

Alterative, diaphoretic, diuretic, astringent, bitter tonic, digestive, mild laxative, antimicrobial, hypo-glycaemic, febrifuge, antitumour.

Indications

Chronic skin problems, fevers, infections, urinary problems, arthritis, gout.

Introduction

An important alterative remedy, *burdock* has a long history of use as a "blood cleanser" and detoxify-ing remedy, hastening the elimination of toxins from the body. Since Medieval times the whole plant has been respected for its cleansing and anti-septic properties. Today it is used particularly for inflammatory skin problems and for chronic inflam-matory conditions such as arthritis and gout. The root is generally the part favoured in Western medicine while in Asian medicine the seeds are also used.

Internal uses

Digestive system

The roots, leaves and seeds are all bitter, stimulat-ing digestion and the function of the liver and pancreas. *Burdock* is reported to have a hypogly-caemic action and so may be helpful in the treat-ment of diabetes (Newall et al 1996). *Burdock* is used to treat symptoms associated with a weak digestion including wind, distension and indiges-tion and works as a mild laxative. It is an effective remedy for bacterial and fungal infections and to help re-establish normal bacteria in the gut. The fructo-oligosaccharides found in *burdock* root have a probiotic effect (Flickinger et al 2002) which may help re-establish intestinal flora following anti-biotic use. Research has demonstrated both anti-bacterial and anticandidal activity (Holetz et al 2002).

Respiratory system

Burdock has been traditionally used to enhance immunity to colds, coughs and used to treat fevers accompanying respiratory infections. It has a par-ticular affinity with the lymphatic system and can be used for sore throats and swollen tonsils. The seeds are also effective for treating sore throats, ton-silitis, colds and coughs.

Reproductive system

The root is reputed to stimulate the uterus, and, perhaps due to its ability to aid liver function and the breakdown of hormones in the liver, it has been used to regulate periods. It has also been used traditionally for prolapse and to give strength before and after childbirth.

Urinary system

Burdock has mild diuretic properties, aiding elim-ination of toxins via the urine. It can be used for cystitis, water retention, stones and gravel.

Immune system

Extracts of the root, flowers and the leaves have all been shown to have antibiotic actions. The leaves are active against Gram-positive and Gram-negative bacteria, the flowers and root against Gram-negative bacteria (Moskalenko 1986). Arctiopicrin also has an antibacterial effect against Gram-negative bacteria. Taken as a hot decoction, it helps to clear toxins from the tissues via the skin as it has a diaphoretic action. *Burdock* helps to bring out eruptions and thus speed recovery from infections such as measles and chickenpox. By pushing toxins from the tissues into the bloodstream, and thence to the gut for elimination, *burdock* makes an effective remedy for skin problems and chronic inflammatory conditions such as gout, arthritis and rheumatism. For this reason it is best taken with a mild laxative to ensure elimination of toxins otherwise it may cause temporary aggravation of symptoms until toxins are cleared. Research has demonstrated that *burdock* possesses antimutagenic effects (Chandler and Osborne 1997) and may have the ability to protect against the toxic effects of chemicals such as food colourings.

Temperature

It can be used to bring down a fever and can be taken at the onset of infections.

Skin

It is excellent for treating chronic skin disease, such as acne, as it improves the action of the sebaceous glands and aids the detoxifying work of the liver.

Precautions

Uterine stimulant actions are contraindicated in pregnancy and lactation. Given *burdock's* effect on blood sugar, care needs to be taken with concomitant use with oral hypoglycaemic medicines (Newall et al 1996).

Drug interactions

Diabetic agents: very large doses of *burdock* may have mild hypoglycaemic effects. Though this effect is minimal with normal use, diabetics should monitor their blood sugar and medications should be adjusted if necessary.

Research

- Chandler F and Osborne F 1997 Can Pharm J Jun; 130: 46–49
- Flickinger EA, Hatch TF, Wofford RC, et al 2002 In vitro fermentation properties of selected fructooligosaccharide-containing vegetables and in vivo colonic microbial populations are affected by the diets of healthy human infants. J Nutr 132(8): 2188–2194
- Holetz FB, Pessini GL, Sanches NR, et al 2002 Screening of some plants used in the Brazilian folk medicine for the treatment of infectious diseases. Mem Inst Oswaldo Cruz 97(7): 1027–1031
- Moskalenko S 1986 Preliminary screening of Far Eastern ethnomedicinal plants for antibacterial activity. J Ethnopharmacol 15: 231–259
- Newall C, Anderson L, Phillipson DJ 1996 Herbal Medicines: A Guide for Health Care Professionals. London. The Pharmaceutical Press, p. 296

Calendula officinalis : Marigold

Family: Compositae
Part used: flowers
Taste/*Rasa*: bitter/*tikta*, pungent/*katu*
Post digestive/*Vipak*: pungent/*katu*
Potency/*Virya*: cooling/*sheeta*
Dosha: PK- V+

Constituents

Flavonoids, including rutin and isoquercetin, volatile oil, terpenoids including lupeol, taraxerol, taraxasterol, saponins, polysaccharides, bitters, beta carotene.

Actions

Alterative, antiseptic, anti-inflammatory, diaphoretic, bitter tonic, digestive, antiulcer, antitumour, antioxidant.

Indications

Inflammatory skin problems, inflammatory digestive problems, fevers, infections, first aid for minor burns, cuts and grazes.

Introduction

Famous today as a first aid remedy, *marigold* has been popular since the Romans who used it for fevers and for applications to warts. In Medieval times it was used for intestinal problems, liver complaints, insect and snake bites. Gerard, in his *Herball* of 1597 and Culpeper, in his *English Physician* written in 1652 recommended *marigold* to comfort the heart and lift the spirits, and for inflammation of the eyes. The Shakers used *marigold* for gangrene. The flowers are edible and can be added to salads. Research has now confirmed that *marigold* flowers have antiseptic and astringent properties provided by the volatile oils, tannins and a yellow resin called calendulin. It has also been shown that triterpenoids have an anti-inflammatory effect (Della Loggia et al 1994) and its antioxidant and free radical scavenging effects may account for its antibacterial and anti-inflammatory properties.

Internal uses

Digestive system

With its anti-inflammatory effects (Mascolo et al 1987) *marigold* makes a good remedy for inflammatory conditions of the gastrointestinal tract including gastritis and peptic ulcers. The tannins with their astringent effect can be used to check diarrhoea and stop bleeding. The bitters stimulate the secretion of digestive enzymes and the actions of the liver and gallbladder, and have a reputation for improving digestion and absorption and preventing gallstones. *Marigold* has a mild laxative effect and has been used for symptoms associated with toxicity or "liverishness" such as headaches, chronic skin problems, nausea, lethargy and irritability. Its antimicrobial and anthelmintic properties help check amoebic infections and intestinal worms. *Marigold* has been used for pelvic and bowel infections, including enteritis and dysentery as well as for viral hepatitis.

Circulatory system

Marigold is employed for its ability to improve venous return for the relief of symptoms related to varicose veins. It enhances the circulation and has a diaphoretic action.

Reproductive system

Marigold has an affinity for the female reproductive system. It has been found to have uterotonic actions in vitro (Shipchlier 1981) and in practice it is found to regulate menstruation, reduce tension in the uterine muscles and relieve menstrual cramps. It is reputed to have a hormone-balancing effect, which can help relieve menopausal symptoms and reduce breast congestion with tenderness and mastitis. Its astringent properties help reduce excessive menstrual bleeding and uterine congestion. *Marigold* has a reputation for treating tumours and cysts of the female reproductive system, such as fibroids and ovarian cysts, as well as cysts in the breast and digestive tract. During childbirth it is used to promote contractions and delivery of the placenta. For this reason it should not be used during pregnancy.

Urinary system

Marigold has a mild diuretic effect and with its antibacterial action it can be used for urinary tract infections and fluid retention.

Immune system

Calendula can enhance the action of the immune system, possibly by enhancing the proliferative response of human lymphocytes (Amirghofran et al 2000). The high-density polysaccharides are reported to have immunostimulant properties in vitro (Wagner 1984). It has been reported to have antibacterial (Dumenil et al 1980) and antiviral activity (Boucaud-Maitre et al 1988) and can be effective in controlling flu and herpes viruses. It is one of the best plants for treating fungal infections such as thrush and is also used to reduce lymphatic congestion and swollen lymph glands. With its diuretic action increasing the elimination of toxins through the urine, and aided by its triterpenoid content which contributes to its anti-inflammatory action *marigold* (Della Loggia et al 1994) has been used to relieve rheumatism, arthritis and gout. It has a reputation as an anticancer remedy and research in which extracts have been found to have in vitro cytotoxicity has backed this up (Boucaud-Maitre et al 1988).

Temperature

Taken in hot infusion *marigold* promotes diaphoresis, and thereby relieves fevers. By bringing blood to the surface of the body it helps the body throw off toxins and bring out eruptions such as measles and chickenpox. It is a good remedy for treating fevers and infections in children, such as colds and flu.

External uses

Externally, *marigold* has pride of place as a first aid remedy to staunch bleeding of cuts and abrasions, as an antiseptic healer for sores and ulcers, and to prevent putrefaction of cuts and wounds. Research has shown it useful as a haemostatic in experimental aerosol preparations (Garg and Sharma 1992). Used in tincture, infusion or simply by crushing a flower, it rapidly resolves inflammation, swelling and exudate due to injuries, promotes tissue repair and minimizes scar formation. Compresses applied to varicose veins, bruises, sprains and strains will reduce swelling and pain. A crushed flower can be rubbed on to insect bites, wasp or bee stings. An infusion can be used as a mouthwash for inflamed gums, a douche for vaginal infections, or an eyewash for inflammatory eye conditions.

Precautions

Contact sensitization has been reported to Calendula (Reider et al 2001). Avoid during pregnancy.

Drug interactions

Sedatives: there are some reports of an additive effect with sedatives.

Research

- Amirghofran Z, Azadbakht M, Karimi MH 2000 Evaluation of the immunomodulatory effects of five herbal plants. J Ethnopharmacol 72(1–2): 167–172
- Boucaud-Maitre Y, Algernon O, Raynaud J 1988 Cytotoxic and antitumoral activity of *Calendula officinalis* extracts. Pharmazie 43: 221–222
- Della Loggia R, Tubaro A, Sosa S, et al 1994 The role of triterpenoid in the topical anti-inflammatory activity of *Calendula officinalis* flowers. Planta Med 60(6): 516–520
- Dumenil G, Chemli R, Balansard G, Guirand H, Lallemand M 1980 Evaluation of antibacterial properties of marigold flowers and homeopathic mother tincture of *Calendula off*. Annales Pharmaceutiques Francaises 36(6): 493–499
- Garg S, Sharma SN 1992 Development of medicated aerosol dressings of chlorhexidine acetate with hemostatics. Pharmazie 47(12): 924–926

- Mascolo N, Autore G, Capasso G 1987 Biological screening of Italian medicinal plants for anti-inflammatory activity. Phytother Res 1(28)
- Reider N, Komericki P, Hausen BM, Fritsch P, Aberer W 2001 The seamy side of natural medicines: contact sensitization to arnica (*Arnica montana* L.) and marigold (*Calendula officinalis* L). Contact Dermatitis 45(5): 269–272
- Shipchlier T 1981 Uterotonic action of extracts from a group of medicinal plants. Vet Med Nauki 18(4): 94–98
- Wagner H 1984 The immune stimulating poly-saccharides and heteroglycans of higher plants. A preliminary communication. Arzneimittel-forschung 34(6): 659–661

Chamomilla recutita syn./Matricaria recutita : German chamomile

ANTHEMIS NOBILIS SYN./CHAMAEMALUM NOBILE: ROMAN CHAMOMILE

Family: Compositae
Part used: flowers
Taste/Rasa: bitter/*tikta*, pungent/*katu*
Post digestive/Vipak: pungent/*katu*
Potency/Virya: cooling/*sheeta*
Dosha: PK- V+ (in excess)

Constituents

Volatile oil, inc. azulene, flavonoids, coumarins, plant acids, fatty acids, cyanogenic glycosides, salicylate derivatives, choline, tannin.

Actions

Anti-inflammatory, antispasmodic, nervine, sedative, antiulcer, antihistamine, digestive, antiseptic, antimicrobial, diaphoretic, febrifuge, anodyne, diuretic, emmenagogue, emetic.

Indications

Inflammatory digestive problems, insomnia, hayfever, eczema, headaches, abdominal pain and spasm, nervous problems of children, inflammatory eye problems, dysmenorrhoea.

Introduction

Two kinds of chamomile are used medicinally: German chamomile (*Matricaria chamomilla/Chamomilla recutita*) and Roman chamomile (*Anthemis nobilis/Chamaemalum nobile*). Their properties are similar but German *chamomile* may be preferable for children as it tastes less bitter. *Chamomile* was recommended by Dioscorides as a cure for fevers as early as 900 BC and was known to the ancient Egyptians who praised it for its ability to cure "ague". It was one of the nine sacred herbs of the Saxons who used it as a calming remedy and to treat stomach problems. In the Middle Ages it was frequently strewn in insanitary halls of castles and great houses to keep infection at bay.

Internal uses

Digestive system

Chamomile is famous for soothing all kinds of digestive upsets, especially those related to stress such as nervous indigestion, heartburn and acidity, and for digestive infections such as gastroenteritis. It has the ability to relax smooth muscle throughout the body. In the digestive tract it relieves tension and spasm and is recommended for colic (particularly in babies), abdominal pain, wind and distension. By regulating peristalsis it can treat both diarrhoea and constipation. Chamazulene in the volatile oil has an anti-inflammatory action, possibly by means of inhibiting leukotriene synthesis (Safayhi et al 1994), and helps to relieve gastritis and peptic ulcers, colitis and irritable bowel syndrome. The bitters in *chamomile* stimulate the flow of bile and the secretion of digestive juices, enhancing the appetite and improving a sluggish digestion. Bisabolol in the volatile oil has been shown to prevent and to speed up the healing of ulcers both internally and externally, making *chamomile* an excellent remedy for gastritis, peptic ulcers.

Nervous system

Chamomile is an excellent relaxant for babies and children, with sedative and mood-enhancing properties (Roberts and Williams 1992). It calms anxiety and nervousness and is particularly useful for tense children who tend to be hyperactive and highly sensitive, prone to digestive problems and allergies. The anxiolytic properties may be due to the affinity of apigenin and other constituents to central benzodiazepine receptors (Viola et al 1995). It is recommended for all stress-related problems, particularly those affecting the digestion, such as acid indigestion, colic, abdominal pain, peptic ulcers, wind, diarrhoea and constipation. It is well known for calming restless babies prone to colic, teething and sleeping problems, as well as overactive, irritable children. Research has shown that infusions of *chamomile* flowers have been used successfully in the treatment of restlessness and in mild cases of insomnia due to nervous disorders (Carle and Gomaa 1992, Gould et al 1973). It promotes sleep and also has pain-relieving properties – it can be taken for headaches, migraine, neuralgia, toothache, aches and pains of flu, cramps, arthritis and gout. It can be used to good effect to relieve period pain and premenstrual headaches and to ease contractions during childbirth.

Respiratory system

Chamomile tea is one of the first remedies to consider for children's fevers and respiratory infections such as sore throats, colds and flu. Its antimicrobial effects enhance the immune system's efforts to throw off infections and allergies and its relaxant effect on the bronchial tubes helps to reduce bronchoconstriction in asthma. Steam inhalations can help relieve asthma, hayfever, catarrh and sinusitis.

Reproductive system

The name Matricaria comes from matrix meaning mother or womb, indicating its historic use going back to Greek and Roman times as a remedy for women's ailments. It is used to relax spasm associated with painful periods, as a digestive remedy for nausea and sickness in pregnancy, to relieve mastitis, premenstrual headaches and migraines and to reduce menopausal symptoms. The tea can be drunk throughout childbirth to relax tension and lessen the pain of contractions. Dilute *chamomile* oil can be used for massage and for inhalation during childbirth and can be effective at transition stage when pain can seem intolerable. It has been prescribed for amenorrhoea due to stress or psychological problems such as anorexia nervosa. It can also be used in infusions and creams for sore nipples and as a douche for vaginal infections including thrush. Sitting in a bowl of *chamomile* tea can be very soothing for cystitis and haemorrhoids.

Urinary system

Its antiseptic oils are excreted via the urinary system where it can soothe an inflamed bladder and relieve cystitis.

Immune system

Chamomile acts to enhance the function of the immune system and is a very useful medicine for all fevers and infections. By inducing a restful sleep it encourages natural recovery, particularly in children for whom rest is probably the best medicine. The volatile oil is a powerful antiseptic, active against bacteria, including *Staphylococcus aureus*, and fungal infections, including thrush (*Candida albicans*) (Carle and Isaac 1987). It has an antiallergic effect, reducing oversensitivity to allergens such as pollen and house dust, making it applicable to the general treatment of allergies. Its relaxing and destressing effect helps in dealing with emotional issues underlying such allergies. The anti-inflammatory properties also help resolve inflammatory problems such as conjunctivitis and tonsillitis.

External uses

Externally the oils exert a soothing, antiseptic and anti-inflammatory effect on the skin, and stimulate tissue repair. In creams and infusion *chamomile* is used for speeding healing of ulcers, sores, burns and scalds and a range of skin disorders. A 2-week placebo-controlled trial on patients using a cream containing *chamomile* extract with atopic eczema demonstrated mild superiority over 0.5% hydrocortisone cream (Patzelt-Wenczler 1985). A small double-blind trial demonstrated a statistically significant decrease in the weeping wound area following dermabrasion of tattoos (Glowania et al 1987).

Chamomile tea makes a good mouthwash for mouth ulcers and inflamed gums, a gargle for sore throats, an antiseptic wash for sore inflamed eyes as in conjunctivitis, and a lotion for inflammatory skin conditions. Dilute oil of *chamomile* when massaged into painful, inflamed joints can bring relief as it will help to relieve pain such as trigeminal neuralgia or sciatica. It can also help repel insects and soothe the pain of bites and stings. Topically it can be an effective treatment for varicose ulcers.

Precautions

There are varied reports of *chamomile* sensitivity in between 1.3 to 7.1% of patients leading to contact eczema (Mills and Bone 2000). Disturbing reports of high levels of pesticides and heavy metals have been reported in chamomile coming out of Eastern Europe. Organic *chamomile* is suggested.

Drug interaction

None known.

Research

- Carl R, Gomaa K 1992 Chamomile: a pharmacological and clinical profile. Drugs of Today 28: 559–565
- Carle R, Isaac O 1987 Zeitschrift für Phytotherapie 8: 67–77
- Glowania H, Raulin Chr, Swoboda M 1987 Effect of chamomile on wound healing – a clinical double blind study. Z Hautkr 62(17): 1262–1271
- Gould L, Reddy CVR, Gomprecht RF 1973 Cardiac effect of chamomile tea. Journal of Clinical Pharmacology 13: 475–479
- Mills S, Bone K 2000 Principles and Practice of Phytotherapy. Churchill Livingstone, London
- Patzelt-Wenczler R 1985 Dtsch Apoth Ztg 125(43 suppl 1): 12–13
- Roberts A, Williams JM 1992 The effect of olfactory stimulation on fluency, vividness of imagery and associated mood: a preliminary study. Br J Med Psychol 65(2): 197–199
- Safayhi H, Sabieraj J, Sailer ER, Ammon HP 1994 Chamazulene: an antioxidant-type inhibitor of leukotriene B4 formation. Planta Med 60(5): 410–413
- Viola H, Wasowski C, Levi de Stein M, et al 1995 Apigenin, a component of *Matricaria recutita* flowers, is a central benzodiazepine receptor-ligand with anxiolytic effects. Planta Med 61: 213–215

Echinacea angustifolia/purpurea : Echinacea

Family: Compositae
Part used: whole herb or root
Taste/Rasa: pungent/*katu*, bitter/*tikta*
Post digestive/Vipak: pungent/*katu*
Potency/Virya: cooling/*sheeta*
Dosha: PK- V+

Constituents

Echinacosides, chlorogenic acid, alkylamides, echinacein, isobutylamides, polyacetylenes, D-acidic arabinogalactan polysaccharide.

Actions

Alterative, antibiotic, diaphoretic, anti-inflammatory, immunostimulant.

Indications

Septic conditions, rheumatoid arthritis, antibiotic resistance, whooping cough in children, flu, chronic respiratory tract infections, gynaecological infections, pelvic inflammatory disease, urinary infections, skin problems and a wide range of complaints including boils and abscesses, blood poisoning, post-partum infection, malaria, typhus and TB problems.

Introduction

Native Americans used *echinacea* to treat wounds, burns, abscesses, insect bites, sore throats, toothaches, and joint pains and as an antidote for poisonous snake bites (Kuhn and Winston 2001). Scientific information on the medicinal benefits of echinacea comes from two fronts. From 1895 to 1930 American doctors demonstrated the immune-enhancing and antimicrobial effects of *echinacea*, and from German studies over the last 50 years much of this research has been validated.

Internal uses

Respiratory system

Research has focused on *echinacea*'s efficacy in treating the common cold and upper respiratory infections. A recent Cochrane review reports that most studies have positive results, though the efficacy of different *echinacea* preparations may vary (Melchart et al 2000).

Immune system

Research into the mode of action of the immune-stimulating effect of *echinacea* suggests many mechanisms, including increased phagocytosis of pathogens by means of macrophage activation (Wildfeuer and Mayerhofer 1994, Barrett 2003). *Echinacea* has an antibiotic and antifungal effect mediated by immune stimulation, an antiviral action (Binns et al 2002) and an antiallergenic action. This means that it can be taken at the first signs of sore throats, colds, chest infections, tonsillitis, and glandular fever as well as for candida and post viral fatigue syndrome (ME). As a blood cleanser it will help to clear the skin of infections, and will help to relieve allergies such as urticaria and eczema. It is particularly useful for people whose deficient immune system makes them prone to one infection after another. It is used in Germany along with chemotherapy in treatment of cancer.

Temperature

Taken in hot infusion, it stimulates the circulation and stimulates sweating, helping to bring down fevers.

Other uses

The anti-inflammatory effect (Clifford et al 2002) of *echinacea* helps relieve arthritis and gout, skin conditions and pelvic inflammatory disease.

External uses

Externally, *echinacea* is a good anti-inflammatory and antiseptic remedy for skin problems, wounds, ulcers, burns, stings and bites. Ten to 20 drops of the tincture diluted in water make a good gargle and mouthwash for sore throats and infected gums and a douche for vaginal infections.

Dosage

Between $\frac{1}{4}$ and $\frac{1}{2}$ a teaspoon in acute infections every 2 hours and in chronic infections three times daily.

Precautions

There are reports of occasional sensitivity to *echinacea*, causing anaphylaxis, asthma or urticaria (Mullins and Heddle 2002). Otherwise, reviews of the literature indicate very few adverse effects and no known drug interactions (Izzo and Ernst 2001). If patients have allergies to Asteraceae family pollen (chrysanthemum, chamomile, ragweed, daisy) avoid products made from *echinacea* flowers. The leaf juice or root products should not provoke an allergic response.

Drug interaction

None known.

Research

- Barrett B 2003 Medicinal properties of Echinacea: a critical review. Phytomedicine 10(1): 66–86
- Binns SE, Hudson J, Merali S, Arnason JT 2002 Antiviral activity of characterized extracts from Echinacea spp against herpes simplex virus. Planta Med 68(9): 780–783
- Clifford LJ, Nair MG, Rana J, Dewitt DL 2002 Bioactivity of alkamides isolated from Echinacea purpurea. Phytomedicine 9(3): 249–253
- Izzo AA, Ernst E 2001 Interactions between herbal medicines and prescribed drugs: a systematic review. Drugs 61(15): 2163–2175
- Kuhn MA, Winston D 2001 Herbal Therapy & Supplements. Lippincott, Philadelphia
- Melchart D, Linde K, Fischer P, Kaesmayr J 2000 Echinacea for preventing and treating the common cold. Cochrane Database Syst Rev (2): CD000530
- Mullins RJ, Heddle R 2002 Adverse reactions associated with echinacea: the Australian experience. 1. Ann Allergy Asthma Immunol 88(1): 42–51
- Wildfeuer A, Mayerhofer D 1994 The effects of plant preparations on cellular functions in body defence. Arzneimittelforschung 44(3): 361–366

Glycyrrhiza glabra : Liquorice

Family: Leguminosae
Part used: peeled roots and runners
Taste/Rasa: sweet/*madhura*, bitter/*tikta*
Post digestive/Vipak: sweet/*madhura*
Potency/Virya: cooling/*sheeta*
Dosha: VP- K+

Constituents

Glycyrrhizin (calcium and potassium salts of gly-cyrrhizic acid), triterpenoid saponins, flavonoids, bitter principle (glycymarin), oestrogenic sub-stances, asparagin, volatile oil, coumarins, tannins.

Actions

Demulcent, expectorant, tonic, laxative, anti-inflammatory, antipyretic, diuretic, adaptogen, anti-tussive, antacid.

Indications

Inflammatory problems, allergies, menstrual and menopausal problems, digestive problems, stress-related problems, constipation, sore throats, respira-tory infections, asthma, viral infections including herpes, hormonal problems.

Introduction

Liquorice is the most remarkable herb with an affin-ity for the endocrine system. Glycyrrhizin has a similar structure to hormones produced by the adre-nal glands, giving *liquorice* an anti-inflammatory (Shibata et al 1996) and antiallergic (Lee et al 1996) effect similar (but without the side effects) of corti-sone. It is useful for people coming off orthodox steroid drugs. Possibly by its action on the adrenal glands, *liquorice* has the ability to improve resist-ance to stress. Its use can be considered during times of physical and emotional stress, after surgery, during convalescence, or nervous exhaustion.

Internal uses

Digestive system

Liquorice has a well-documented reputation for healing ulcers (Baker 1994). It lowers stomach acid levels and relieves heartburn and indigestion. It also acts as a mild laxative. Through its beneficial action on the liver, it increases bile flow and lowers cholesterol levels. Its antihepatoxic effects make *liquorice* useful in treating chronic hepatitis and possibly cirrhosis (Tillotson et al 2001).

Nervous system

Liquorice is an adaptogen that improves resilience to stress.

Respiratory system

In the respiratory system its demulcent action reduces irritation and inflammation. It is one of the best remedies for soothing sore throats and dry coughs and it also has an expectorant effect (Barnett 1997), making it useful in treatment of irritating coughs, asthma and chest infections. Its antialler-genic effect is useful for hayfever, allergic rhinitis, conjunctivitis and bronchial asthma.

Immune system

A number of trials have demonstrated an antiviral effect including anticytomegalovirus (Numazake et al 1994) and antiherpes simplex (Pompei et al 1980) properties. Its anti-inflammatory effects can be applied for the relief of a wide variety of condi-tions including arthritis, skin problems such as eczema and psoriasis, headaches, hayfever and asthma. *Liquorice* is classed as a desmutagen, due to its ability to bind to toxic chemicals and carcinogens. The polyphenol flavonoids known as isoflavones may reduce the negative effect of LDL cholesterol and reduce atherosclerotic lesions (Tillotson et al 2001).

Reproductive system

The steroid-like compounds in *liquorice* can change to oestradiol and oestrone, which are oestrogen precursors, giving *liquorice* mild oestro-genic properties.

Temperature

Its cooling and anti-inflammatory properties are helpful in relieving fevers and soothing pain such as headaches.

External uses

Liquorice can be applied to wounds as an ointment made by mixing fine root powder with ghee.

Precautions

Side effects have been noted in cases of prolonged use of excessive intake, though generally through consumption of *liquorice* sweets (Heldal and Midtvedt 2002). These include hyperkalaemia, pseudo-aldosteronism and hypertension. *Liquorice* is contraindicated if there is a history of hypertension, and may result in excessive potassium loss if combined with diuretics or laxatives. *Liquorice* may potentiate the effects of prednisolone and should not be used during pregnancy (Mills and Bone 2000).

Drug interactions

Avoid use with diuretics as *liquorice* inhibits fluid loss and increases potassium loss. Do not use with digitalis as it decreases effectiveness and increases side effects related to K+ and Na+. Use cautiously with antihypertensives as may inhibit activity. Use cautiously with corticosteroids as it can potentiate effects. Dosage of medication may need to be adjusted. Use cautiously with laxatives as may increase potassium loss and cause hypokalaemia (Kuhn and Winston 2001).

Research

- Baker ME 1994 Liquorice and enzymes other than 11 beta-hydroxysteroid dehydrogenase: an evolutionary perspective. Steroids 59(2): 136–141
- Barnett RA 1997 Tonics. HarperPerennial, HarperCollins, New York
- Lee YM, Hirota S, Jippo-Kanemoto T 1996 Inhibition of histamine synthesis by glycyrrhetinic acid in mast cells cocultured with Swiss 3T3 fibroblasts. Int Arch Allergy Immunol 110(3): 272–277
- Heldal K, Midtvedt K 2002 Liquorice – not just candy. Tidsskr Nor Laegeforen 122(8): 774–776
- Kuhn MA, Winston D 2001 Herbal Therapy & Supplements. Lippincott, Philadelphia
- Mills S, Bone K 2000 Principles and Practice of Phytotherapy. Churchill Livingstone, London
- Numazake K, Umetsu M, Chiba S 1994 Effect of glycyrrhizin in children with liver dysfunction associated with cytomegalovirus infection. Tohoku J Exp Med 172(2): 147–153
- Pompei R, Pani A, Flore O 1980 Antiviral activity of glycyrrhizic acid. Experimentia 36(3): 304
- Shibata T, Morimoto T, Suzuki A 1996 The effect of Shakuyaku-kanzo-to on prostaglandin production in human uterine myometrium. Nippon Sanka Fujinka Gakkai Zasshi 48(5): 321–327
- Tillotson AK, Tillotson NH, Robert A Jr 2001 The One Earth Herbal Sourcebook. Kensington Publishing Corps, New York

Hamamelis virginiana : Witch hazel

Family: Hamamelidaceae
Part used: leaves, bark and twigs
Taste/*Rasa*: bitter/*tikta*, astringent/*kashaya*, pungent/*katu*
Post digestive/*Vipak*: pungent/*katu*
Potency/*Virya*: cooling/*sheeta*
Dosha: PK- V+

Constituents

Tannins, saponins, choline, resins, flavonoids.

Actions

Astringent, haemostatic, vulnerary, slightly sedative, anodyne.

Indications

Skin problems, sore throat, burns, bruising, cold sores, haemorrhoids, varicose veins.

Introduction

Extracts of *witch hazel* used to be popular as a household first aid remedy for scalds and burns, bleeding and bruising. Its main action is astringent due to the high levels of tannins that occur in the plant, making it an effective remedy to staunch bleeding. *Witch hazel* was a favourite herb of the Native Americans, who dried it and used it as snuff for nose bleeds and mixed it with flax seed to apply to painful swellings and tumours. The branches used to be valued as divining rods for finding underground water and metals.

Internal uses

Digestive system

Witch hazel has a traditional use in treatment of diarrhoea, dysentery, colitis and respiratory catarrh, but is not generally used internally in present practice.

Reproductive system

Due to its astringent properties *witch hazel* used to be prescribed for uterine prolapse and a debilitated state after miscarriage or childbirth, to tone up the uterine muscles.

External uses

Externally, either as a decoction, tincture or in distilled form, *witch hazel* can be applied to cuts and wounds and used as a mouthwash for bleeding gums. The tannins not only stop bleeding, but also speed healing, reduce pain, inflammation and swelling, and provide a protective coating on wounds to inhibit the development of infection. A small human trial demonstrated the efficacy of a 10% *Hamamelis* lotion as an anti-inflammatory in a UVB erythema test (Hughes-Formella et al 1998). In vitro research indicates that inhibition of tumour necrosis factor-alpha may explain its protective effect against UV radiation and its anti-haemorrhagic effect (Habtemariam 2002). As a lotion or ointment *witch hazel* can relieve the pain and swelling of varicose veins and phlebitis, the itching of haemorrhoids (MacKay 2001), and speed the healing of varicose ulcers. A poultice or compress can relieve burns, swollen inflammatory skin problems, such as boils, insect bites and stings, swollen engorged breasts, bed sores, bruises, sprains and strains.

As a lotion it can be applied to soothe the pain, irritation and swelling of insect and mosquito bites and stings, to relieve tender aching muscles, as a toning skin lotion to tighten the tissues and to reduce broken capillaries. Mixed with rosewater it makes a refreshing eyebath, and eye pads soaked in witch hazel will relieve sore, tired or inflamed eyes, including conjunctivitis. The potent oxygen-scavenging properties of *Hamamelis* have led to suggestions it may be used in antiageing/antiwrinkle preparations for the skin (Masaki et al 1995).

Other uses

As a lotion, decoction or tincture it can be used as a douche for vaginal discharge and irritation; or as a gargle for sore throats and infections, such as tonsillitis and laryngitis, and a mouthwash for an inflamed mouth and mouth ulcers.

Precautions

Avoid in pregnancy and during breast feeding.

Drug interactions

May impair the absorption of ephedrine, codeine, theophylline, atropine or pseudoephedrine taken by mouth.

Research

- Habtemariam S 2002 Hamamelitannin from *Hamamelis virginiana* inhibits the tumour necrosis factor-alpha (TNF)-induced endothelial cell death in vitro. Toxicon 40(1): 83–88
- Hughes-Formella BJ, Bohnsack K, Rippke F, et al 1998 Anti-inflammatory effect of hamamelis lotion in a UVB erythema test. Dermatology 196(3): 316–322
- MacKay D 2001 Hemorrhoids and varicose veins: a review of treatment options. Altern Med Rev 6(2): 126–140
- Masaki H, Sakaki S, Atsumi T, Sakurai H 1995 Active-oxygen scavenging activity of plant extracts. Biol Pharm Bull 18(1): 162–166

Lavandula spp. : Lavender

Family: Labiatae
Part used: flowers
Taste/*Rasa*: pungent/*katu*
Post digestive/*Vipak*: pungent/*katu*
Potency/*Virya*: cooling/*sheeta*
Dosha: PK- Vo

Constituents

Volatile oil: including linalool, geraniol, nerol, cineole, limonene; tannins; coumarins; flavonoids: antioxidant – rosmarinic acid; triterpenoids.

Actions

Carminative, diuretic, antispasmodic, tonic, analgesic, stimulant, digestive, sedative, antimicrobial, antioxidant.

Indications

Anxiety, insomnia, colds, catarrh, coughs, asthma, croup, pain, headaches, migraine, muscle tension, colic, gastrointestinal tract infections, first aid, burns, slow skin healing, insect repellent.

Introduction

During the Middle Ages and the Renaissance *lavender* was very popular as a strewing herb, to perfume and sanitize the floors of houses and churches and to ward off the plague. It was hung in rooms to keep away germ-carrying flies and mosquitos, much as it was hung in linen cupboards by our grandmothers to scent the clothes and deter moths. In the 16th and 17th centuries herbalists used *lavender*'s analgesic properties for treating migraine, faintness and "the panting and passion of the heart", while Mattioli, the 16th century Italian herbalist, recommended it for "disorders of the brain due to coldness, such as epilepsy, apoplexy, spasms and paralysis". Today we have verified the antimicrobial and relaxant properties of *lavender* and *lavender* oil is again becoming a household name for treatment of minor infections and as a first aid remedy. It appears that the volatile oils in *lavender* account for the major part of its medicinal action.

Internal uses

Digestive system

Lavender relaxes the digestive tract by means of an antispasmodic effect on smooth muscle (Lis-Balchin and Hart 1999), releasing spasm and colic wind and bowel problems related to tension and anxiety. Its antiseptic volatile oils have been shown in vitro to be active against bacteria, yeasts and fungi (Larrondo et al 1995). The tea or tincture can also be taken for stomach and bowel infections causing vomiting and diarrhoea.

Nervous system

Lavender makes an excellent remedy for anxiety and nervousness, and stress-related symptoms such as tension headaches, migraines, neuralgia, palpitations and insomnia. A few drops of oil in the bath will help soothe a fractious child into restful sleep. A number of trials support the relaxing effect of *lavender* including a demonstration of a modest effect on agitated behaviour in severe dementia (Holmes et al 2002), indications of changes in parasympathetic nervous activity (Saeki 2000) and changes in alpha wave fluctuation (Lee et al 1994) on exposure to the oil. It lifts the spirits, and has a stimulating edge, recommended for restoring energy in tiredness and nervous exhaustion.

Respiratory system

The antimicrobial properties of *lavender* can be used to increase resistance to respiratory tract infections. *Lavender* is used for colds, coughs, chest infections, flu, tonsillitis and laryngitis. Its decongesting and expectorant action helps to clear phlegm, making it a useful remedy for asthma.

Reproductive system

Midwives have valued the pain-killing and antiseptic properties of lavender since medieval times. *Lavender* was burned in delivery rooms as a disinfectant and used in baths to speed healing and relieve pain after childbirth. Recent research indicates that *lavender* oil added to bath water can do just this (Cornwell and Dale 1995).

Immune system

The volatile oils in *lavender* are antibacterial, antifungal and antiseptic (Foster 1997). Rosmarinic acid has an antioxidant action, protecting the body against free radicals and exerting an anti-inflammatory effect.

Temperature

When taken as hot tea *lavender* promotes diaphoresis and reduces fevers. It increases elimination of toxins through the skin and the urine.

External uses

Externally, the antiseptic oils in *lavender* make it an extremely useful disinfectant for applying (as a dilute oil, strong infusion or tincture) in inflammatory and infective skin problems, including eczema, acne and varicose ulcers. It can be used for nappy rash and minor infections on the skin. It stimulates tissue repair and minimizes scar formation when the oil is applied neat to burns, cuts and wounds, sores and ulcers. The oil repels insects and relieves insect bites and stings. Diluted it soothes the pain and swelling of bruises, sprains, gouty and arthritic pain, and when used as a massage oil or added to the bath, reduces muscle tension and spasm. It can be rubbed on the chest and inhaled for chest infections, coughs, colds and catarrh. The tea or dilute tincture makes a gargle for sore throats, tonsillitis and hoarseness, a mouthwash for mouth ulcers and inflamed or infected gums, and a douche for leucorrhoea.

Precautions

One report indicates dermatitis caused by airborne exposure to *lavender* oil from an aromatherapy burner (Schaller and Korting 1995).

Drug interactions

None known.

Research

- Cornwell X, Dale A 1995 Lavender oil and perineal repair. Mod Midwife 5(3): 31–33
- Foster S 1997 Herbal Renaissance. Gibbs-Smith, Utah, p. 116
- Holmes C, Hopkins V, Hensford C 2002 Lavender oil as a treatment for agitated behaviour in severe dementia: a placebo controlled study. Int J Geriatr Psychiatry 17(4): 305–308
- Larrondo JV, Agut M, Calvo-Torras MA 1995 Antimicrobial activity of essences from labiates. Microbios 82(332): 171–172
- Lee CF, Katsuura T, Shibata S 1994 Responses of electroencephalogram to different odors. Ann Physiol Anthropol 13(5): 281–291
- Lis-Balchin M, Hart S 1999 Studies on the mode of action of the essential oil of lavender (*Lavandula angustifolia* P. Miller). Phytother Res 13(6): 540–542
- Saeki Y 2000 The effect of foot-bath with or without the essential oil of lavender on the autonomic nervous system: a randomized trial. Complement Ther Med 8(1): 2–7
- Schaller M, Korting HC 1995 Allergic airborne contact dermatitis from essential oils used in aromatherapy. Clin Exp Dermatol 20(2): 143–145

Melissa officinalis : Lemon balm

Family: Labiatae
Part used: aerial parts
Taste/*Rasa*: pungent/*katu*, sweet/*madhur*
Post digestive/*Vipak*: pungent/*katu*
Potency/*Virya*: cooling/*sheeta*
Dosha: PK- Vo

Actions

Diaphoretic, carminative, nervine, antispasmodic, antimicrobial, sedative, antiemetic, antiviral, antioxidant.

Constituents

Volatile oils including: citronellal, geraniol, linalool, nerol; polyphenols; tannins; flavonoids including: isoquercetin; phenylpropanoids including: rosmarinic acid and triterpenoids.

Indications

Herpes, insomnia, stress-related problems, anxiety, colds, fevers, digestive problems, headaches, tiredness, nervous exhaustion, exam nerves, poor concentration, depression.

Introduction

Its refreshing lemon scent and taste make *lemon balm* an attractive herb for treating children. *Lemon balm* was brought to Britain by the Romans who praised it as a medicine to clear the mind, improve memory and lift the spirits. It was recommended to Oxford students in the 16th century to drive away "heaviness of mind" and sharpen the understanding. It was a favourite of Arabs in the Middle Ages in their elixirs of life and Carmelite nuns made it into Carmelite tea and water, in 17th century Paris, to promote longevity. This can now be explained by the presence of antioxidant substances in the plant, most likely rosmarinic acid.

Internal uses

Digestive system

Lemon balm has particular affinity with the digestive system, calming and soothing stress-related problems. The bitters provide tonic support and gently stimulate the liver and gallbladder. A mild infusion is excellent for children's nervous tummy upsets.

Nervous system

Lemon balm influences the limbic system in the brain, which is concerned with mood and temperament. Its key effect is as a sedative, demonstrated in a double-blind placebo-controlled trial on patients with severe dementia where it produced a "safe and clinically significant reduction in agitation" (Ballard et al 2002). Research has also demonstrated the sedative and analgesic effects of *lemon balm* and its use in the treatment of insomnia. One study showed that when combined with valerian it promoted sleep as effectively as triazolam (Dressing et al 1992). While being sedative, enhancing relaxation and inducing natural sleep, calming tension and anxiety, and even mania and hysteria, *lemon balm* is also restoring. It lifts the spirits, may improve memory (Wake et al 2000) and helps tired brains to concentrate. It can be given to relieve headaches, migraine, vertigo and buzzing in the ears.

Circulatory system

Lemon balm also influences the heart and has been used to calm nervous palpitations and hypertension. Carmelite water, made from *lemon balm* with lemon peel, nutmeg and angelica root was a traditional remedy when nervousness, agitation or depression cause heart pains, palpitations or an irregular heartbeat.

Respiratory system

The relaxant effects and mucus-reducing properties of *lemon balm* are exerted in the chest where they are helpful in the treatment of chest infections, dry irritating coughs and asthma.

Reproductive system

In the reproductive system, *lemon balm* is used for dysmenorrhoea and to relieve irritability associated with premenstrual tension. It also helps to regulate periods. During the weeks prior to childbirth it helps prepare for the birth, to ease and speed the process and reduce pain. *Lemon balm* can help relieve menopausal depression. Genital herpes responds well to internal and topical application (Koytchev et al 1999).

Urinary system

Lemon balm is reputed to have an antispasmodic effect in the urinary tract.

Immune system

Lemon balm's antiviral action has been demonstrated in a number of trials and has been found to be effective against herpes simplex, mumps and other viruses, possibly including HIV (Dimitrova et al 1993, Yamasaki et al 1998). Intriguingly one trial suggests the mechanism of action may counteract the development of viral resistance through prolonged use (Koytchev et al 1999). The oil is antibacterial (Larrondo et al 1995) antifungal (Leung and Foster 1996) and antihistamine, helpful for treating hayfever and allergic rhinitis. Rosmarinic acid has also been shown to influence complement activity and has an anti-inflammatory effect (Englberger et al 1988).

Temperature

Taken in hot infusion, its diaphoretic action helps reduce fevers and makes a good remedy for childhood infections, colds and flu, coughs and catarrh.

Other uses

Extracts of *lemon balm* have long been documented for their thyroid inhibitory effect and *lemon balm* has been used historically for the management of hyperthyroidism.

External uses

A strong infusion in a warm bath or inhalation of the essential oil at night will help calm excitable children. Part of the effect of *lemon balm* may be on account of the affinity of the constituent apigenin on benzodiazepine receptors (Viola et al 1995). Its ability to destroy bacteria makes it useful for surgical dressings. When diluted, the essential oil can be massaged into the lower abdomen to relieve period pains, and into muscles to ease tension and pain. It will help joint pain and neuralgia. As an antiviral remedy the dilute oil is effective topically for mumps and cold sores and also relieves wasp and bee stings. Its antihistamine action is helpful for allergy sufferers and it can be used in creams for allergic skin conditions. The dried leaves are a frequent component in sleep pillows. The oil can be used in eardrops for infections and in mouthwashes for gum infections and toothache.

Drug interactions

Avoid use with thyroid drugs. Large doses may act as a thyroxin antagonist.

Research

- Ballard CG, O'Brien JT, Reichelt K, Perry EK 2002 Aromatherapy as a safe and effective treatment for the management of agitation in severe dementia: the results of a double-blind, placebo-controlled trial with Melissa. J Clin Psychiatry 63(7): 553–558
- Dimitrova Z, Dimov B, Manolova N, Pancheva S, Ilieva D, Shishkov S 1993 Antiherpes effect of *Melissa officinalis* L. extracts. Acta Microbiol Bulg 29: 65–72
- Dressing H, Riemann D, Low H, et al 1992 Insomnia: Are valerian/balm combination of equal value to benzodiazepine? Therapiewoche 42: 726–736
- Englberger W, Hadding V, Etschenberg E, et al 1988 Rosmarinic acid; A new inhibitor of complement C3-convertase with anti-inflammatory activity. Intern J Immunopharmacol 10(6): 729–737
- Koytchev R, Alken RG, Dundarov S 1999 Balm mint extract (LO-701) for topical treatment of

recurring herpes labialis. Phytomedicine 6(4): 225–230

- Larrondo JV, Agut M, Calvo-Torras MA 1995 Antimicrobial activity of essences from labiates. Microbios 82(332): 171–172
- Leung A, Foster S 1996 Encyclopedia of Common Natural Ingredients used in Food, Drugs and Cosmetics. John Wiley and Sons, New York, NY, p. 649
- Viola H, Wasowski C, Levi de Stein M et al 1995 Apigenin, a component of *Matricaria recutita* flowers, is a central benzodiazepine receptor-ligand with anxiolytic effects. Planta Med 61: 213–215
- Wake G, Court J, Pickering A, Lewis R, Wilkins R, Perry E 2000 CNS acetylcholine receptor activity in European medicinal plants traditionally used to improve failing memory. J Ethnopharmacol 69(2): 105–114
- Yamasaki K, Nakano M, Kawahata T, et al 1998 Anti-HIV-1 activity of herbs in Labiatae. Biol Pharm Bull 21(8): 829–833

Mentha piperita : Peppermint

Family: Laminaceae
Part used: aerial part
Taste/*Rasa*: pungent/*katu*
Post digestive/*Vipak*: pungent/*katu*
Potency/*Virya*: cooling/*sheeta*
Dosha: PK- Vo

Actions

Diaphoretic, carminative, nervine, antispasmodic, antiemetic, antiseptic, digestive, circulatory stimulant, analgesic, antimicrobial.

Constituents

Volatile oil: menthol and its derivatives, flavonoids, phytol, carotenoids, choline, rosmarinic acid and tannins.

Indications

Irritable bowel disease, spastic colon, gastritis, catarrhal congestion, colds, flu, fevers, poor circulation, headaches, gastrointestinal tract infections.

Introduction

Peppermint with its refreshing taste and stimulating action has a long history as a popular herb for culinary and medicinal use and for perfumes and flavouring. It is traditionally used as a carminative and digestive for a wide range of digestive problems and as an analgesic and decongestant for colds, catarrh, headaches and cramps. *Peppermint* is both cooling and warming, depending on how and where it is used. As a hot tea it makes an excellent warming remedy to ward off and relieve colds and flu and enhance resistance to infection while a liniment or massage oil with the essential oil will cool sore inflamed joints and aching muscles.

Internal uses

Digestive system

Its relaxant effect on smooth muscle can relieve conditions associated with pain and spasm: stomach aches, colic, flatulence, heartburn and indigestion, hiccoughs, constipation, IBS and diarrhoea. Its digestive properties enhance appetite and digestion and by settling the stomach *peppermint* helps relieve nausea and travel sickness. The tannins help protect the gut lining from irritation and infection and may have a protective effect on Crohn's disease and ulcerative colitis. The bitters account for its traditional use for liver problems and gallstones. Eight trials have been reviewed investigating the effect of *peppermint* oil in IBS. "Collectively they indicate that peppermint oil could be efficacious for symptom relief in IBS", though the authors conclude that more trials are needed to confirm this well-known effect (Pittler and Ernst 1998). It is used as an adjunctive therapy for colonoscopy and barium enema. General studies here indicated that the volatile oils in *peppermint* need to reach the colon in its unmetabolized state to exert its beneficial effect in the treatment of IBS and spastic colon (Somerville et al 1984). As a result many *peppermint* products for the digestion are sold enteric coated.

Nervous system

The name mint comes from the Latin *mente* meaning "thought", in reference to the Roman's respect for mint as a brain tonic. It was used by Greek and Romans alike to clear the mind and improve concentration and to give inspiration. Today it can still be used to keep the mind clear and alert, especially after eating. *Peppermint* also has a relaxing effect, helpful in calming anxiety and tension. Its analgesic and antispasmodic effects can be applied to headaches, joint and muscle pain, menstrual pain and spasm as in the bronchial tubes in asthma. In a trial on healthy volunteers, exposure to peppermint oil was associated with a decrease in beta waves and a decrease in arousal response (Satoh and Sugawara 2003). This may be part of the action involved in its effect as an analgesic for headaches. A randomized placebo-controlled double-blind crossover trial of 41 patients indicated that *peppermint* oil was effective for tension headaches (Mills and Bone 2000).

Circulatory system

Taken as a warm infusion *peppermint* induces heat and improves the circulation. Its diaphoretic action dispersing blood to the surface of the body, causes sweating.

Respiratory system

Taken in hot infusion *peppermint* will help decongest the airways and enhance resistance to respiratory infections. A Russian trial suggests inhalation of *Mentha* essential oil may help as an adjunct to multidrug treatment of TB (Shkurupii et al 2002). Together peppermint's antispasmodic and decongestant effects can also be helpful in the relief of bronchospasm and wheezing.

Reproductive system

Its antispasmodic effect may help relieve dysmenorrhoea.

Immune system

The volatile oils are antiseptic, antiviral and antifungal, and explain why *peppermint* has been used to treat herpes simplex and ringworm. *Peppermint* oil is a good inhalant for colds, catarrh and sinusitis. Its stimulant action makes a good general tonic to recharge vital energy and dispel lethargy, useful during chronic illness and convalescence. *Peppermint* has been shown in vitro to be active against a wide range of bacteria including *H. pylori*, *Salmonella enteritidis* and *E. coli* (Imai et al 2001). The flavonoid luteolin-7-O-rutinoside has shown a potent inhibitory effect on histamine release in vitro (Inoue et al 2002). *Peppermint* is also reported to be active against a variety of fungi including *Candida albicans*.

Temperature

An excellent remedy for children's fevers when taken in warm infusion.

External uses

The fresh bruised leaf is applied or the oil added to lotions for relief of muscular aches and pains and hot, aching feet. *Peppermint* makes a useful gargle for sore throats and a mouthwash for gum infections and mouth ulcers. As an analgesic it can relieve toothache and earache. It is used extensively as an antiseptic and flavouring in toothpastes, cough and cold preparations, throat lozenges and indigestion remedies.

Precautions

Caution in infants and young children as well as patients with achlorhydria and hiatus hernia. Essential oil should not be used on the face or mucous membranes. Do not give to or apply directly to the nose or chest of small children due to risk of laryngeal or bronchial spasm.

Drug interactions

None known.

Research

- Imai H, Osawa K, Yasuda H, Hamashima H, Arai T, Sasatsu M 2001 Inhibition by the essential oils of peppermint and spearmint of the growth of pathogenic bacteria. Microbios 106(Suppl 1): 31–39
- Inoue T, Sugimoto Y, Masuda H, Kamei C 2002 Antiallergic effect of flavonoid glycosides obtained from *Mentha piperita*. Biol Pharm Bull 25(2): 256–259
- Mills S, Bone K 2000 Principles and Practice of Phytotherapy. Churchill Livingstone, London
- Pittler MH, Ernst E 1998 Peppermint oil for irritable bowel syndrome: a critical review and meta-analysis. Am J Gastroenterol 93(7): 1131–1135
- Satoh T, Sugawara Y 2003 Effects on human elicited by inhaling the fragrance of essential oils: sensory test, multi-channel thermometric study and forehead surface potential wave measurement on basil and peppermint. Anal Sci 19(1): 139–146
- Shkurupii VA, Kazarinova NV, Ogirenko AP, Nikonov SD, Tkachev AV, Tkachenko KG 2002 Efficiency of the use of peppermint essential oil inhalation in the combined multi-drug therapy for pulmonary tuberculosis. Probl Tuberk 4: 36–39
- Somerville KW, Richmond CR, Bell GO 1984 Delayed release of peppermint oil capsules (colpermin) for the spastic colon syndrome. A pharmacokinetic study. Br J Clin Pharmacol 18: 638–640

Ocimum basilicum : Basil

Family: Labiatae
Part used: leaves
Taste/*Rasa*: pungent/*katu*
Post digestive/*Vipak*: pungent/*katu*
Potency/*Virya*: heating/*ushna*
***Dosha*:** VK- P+

Constituents

Essential oil including linalool, methylchavicol, eugenol, borneol, camphor, geraniol (depending on the species). Tannins, flavonoid glycosides.

Actions

Diaphoretic, febrifuge, nervine, antispasmodic, antimicrobial, fungasitic, insecticidal, anodyne, galactagogue, digestive, aperient, anthelmintic, antioxidant.

Indications

Fevers, digestive problems, colds and flu, coughs, asthma, anxiety, insomnia.

Introduction

Sweet basil has been valued for centuries all over the world for its ability to protect against infection and its strengthening properties have been associated with giving courage in times of difficulty. Research has now confirmed that basil has antioxidant and antibacterial properties to validate its traditional use. As a nervine and antispasmodic it can help a variety of stress-related symptoms including headaches, nerve pain and digestive disorders.

Internal uses

Digestive system

The volatile oils in *basil* have an antispasmodic effect particularly in the digestive system, making it a good remedy for stomach cramps, wind, nausea, diarrhoea and vomiting and constipation related to tension. Its pungent taste and warming effect aids digestion and can be used to relieve indigestion, nausea, colic and flatulence related to low digestive

fire. *Basil* also has a useful anti-ulcer effect. The antimicrobial action is helpful in the treatment of stomach and bowel infections and some species have been used for expelling worms. Chewing *basil* leaves or drinking the sweet-tasting tea is an excellent remedy for children's stomach aches and travel sickness.

Nervous system

Basil has an affinity for the nervous system and helps increase energy and vitality, enhance resilience to stress, release tension and lift the spirits. It helps to calm and clear the mind, improves concentration and sharpens the memory. *Basil* can be used to relieve headaches and neuralgia and for other stress-related problems such as indigestion, exhaustion, muscle and back pain and migraine. It is refreshing and reviving when feeling tired and yet calming when feeling tense or anxious. It is particularly helpful for those studying for exams as it relieves intellectual fatigue and exam nerves.

Respiratory system

Basil has antimicrobial properties enhancing immunity to respiratory infections. With decongestant properties it helps clear phlegm from the nose and chest. It is best in hot infusions for colds, flu, catarrh, sinusitis and as an expectorant for coughs. It relaxes spasm in the bronchi and is used for whooping cough and asthma. *Basil* has diaphoretic properties, bringing blood to the surface of the skin and releasing heat and makes a good remedy for reducing fevers.

Reproductive system

Basil is used as an antispasmodic to relieve dysmenorrhoea and the pain of uterine contractions during childbirth. In China *basil* is used to relieve spasm and to promote the circulation before and after childbirth (Foster 1997).

Immune system

Trials have also shown *basil* to be a potent antioxidant (Maulik et al 1997) and to have antimicrobial and antiseptic properties (Omoregbe et al 1996, Lachowicz et al 1998), which can help protect against infection. Recent research has indicated encouraging potential of *basil* as an antibiotic against resistant bacteria (Opalchenova and Obreshkova 2003).

External uses

Externally the essential oil can be used in base massage oils such as sesame oil for muscle and joint pain and it makes a good insect repellent. With its antiseptic and anodyne properties the herbal oil (steeping the leaves in olive oil for 2 weeks) has been used in relief of earache. The leaves can be rubbed on to minor cuts and grazes and bites and stings for antiseptic first aid.

Research

- Foster S 1997 Herbal Renaissance. Gibbs Smith, Layton, UT, p. 43

- Lachowicz KJ, Jones GP, Briggs DR, et al 1998 The synergistic preservative effects of the essential oils of sweet basil (*Ocimum basilicum* L.) against acid-tolerant food microflora. Lett Appl Microbiol 26(3): 209–214
- Maulik G, Maulik N, Bhandari V, et al 1997 Evaluation of antioxidant effectiveness of a few herbal plants. Free Radic Res 27(2): 221–228
- Omoregbe RE, Ikuebe OM, Ihimire IG 1996 Antimicrobial activity of some medicinal plants extracts on *Escherichia coli*, *Salmonella paratyphi* and *Shigella dysenteriae*. Afr J Med Sci 25(4): 373–375
- Opalchenova G, Obreshkova D 2003 Comparative studies on the activity of basil – an essential oil from *Ocimum basilicum* L. – against multidrug resistant clinical isolates of the genera *Staphylococcus*, *Enterococcus* and *Pseudomonas* by using different test methods. J Microbiol Methods 54(1): 105–110

Plantago major : Plantain

Family: Plantaginaceae
Part used: leaves
Taste/Rasa: bitter/*tikta*, astringent/*kashaya*
Post digestive/Vipak: pungent/*katu*
Potency/Virya: cooling/*sheeta*
Dosha: PK- V+

Constituents

Leaves: mucilage, glycosides, tannins, silica.
Seeds: 30% mucilage, monoterpene alkaloids, glycosides, fixed oil, fatty acids, tannins, sugars.

Actions

Astringent, alterative, diuretic, vulnerary, demulcent, refrigerant, detoxifying, decongestant, expectorant, antiseptic, antispasmodic.

Indications

Diarrhoea, catarrh, allergies including hayfever, insect bites, gastritis, bronchitis, gastrointestinal tract infections, urinary tract infections.

Introduction

Historically *plantain* leaf was famous as a wound healer and an antidote to poisons. The Greeks and Romans used it for skin infections. Its soothing action particularly in the respiratory, urinary and digestive tract has made it a popular remedy for relief of a range of inflammatory conditions.

Internal uses

Digestive system

The astringent effect of *plantain* is useful for countering irritation and inflammation in the stomach and bowels, and for treatment of gastritis, diarrhoea and colitis. It has been used to treat stomach and bowel infections, as well as urinary tract infections, and its demulcent and antispasmodic properties can be put to good use for soothing irritation and reducing spasm contributing to colic in babies and children.

Respiratory system

Plantain depresses the secretion of mucus, particularly in the respiratory system which is useful when treating colds, catarrh, sinusitis, bronchial congestion and allergic conditions such as hayfever and asthma. In vitro research suggests that the antiallergic effect may be due to the effect of *Plantago major* on inhibiting mast cell degranulation (Ikawati et al 2001). Its mucilage has a soothing effect protecting the mucous linings from irritation and helps prevent spasm in asthma; it soothes the cough reflex, relieving harsh, tickly and nervous coughs. The tannins are astringent, useful to reduce swelling and inflammation (Ringborn et al 1998), staunching bleeding and encouraging healing, explaining its traditional use for TB. A review of trials in Germany recommends *plantain* for moderate chronic irritating coughs, especially in children on account of its anti-inflammatory, spasmolytic and immunostimulatory properties (Wegener and Kraft 1999). Its decongestant and expectorant action helps clear phlegm from the chest and catarrhal congestion in the middle ear, predisposing to glue ear and ear infections. The antiseptic action of *plantain* (Holetz et al 2002) augments its success as a remedy for respiratory complaints such as colds, sore throats, tonsillitis and chest infections.

Reproductive system

The tannins exert an astringent action useful for excessive menstrual bleeding. *Plantain* is a useful remedy for prostatitis enlargement.

Immune system

Plantain is famous as a wound healer and an antidote to poisons. It clears heat, congestion and toxins from the body, useful in treating fevers, infections and skin problems. The wound-healing properties may be due to the polysaccharide component acting as a potent complement activator (Michaelsen et al 2000). The polysaccharides appear to have an immunomodulating effect in vitro which may account for the use in infectious conditions (Ebringerova et al 2003). In vitro research also indicates a useful antiviral action against herpes viruses and adenoviruses (Chiang et al 2002).

Other uses

Seeds of the *Plantago psyllium* are used as bulk laxative.

External uses

Used for stings and cuts and insect bites.

Precautions

Always take psyllium seeds with plenty of fluid to prevent bowel obstruction. They can lower blood sugar. Practitioners should be aware of this for patients on insulin.

Drug interactions

Seeds may interfere with digoxin (Miller 1998). Separate by 2 hours from all other drugs as may inhibit absorption.

Research

- Chiang LC, Chiang W, Chang MY, Ng LT, Lin CC 2002 Antiviral activity of *Plantago major* extracts and related compounds in vitro. Antiviral Res 55(1): 53–62
- Ebringerova A, Kardosova A, Hromadkova Z, Hri-balova VV 2003 Mitogenic and comitogenic activities of polysaccharides from some European herbaceous plants. Fitoterapia 74(1–2): 52–61
- Holetz FB, Pessini GL, Sanches NR, Cortez DA, Nakamura CV, Filho BP 2002 Screening of some plants used in Brazilian folk medicine for the treatment of infective diseases. Mem Inst Oswaldo Cruz 97(7): 1027–1031
- Ikawati Z, Wahyuono S, Maeyama K 2001 Screening of several Indonesian medicinal plants for their inhibitory effect on histamine release from RBL-2H3 cells. J Ethnopharmacol 75(2–3): 249–256
- Michaelsen TE, Gilje A, Samuelsen AB, Hogasen K, Paulsen BS 2000 Interaction between human complement and a pectin type polysaccharide fraction, PMII, from the leaves of *Plantago major* L. Scand J Immunol 52(5): 483–490
- Miller LG 1998 Herbal medicinals: selected clinical considerations focusing on known or potential drug–herb interactions. Arch Intern Med 158(20): 2200–2211
- Ringborn T, Segura L, Noreen Y, Perera P, Bohlin L 1998 Ursolic acid from *Plantago major*, a selective inhibitor of cyclooxygenase-2 catalyzed prostaglandin biosynthesis. J Nat Prod 61(10): 1212–1215
- Wegener T, Kraft K 1999 Plantain (*Plantago lanceolata* L.): anti-inflammatory action in upper respiratory tract infections. Wien Med Wochenschr 149(8–10): 211–216

Rosa spp. : Rose

Family: Rosaceae
Part used: hips, leaves and flowers
Taste/*Rasa*: bitter/*tikta*, pungent/*katu*, sweet/*madhur*, astringent/*kashaya*
Post digestive/*Vipak*: sweet/*madhur*
Potency/*Virya*: cooling/*sheeta*
Dosha: V- PK-

Constituents

Tannins, pectin, carotene, fruit acids, fatty oil, nicotinamide, vitamins C, B, E, K.

Actions

Diaphoretic, carminative, stimulant, emmenagogue, laxative, decongestant, febrifuge, nervine, anti-inflammatory, astringent, antimicrobial, thymoleptic, analgesic.

Indications

Headaches, catarrh, GI tract infection, acidity, gastritis, diarrhoea, stress-related disorders, respiratory infections, dysmenorrhoea, hormonal problems, inflammatory problems, insomnia.

Introduction

Roses have been praised since Greek and Roman times not only for their beauty but also for their benefits as medicine. The Roman Pliny listed at least 32 different preparations of *roses* for a variety of ailments including the bites of mad dogs. John Gerard said they had cooling properties and the distilled water of roses "mitigateth the paine of the eies proceeding from a hot cause, bringeth sleep", and he also said it was good for strengthening the heart and refreshing the spirit. Today rose is still one of the best herbs for cooling hot and inflammatory conditions.

Internal uses

Digestive system

Due to its antimicrobial properties rose combats infection in the digestive tract and help re-establish the normal bacterial population of the gut after disruption by antibiotics or faulty diet. The astringent tannins and their cooling effect help reduce hyperacidity and stomach over-activity causing excessive hunger, thirst and mouth ulcers. An infusion makes a useful remedy for diarrhoea, enteritis and dysentery.

Nervous system

Rose hips, *rose* petals and *rose* oil have an uplifting and restoring effect on the nervous system. They are calming and can be used in insomnia, depression, mental and physical fatigue. In children they are particularly useful for calming irritability and anger.

Respiratory system

An infusion of the petals or hips enhances resistance to a range of respiratory infections. By enhancing the action of the mucociliary escalator they may help to prevent chest infections and through their antimicrobial and decongestant action they can be given to bring relief in cold and flu symptoms, sore throat, runny nose, as well as blocked bronchial tubes.

Reproductive system

Rose petals have long been used to relieve uterine congestion causing pain and heavy periods, as well as for irregular periods.

Urinary system

Like the seeds, *rose* petals have a diuretic effect, relieving fluid retention and hastening elimination of wastes through the urinary system. They have been used for stones and gravel in the kidneys and bladder.

Immune system

Rose is reputed to help restrain the development of infections by its antimicrobial effects and by clearing heat and toxins from the system. *Rose* hips have been shown to have anti-inflammatory effect (Yesilada et al 1997) and a small trial indicates a positive effect on reducing pain and increasing flexibility in osteoarthritis (Rossnagel and Willich 2001). An infusion of *rose* petals in wine or vinegar added to the bath was a traditional remedy to relieve arthritis and rheumatism. An infusion of *rose* petals can relieve cold and flu symptoms, sore throat, runny nose, as well as blocked bronchial tubes. The hips of the wild *rose*, *R. canina*, were found just before the Second World War to contain one of the most abundant sources of vitamin C in the plant kingdom. They are also rich in vitamins A, B and K. They were made into *rose* hip syrup, which was then rationed in Britain in wartime to ensure children's resistance to infection. This syrup or a decoction made from the empty seed cases makes a remedy for diarrhoea, stomach and menstrual cramps, nausea and indigestion.

Temperature

Both the leaves and petals of roses have a cooling effect and have been used in tea to bring down fevers and to clear toxins and heat from the body, which produces rashes and inflammatory problems.

External uses

Rose water has been used to cleanse and tone the skin, to prevent and smooth out wrinkles, to clear skin blemishes and inflammation such as acne and spots, boils and abscesses. It can be used to bathe sore, tired or inflamed eyes, and to promote tissue repair. The astringent tannins and antiseptic volatile oils help to prevent infection of minor cuts and wounds, and to reduce the swelling of bruises and sprains. An infusion of *rose* petals can be used as a mouthwash for mouth ulcers or inflamed, bleeding gums, a gargle for sore throats and a douche for vaginal discharge.

Drug interactions

None known.

Research

- Rossnagel K, Willich SN 2001 Value of complementary medicine exemplified by rose-hips. Gesundheitswesen 63(6): 412–416
- Yesilada E, Ustun O, Sezik E, Takaishi Y, Ono Y, Honda G 1997 Inhibitory effects of Turkish folk remedies on inflammatory cytokines: interleukin-1alpha, interleukin-1beta and tumor necrosis factor alpha. J Ethnopharmacol 58(1): 59–73

Rosmarinus officinalis : Rosemary

Family: Labiatae
Part used: aerial parts
Taste/*Rasa*: pungent/*katu*, bitter/*tikta*
Post digestive/*Vipak*: pungent/*katu*
Potency/*Virya*: heating/*ushna*
Dosha: KV- P+

Constituents

Volatile oils, flavonoids, phenolic acids, tannins, bitters, resins.

Actions

Diaphoretic, carminative, stimulant, emmenagogue, nervine, digestive, antioxidant, cholagogue, thymoleptic, decongestant, antispasmodic, antimicrobial, circulatory stimulant, febrifuge.

Indications

Headaches, migraine, colds and flu, coughs, GI tract infections, arthritis, gout, poor memory and concentration, fevers, liver problems.

Introduction

Since the time of the ancient Egyptians *rosemary* has been considered excellent for the brain, to dispel melancholy and make one "light and merrie". It was grown in the early physic and apothecary's gardens, and was considered a rejuvenating tonic by many herbalists including Bankes who said of it "to smell the scent of the leaves kept one youngly". The presence of antioxidants goes some way to explaining its ancient reputation. It has been most popular as a remedy for headaches and migraines from a variety of different causes, as it is still among professional herbalists.

Internal uses

Digestive system

The tannins in *rosemary* are astringent, checking bleeding, explaining its use for reducing diarrhoea and heavy periods. It has a protective effect on mucous membranes helping to prevent irritation and inflammation. *Rosemary* has a stimulating effect on the digestion, enhancing the appetite and increasing the flow of digestive juices, relieving flatulence and distension. It helps move food and wastes efficiently through the system, removes stagnant food, improves sluggish digestion and helps the absorption of nutrients so that maximum benefit is derived from the diet. The bitters in *rosemary* stimulate the action of the liver and gallbladder, increasing the flow of bile and aiding digestion of fats. By enhancing liver function *rosemary* will help to clear toxins from the system that may account for headaches, lethargy, irritability and general malaise. It used to be sold in apothecaries as a cure for hangovers, and was considered excellent for jaundice, gallstones, "liverishness", and for gout, arthritis and as a remedy to clear the skin.

Nervous system

Rosemary has long been held to have an affinity to the brain and nervous system. By increasing blood flow to the brain, it helps to clear the mind, heighten concentration and this may account for the belief that *rosemary* improves the memory. A small trial of the effect of essential oils on mood demonstrated that those in the *rosemary* group showed decreased frontal alpha and beta power, suggesting an increase in alertness. Subjects showed greater accuracy at maths computations and reported feeling more relaxed (Diego et al 1998). A larger trial of 144 healthy adults came to similar conclusions, particularly that *rosemary* increased alertness and quality (although not speed) of memory (Moss et al 2003). Not surprisingly it is popular among nervous exam students and interviewees. *Rosemary* is also used for its relaxing and thymoleptic properties for nervousness, anxiety, exhaustion, lethargy, depression and insomnia.

Circulatory system

By stimulating blood flow to the head, reducing inflammation and relaxing tense muscles, *rosemary* can be used for preventing migraines and headaches. It also stimulates general circulation, improving peripheral blood flow. It has been used for varicose veins, a tendency to bruising, and to prevent chilblains and arteriosclerosis.

Respiratory system

The volatile oils in *rosemary* have an antimicrobial effect and taken as a hot tea rosemary can help relieve sore throats, colds, flu and chest infections. It used to be *the* remedy for tuberculosis, and smoked for coughs and flu. Its decongestant action helps clear phlegm while its relaxant effects on smooth muscle help relieve spasm in the bronchial tubes (Aqel 1991), helpful in the prevention and treatment of asthma.

Reproductive system

The tannins in *rosemary* have an astringent effect, which explains its use for reducing heavy menstrual bleeding. Its relaxant effect in the uterus can help relieve dysmenorrhoea.

Urinary system

Rosemary enhances elimination of wastes through its diuretic action.

Immune system

The antimicrobial properties of *rosemary* have long been used to enhance resistance to infection. Nurses used to brew *rosemary* tea as an antiseptic wash in delivery rooms to protect mother and baby from infection and to sterilize the instruments. Tubs full of dried *rosemary* leaves mixed with juniper berries were burnt to fumigate hospitals and dispel the foul air of disease and death there and in the homes of the sick. In the streets ladies of delicate health carried fresh *rosemary* to disguise bad odours and protect against disease. Like other aromatic herbs, *rosemary* contains volatile oils, which are antiseptic with antibacterial, antifungal and antiviral properties (Mangena and Muyima 1999, Mazumder et al 1997), and which enhance the function of the immune system. The antioxidant effect (Hay et al 1998) of a number of constituents in *rosemary* may account for its reputation as a rejuvenative, enhancing concentration and memory. Oxidative stress is implicated in cancer and since *rosemary* has been

shown to protect biological systems against oxidative stress it may have potential as an anticancer remedy (Barnett 1997). It has been reported that *rosemary*'s antioxidant effects stimulate liver enzymes that detoxify poisons including carcinogens and xenobiotics. As an anti-inflammatory, *rosemary* helps relieve pain and swelling in arthritis and gout.

Temperature

Rosemary's diaphoretic action increases circulation to the skin, and helps bring down fevers.

External uses

The diluted essential oil rubbed on to the skin has an anti-inflammatory effect. A bath with a few drops of *rosemary* oil makes a good "pick you up" when tired. It is stimulating and relaxing at the same time, so it makes a good early morning bath too. It can be used for cuts, wounds, sores, chilblains, scalds and burns. Rubbed into the scalp it will check hair fall and condition the hair. A randomized, double-blind, controlled trial of 86 patients with alopecia areata tested the effects of rubbing a mix of thyme, *rosemary*, lavender and cedarwood into the scalp. The researchers concluded that this was a safe and effective treatment (Haraguchi et al 1995). It is frequently made into shampoos and hair conditioners for this reason. It has been used to treat scabies and lice. *Rosemary* tea can be used as a douche for vaginal infections and as a mouthwash for bleeding gums. The fresh leaves can be chewed to sweeten the breath and to combat infection of the teeth and gums. A wreath of rosemary was often worn round the heads of students to enhance memory and concentration. The oil rubbed into the temples relieves tension and headaches and can be inhaled to dispel drowsiness and increase concentration.

Precautions

Rosemary should only be taken for a few days at a time. It should not be taken in pregnancy. Side effects of contact dermatitis. Kidney irritation and gastrointestinal disturbances may occur with large internal doses.

Drug interactions

None known.

Research

- Aqel MB 1991 Relaxant effect of the volatile oil of *Rosmarinus officinalis* on tracheal smooth muscle. J Ethnopharmacol 33(1–2): 57–62
- Barnett R 1997 Tonics. Harper Collins, New York, NY, p. 232
- Diego MA, Jones NA, Field T, et al 1998 Aromatherapy positively affects mood, EEG patterns of alertness and math computations. Int J Neurosci 96(3–4): 217–224
- Haraguchi H, Saito T, Okamura N, Yagi A 1995 Inhibition of lipid peroxidation and superoxide generation by diterpenoids from *Rosmarinus officinalis*. Planta Med 61(4): 333–336
- Hay IC, Jamieson M, Ormerod AD 1998 Randomized trial of aromatherapy. Successful treatment for alopecia areata. Arch Dermatol 134(11): 1349–1352
- Mangena T, Muyima NY 1999 Comparative evaluation of the antimicrobial activities of essential oils of *Artemisia afra, Pteronia incana* and *Rosmarinus officinalis* on selected bacteria and yeast strains. Lett Appl Microbiol 28(4): 291–296
- Mazumder A, Neamati N, Sunder S, et al 1997 Curcumin analogs with altered potencies against HIV-1 integrase as probes for biochemical mechanisms of drug action. J Med Chem 40(19): 3057–3063
- Moss M, Cook J, Wesnes K, Duckett P 2003 Aromas of rosemary and lavender essential oils differentially affect cognition and mood in healthy adults. Int J Neurosci 113(1): 15–38

Sambucus nigra : Elder

Family: Caprifoliaceae
Part used: flowers, leaves, berries
Taste/*Rasa*: bitter/*tikta*, pungent/*katu*
Post digestive/*Vipak*: pungent/*katu*
Potency/*Virya*: cooling/*sheeta*
Dosha: KP- Vo

Constituents

Flowers: tannins, flavonoids, essential oil, mucilage, triterpenes.
Berries: sugar, vitamin C, bioflavonoids, fruit acids.
Leaves: cyanogenic glycosides, vitamins, tannins, resins, fats, sugars.

Actions

Relaxant, decongestant, diuretic, immune enhancer, diaphoretic, alterative, astringent, anti-inflammatory, antimicrobial.

Indications

Colds, flu, catarrh, coughs, diarrhoea, skin problems, fevers, lowered immunity, inflammatory problems, eruptions, insomnia.

Introduction

The *elder* is a legendary tree, considered sacred and magical in folklore and myths and deserving of great respect. It has been called the "medicine chest of the country people" and described by the 17th century diarist, John Evelyn, as a tree providing a remedy for almost every ill. The flowers were used particularly for fevers and infections as well as dispelling melancholy and anxiety, while hot elderberry wine on cold winter's nights made a delicious cold cure.

Internal uses

Nervous system

Elderflowers also have a long history of use as a relaxant, soothing nerves, allaying anxiety and lifting depression. A hot infusion at night-time will induce a restful sleep and is particularly useful for restless or irritable children at the onset of infections, to encourage healing rest, allowing the body to carry out its recuperative work.

Respiratory system

The flowers are principally used therapeutically and when taken in hot infusion they make a good remedy for the onset of upper respiratory infections, colds, fevers, tonsillitis, laryngitis and flu. Their decongestant and relaxant effects are helpful in catarrh, bronchial congestion, as well as asthma and tight coughs.

Urinary system

Elderflowers enhance the action of the kidneys, relieving fluid retention, eliminating toxins and clearing heat from the system via the urinary system.

Immune system

Elderflowers and elderberries have antimicrobial and decongestant actions. A placebo-controlled double-blind trial of individuals during an outbreak of influenza found that the group that received a standardized extract of *Sambucus* were cured within 2 to 3 days compared to 6 days in the placebo group. The researchers suggest that the efficacy, low cost and absence of side effects make *Sambucus* a promising treatment for influenza A and B (Zakay-Rones et al 1995). "Sambucol" a preparation of elderberry has been found to activate the immune system by increasing inflammatory and anti-inflammatory cytokine production in healthy donors (Barak et al 2002). *Elderflowers* with their diaphoretic action, are recommended at the onset of eruptive diseases such as measles and chickenpox to bring out the rash and speed recovery.

Temperature

When hot, *elderflower* tea increases the circulation and causes sweating, helping to eliminate toxins and bring down fevers.

External uses

An infusion of *elderflower* can be used as a gargle for sore throats, a mouthwash for mouth ulcers and inflamed gums, and an eyewash for conjunctivitis and sore, tired eyes. It also makes a good lotion for chilblains, skin eruptions, sunburn, any irritable skin condition and itching piles. An infusion can be used as a lotion to keep away midges and mosquitoes, and as an astringent remedy for wounds, bruises, burns, sprains, swollen joints and haemorrhoids.

Precautions

Sometimes the leaves can cause a reaction on sensitive skins. Avoid use of root and bark.

Drug interactions

None known.

Research

- Barak V, Birkenfeld S, Halperin T, Kalickman I 2002 The effect of herbal remedies on the production of human inflammatory and anti-inflammatory cytokines. Isr Med Assoc J 4(11 Suppl): 919–922
- Zakay-Rones Z, Varsano N, Zlotnik M, et al 1995 Inhibition of several strains of influenza virus in vitro and reduction of symptoms by an elderberry extract (*Sambucus nigra* L.) during an outbreak of influenza B Panama. J Altern Complement Med 1(4): 361–369

Taraxacum officinale : Dandelion

Family: Compositae
Part used: leaves (as diuretic), root (digestive)
Taste/Rasa: bitter/*tikta*, sweet/*madhur*
Post digestive/Vipak: pungent/*katu*
Potency/Virya: cooling/*sheeta*
Dosha: PK- V+

Constituents

Terpenoids, acids (chlorogenic acid, caffeic acid), carbohydrates, vitamins and minerals (potassium and vitamin A and C also B complex and zinc and manganese, phytosterols and flavonoid glycosides.

Actions

Digestive, bitter tonic, diuretic, mild laxative, cholagogue.

Indications

Skin problems, arthritis, gout, fluid retention, urinary infections, indigestion, liver and gallbladder problems, liver disease, jaundice, hepatitis.

Introduction

This cheerful weed has been respected as a medicine for thousands of years. It is most famous as a gently detoxifying bitter tonic, increasing elimination of toxins, wastes and pollutants through the liver and kidneys, thereby cleansing the blood. The leaves are eaten young in the spring as a bitter detoxifying tonic to cleanse the body of wastes from the heavy clogging food, and more sedentary habits of winter.

Internal uses

Digestive system

Today *dandelion* is still popular as a bitter digestive and liver tonic, enhancing appetite and promoting digestion. The bitter taste of both root and leaf stimulates the bitter receptors in the mouth and by reflex this activates the whole of the digestive tract and the liver. *Dandelion* increases the flow of digestive juices, regulating the appetite and digestion. By increasing bile production and flow, it supports the work of the liver as the major detoxifying organ of the body. It is taken for problems associated with a sluggish liver such as tiredness and irritability, headaches and skin problems. The root is also mildly laxative.

Urinary system

Dandelion, particularly the leaves, is an effective diuretic as the traditional names "piss-a-bed" or in French *pis-en-lit* tell us, useful in water retention, cellulite and urinary tract infections. While diuretic drugs leach potassium from the body and require a potassium supplement, *dandelion* comes complete with its high potassium content replacing that lost through increased urination. A decoction of the root and leaves is a traditional remedy for dissolving urinary stones and gravel. Since *dandelion* leaves improve elimination of uric acid, it makes a useful remedy for gout.

Immune system

Dandelion root has anti-inflammatory properties (Bradley 1992). Combined in a tea with celery seed and taken regularly it is used for arthritis and rheumatism. The effect of *dandelion* extends to the pancreas where it is reputed to increase insulin secretion, which could be helpful in the treatment of diabetes.

External uses

The white juice from the stems can be applied to warts. Tea of the leaves and flowers makes a good wash for ulcers and skin complaints, and a decoction has been used as a lotion for freckles.

Precautions

Avoid in obstructions of the bile ducts and gallbladder (Bisset 1996). Milky latex in leaves can cause dermatitis.

Drug interactions

Diuretic properties of the leaf can interact with orthodox diuretics and hypotensives.

Research

- Bisset N 1996 Herbal Drugs and Phytopharmaceutical. Stuttgart, Scientific Publishers
- Bradley P (ed) 1992 British Herbal Compendium, Vol 1. Dorset, British Herbal Medicine Association

Thymus vulgaris : Thyme

Family: Labiatae
Part used: flowering aerial parts
Taste/Rasa: bitter/*tikta*, pungent/*katu*
Post digestive/Vipak: pungent/*katu*
Potency/Virya: heating/*ushna*
Dosha: VK- P+

Constituents

Tannins, bitters, essential oil, terpenes, flavonoids, saponins.

Actions

Antispasmodic, carminative, digestive, antiseptic, antibacterial, decongestant, circulatory stimulant, relaxant, immunostimulant, antioxidant.

Indications

Coughs, asthma, chest infections, colds, fevers, sore throats, nervous disorders, digestive problems, lowered immunity, poor circulation.

Introduction

Thyme's name comes from the Greek *Thumos*, to smoke, as the Greeks burnt it on their altars in classical times when making sacrifices to the Gods and burnt it as incense to dispel insects and contagion. The Romans slept on *thyme* to cure melancholy and later John Gerard said *thyme* was "profitable for such as are ferfull melancholic and troubled in mind". It was considered a strengthening tonic to the brain and to increase longevity. Today *thyme* is most famous as a powerful antibacterial and antifungal for both internal and external use (Hammer et al 1999, Pina-Vaz et al 2004). The main component of its volatile oil, thymol, has long been used in antiseptic cream, lotion, mouthwash and toothpaste. It is an excellent remedy for the treatment of infections of the respiratory, digestive and genito-urinary system such as colds, coughs, flu, gastroenteritis, candida and cystitis.

Internal uses

Digestive system

Thyme makes an excellent digestive herb, enhancing appetite, digestion and stimulating the liver. Its relaxing effects can be used to good effect for relief of wind and colic, irritable bowel syndrome and spastic colon. The spasmolytic activity has been demonstrated in vitro and may be due to the action of flavonoids on calcium ion influx (Mills and Bone 2000). The astringent tannins help to protect the gut from irritation and reduce diarrhoea, while the antiseptic oils fight infections such as gastroenteritis and dysentery and help re-establish a normal bacterial population in the bowel. This is a great help to those taking antibiotics and those suffering with candida. A teaspoonful of tincture half an hour before breakfast has been used traditionally with castor oil for worms. In France, *thyme* is used particularly as a cleansing liver tonic, stimulating the digestive system and liver function to treat indigestion, poor appetite, anaemia, liver and gallbladder complaints, skin complaints and lethargy.

Nervous system

Thyme's tonic action on the nervous system makes it excellent for physical and mental exhaustion, and for relieving tension, anxiety and general depression.

Circulatory system

Thyme's pungent taste and warming properties stimulate the circulation and can be used to prevent chilblains and the effects of cold in the winter.

Respiratory system

Thyme makes a good remedy for colds, sore throats, flu, and chest infections. It is excellent for children's coughs, whether they are caused by nerves and anxiety or an infection such as bronchitis, pneumonia or pleurisy. Its relaxant effect on the bronchial tubes relieves asthma and whooping cough, while its expectorant action increases the production of fluid mucus and helps shift phlegm – particularly useful for dry, hacking coughs. A double-blind trial of 60 patients with productive coughs reported equivalent results with either syrup of thyme or bromhexine (Knols et al 1994).

Reproductive system

Thyme's relaxant effect can be helpful for dysmenorrhoea, while the antimicrobial action can help infections of the reproductive tract.

Urinary system

As a diuretic it helps combat water retention, and it is used for infections of the urinary tract.

Immune system

The volatile oils in *thyme* are highly antiseptic and support the immune system's fight against infections of all kinds, particularly in the respiratory, digestive and genito-urinary systems. *Thyme* acts as an anti-inflammatory, possibly by inhibition of prostaglandin synthesis (Wagner et al 1986). It has an antioxidant effect, protecting the body against a range of degenerative problems.

Temperature

By virtue of its sudorific properties, *thyme* also helps to increase perspiration and bring down fevers.

External uses

Externally it can be used in liniments and lotions to relieve aching joints, muscular pain, to disinfect cuts and wounds and as a gargle for sore throats, an antiseptic mouthwash and a douche for thrush and other vaginal infections. It can also be used daily for friction of the hair and as a hair lotion, giving it a healthy lustre and arresting hair fall. *Thyme* makes an excellent inhalant for chesty conditions, asthma, colds, catarrh and sinusitis. Vinegar of thyme is an old folk remedy used like smelling salts for nervous headaches.

Other uses

It is used in some parts of the world for intestinal parasites and head lice.

Precautions

Avoid large amounts in pregnancy. No adverse effects expected in lactating women.

Drug interactions

None known.

Research

- Hammer KA, Carson CF, Riley TV 1999 Antimicrobial activity of essential oils and other plant extracts. J Appl Microbiol 86(6): 985–990
- Knols G, Stal PC, Van Ree JW 1994 Productive coughing complaints: Sirupus Thymi or Bromhexine? A double blind randomized study. Huisarts Vet 37: 392–394
- Mills S, Bone K 2000 Principles and Practice of Phytotherapy. Churchill Livingstone, London
- Pina-Vaz C, Goncalves Rodrigues A, Pinto E, et al 2004 Antifungal activity of Thymus oils and their major compounds. J Eur Acad Dermatol Venereol 18(1): 73–78
- Wagner H, Wierer M, Bauer R 1986 In vitro inhibition of prostaglandin biosynthesis by essential oils and phenolic compounds. Planta Med 3: 184–187

Urtica dioica/urens : Stinging/annual nettle

Family: Urticaceae
Part used: aerial parts of the young plants (roots and seeds are also used)
Taste/*Rasa*: astringent/*kashaya*
Post digestive/*Vipak*: pungent/*katu*
Potency/*Virya*: cooling/*sheeta*
***Dosha*:** PK- V+

Constituents

Amines including: histamine, serotonin; minerals including: potassium, iron, calcium; rutin; quercetin; malic acid and formic acid and high levels of chlorophyll.

Actions

Alterative, astringent, haemostatic, galactagogue, diuretic, blood building.

Indications

Convalescence, anaemia, worms, colds, chest infections, arthritis, allergic rhinitis, asthma, lactating mothers, cystitis and urethritis, eczema, urticaria, fevers, cuts.

Introduction

The familiar *nettle*, much maligned for its cruel sting and tiresome tendency to invade gardens, is a highly versatile medicinal herb. It was brought to England by the Romans, under Julius Caesar, who used a particularly cruel *nettle*, *Urticaria pilulifera*, to flog themselves to keep themselves warm and ward off illness caused by the cold and damp, such as chest infections, colds and arthritis. *Nettle* is highly nutritious, rich in vitamins A and C, and minerals, particularly iron, silica and potassium. *Nettle* tops in food and drinks have been used throughout history as a nourishing spring tonic for weakness and debility, convalescence and anaemia.

Internal uses

Digestive system

The astringent action of *nettle* can help protect the gut lining from irritation and infection and can be used in the treatment of diarrhoea. By stimulating the action of the liver and kidneys, *nettle* helps to aid elimination of body toxins and wastes.

Respiratory system

The astringent effect of *nettle* helps to clear catarrhal congestion and is useful in relieving allergies such as hayfever, bronchitis and asthma. A randomized double-blind trial of freeze-dried *Urtica* for treatment of allergic rhinitis indicated a significant improvement compared to placebo (Mittman 1990). A tincture of the seeds used to be a traditional remedy for fevers and lung disorders and a decoction of the root was a well-known remedy for pleurisy. Fresh *nettle* juice is equally effective. Smoke inhaled from burning the leaves is an old remedy for asthma and bronchitis.

Reproductive system

Nettle has long been used to stimulate milk production in nursing mothers and to help to regulate periods. The astringent effect of *nettle* can help lessen heavy menstrual bleeding and help raise haemoglobin levels by its rich iron level.

Urinary system

The diuretic properties of *nettle* can be used to relieve fluid retention, cystitis and urethritis. It has a reputation for softening and expelling kidney stones and gravel, and as a remedy for bedwetting and incontinence. *Nettle* enhances the excretion of uric acid through the kidneys, making nettle a good remedy for gout and all other arthritic conditions. The traditional use of *nettle* sting for arthritic pain is supported by a small trial indicating significant benefit over placebo for osteoarthritic pain at the base of the thumb (Randall et al 2000). The root has long been used in treatment of urinary problems.

Immune system

Research has demonstrated that *nettle* makes a good remedy for allergies such as eczema, asthma and hayfever. An in vitro trial suggests flavonoids in *urtica* extract have an immunostimulatory effect (Akbay et al 2003). Extracts of water-soluble fractions of nettle have antibacterial activity against *Staph. aureus* and *Staph. albus* (Foster 1997).

Skin

By its depurative action, *nettle* helps clear the skin in eczema, urticaria and other chronic skin problems. The anti-inflammatory effect of *nettle* has been extensively investigated, suggesting caffeic acids and other constituents act on a number of enzymatic targets including inhibiting biosynthesis of arachidonic acid metabolites (Obertreis et al 1996, Riehemann et al 1999).

Temperature

Nettle has a diaphoretic effect and can be used to reduce fevers when taken as a hot tea.

External uses

Fresh juice or tea can be applied to cuts and wounds, haemorrhoids, burns and scalds, to stop bleeding and speed healing. *Nettle* juice can be applied to relieve bites and stings as well as the sting of the *nettle* (dock, sage and rosemary are also effective for this). Made into an ointment, *nettle* can help to relieve irritating skin conditions such as eczema. "Urtication" is a rather painful therapy involving stinging the skin with fresh *nettle* to produce a counter irritant effect. This has been found to be useful for stimulating the circulation in conditions associated with poor peripheral circulation and for relief of pain and swelling of arthritis.

Other uses

The astringent properties of *nettle* help stem bleeding internally and externally. It may also help reduce blood sugar.

Precautions

Contact dermatitis can occur with fresh leaf. The German Commission E contraindicates the use of *nettle* leaf if oedema is due to impaired cardiac or renal function.

Drug interactions

Diuretics: patients taking prescription diuretics should be monitored for additive effects. Antihypertensives: there may be an additive effect if sufficient quantities are taken with antihypertensive medications.

Research

- Akbay P, Basaran AA, Undeger U, Basaran N 2003 In vitro immunomodulatory activity of flavonoid glycosides from *Urtica dioica* L. Phytother Res 17(1): 34–37
- Foster S 1997 Herbal Renaissance. Gibbs-Smith, Utah, p. 155
- Mittman P 1990 Randomized, double blind study of freeze-dried *Urtica dioica* in the treatment of allergic rhinitis. Planta Med 56(1): 44–47
- Obertreis B, Giller K, Teucher T, Behnke B, Schmitz H 1996 Anti-inflammatory effect of *Urtica dioica* folia extract in comparison to caffeic malic acid. Arzneimittelforschung 46(1): 52–56
- Randall C, Randall H, Dobbs F, Hutton C, Sanders H 2000 Randomized controlled trial of nettle sting for treatment of base-of-thumb pain. J R Soc Med 93(6): 305–309
- Riehemann K, Behnke B, Schulze-Osthoff K 1999 Plant extracts from stinging nettle (*Urtica dioica*), an antirheumatic remedy, inhibit the proinflammatory transcription factor NF-kappaB. FEBS Lett 442(1): 89–94

Verbascum thapsus : Mullein

Family: Scrophulariaceae
Part used: leaves, flowers and root
Taste/Rasa: bitter/*tikta*, astringent/*kashaya*, sweet/*madhur*
Post digestive/Vipak: pungent/*katu*
Potency/Virya: cooling/*sheeta*
Dosha: PK- V +

Constituents

Mucilage, volatile oil, saponins, resins, flavonoids, glycosides.

Actions

Expectorant, astringent, vulnerary, sedative, diuretic, anodyne, antispasmodic, antimicrobial.

Indications

Coughs, sore throats, ear infections, headaches, arthritis, gout, asthma, anxiety.

Introduction

Mullein has a long history of use as a cough remedy and it used to be cultivated widely in Ireland for its efficacy in treating tuberculosis and the leaves smoked to relieve irritating coughs. The saponins have an expectorant action, the mucilage is soothing and cooling and is used today for the treatment of irritated and inflammatory conditions of the respiratory tract. It is also one of the best remedies for earache in children.

Internal uses

Nervous system

As a pain-killer *mullein* can be used for headaches and neuralgia, arthritis and rheumatism. The relaxant and anodyne properties, particularly of the flowers, help to encourage restful sleep, particularly for those disturbed by coughing and pain. *Mullein* is used specifically for pain in the ears, and can be applied locally as well as taken internally for catarrhal deafness and tinnitus, ear infections, wax accumulation and head pain caused by congestion in the ears. *Mullein* will also relieve tension and anxiety, and has a history of use for nervous palpitations, heart irregularities, cramp and nervous colic. Its astringent properties are useful to treat diarrhoea, particularly when it is related to nerves. A decoction of the root was an old remedy to relieve toothache, cramps and convulsions.

Respiratory system

Mullein is indicated for harsh, irritating and dry coughs, sore throats and bronchitis. Its relaxing and antiseptic properties help to relieve asthma and croup as well as chest and throat infections. It has a history of use in treating whooping cough and pleurisy. As a decongestant it helps clear phlegm in chronic catarrh, sinusitis and hayfever.

Urinary system

As a soothing diuretic, *mullein* can be used for burning and frequency of urination in cystitis, and for fluid retention. By increasing elimination of toxins via the kidneys, it is useful in treatment of arthritis, rheumatism and gout.

Immune system

The antimicrobial properties enhance the efforts of the immune system to fight off infection and the anti-inflammatory actions help relieve pain of swollen glands and mumps. Antibacterial activity against a number of organisms has been demonstrated in vitro (Turker and Camper 2002) whilst antiviral activity has been demonstrated against various influenza strains and herpes simplex (McCutcheon et al 1995, Zgorniak-Nowosielska et al 1991).

External uses

Externally, a compress or poultice of *mullein* leaves can be applied to painful arthritic joints and aching muscles, and used to speed healing of wounds, burns, sores, ulcers and piles. The flowers can be used for ringworm and other skin infections. The leaves once boiled used to be applied to the chest for asthma, to the head for headaches, and to the throat for sore throats, swollen glands and mumps.

Mullein oil prepared from the flowers is excellent used as eardrops or massaged around the ears for earache, and eczema of the outer ear.

Precautions

None reported.

Drug interactions

None known.

Research

- McCutcheon AR, Roberts TE, Gibbons E 1995 Antiviral screening of British Columbian medicinal plants. J Ethnopharmacol 49(2): 101–110

- Turker AU, Camper ND 2002 Biological activity of common mullein, a medicinal plant. J Ethnopharmacol 82(2–3): 117–125
- Zgorniak-Nowosielska I, Grzybek J, Manolova N, Serkedijieve J, Zawilinska B 1991 Antiviral activity of *Flos verbasci* infusion against influenza and herpes simplex viruses. Arch Immunol Ther Exp (Warsz) 39(1–2): 103–108

Chapter 3

The principles of Ayurveda

WHAT IS AYURVEDA?

Ayurveda is an ancient philosophy based on a deep understanding of eternal truths about the human body, mind and spirit. The traditional natural healing system of India, Ayurveda, is rapidly growing in popularity in the West today. A thoroughly comprehensive system of healing, it embraces medical science, philosophy, psychology, spiritual understanding as well as astrology and astronomy. It is based on the accumulated knowledge and understanding of millennia and yet it is very up to date, offering practical and effective treatment for many modern disorders such as asthma, IBS, anxiety and skin disease. Clinical trials are being carried out at major Ayurvedic institutions all over the world as the search continues for treatments that are safe and effective through reviews of Eastern as well as Western medicine. Ancient wisdom is constantly being verified by modern research.

The roots of Ayurveda are lost in the mists of time and there has been much speculation about its true origins. A study by Zysk (1991) provides evidence in early literature preserved by Buddhist monks for Ayurveda evolving as a medical tradition from the deep wisdom of spiritually enlightened prophets, known as Rishis, living in North India in the 5th century BC. Their wisdom was apparently transmitted orally from teacher to disciple and eventually set down in Sanskrit poetry known as the Vedas. These writings, dating from approximately 1500 BC, distilled the prevailing historical, religious, philosophical and medical knowledge and form the basis of Indian culture. At approximately the beginning of the first century AD, the first and most important of Ayurvedic texts appeared written by the famous physician Caraka. His work, the Charaka Samhita, is still considered the main authority of Ayurveda today and is referred to constantly in both the teaching and practice of Ayurveda.

The name Ayurveda derives from two Sanskrit words: "Ayur" meaning life and "Veda" meaning knowledge or science. This conveys that Ayurveda is more than a system of medicine, it is a complete way of life that aims to enhance health and well-being and increase longevity, through a union of physical, emotional and spiritual balance, as a prerequisite for attaining Moksha or self-realization.

According to Vedic philosophy, there are four rightful goals in life and all human beings aspire to one or more of them: *Kama* (enjoyment), *Artha* (prosperity), *Dharma* (career) and *Moksha* (liberation).

Kama/enjoyment is our most basic goal. We all have a basic desire to be happy and avoid suffering, to enjoy the world of sensory experience and the satisfaction of emotional desires.

Artha/prosperity refers to acquirement of wealth and possessions in the material world. We all need vital possessions like food, clothing and shelter to be able to stay alive.

Dharma/career or vocation refers to the attainment of status, recognition for our abilities, gifts, skills or talents, so that we can fulfil our role in life.

Moksha/enlightenment, bliss, spiritual liberation and recognition of our own true nature. The fundamental purpose in life is true inner knowledge and liberation from suffering, to enable us to reach our full potential. The other three goals are outer or secondary.

When the lower three goals become ends in themselves, they give rise to attitudes, beliefs and behaviour that predispose to physical and mental imbalance and disease. *Kama* as a primary goal is said to lead to over-indulgence and dissipation of vital energy; *Artha* can lead to greed and selfish acquisitiveness; *Dharma* can lead to the pursuit of fame, power and control. *Moksha* is freedom from attachment to the first three gross states and a state of inner peace and joy.

At the heart of Ayurveda lies the understanding that everything is One, that everything exists in relation, not in isolation. Body affects mind and vice versa, feelings and thought processes have physical effects as disorders of the body affect our psychological state. *Moksha*/enlightenment can be attained by those who enjoy good physical and mental health, and this is the goal of Ayurveda.

I started to use this ancient system of Ayurveda in my own practice as a herbalist almost 15 years ago. As my knowledge of Ayurveda has increased through the years of study and practice, I have found it an invaluable tool for helping me understand how to prevent and treat disease. The Ayurvedic approach emphasizes the importance of addressing the roots of health and disease rather than the thousands of disease symptoms which arise from these roots. It is an approach which is simple without being simplistic, and can be grasped by any of us wanting to maximize our healing potential through an understanding of ourselves and the universe around us.

THE FIVE ELEMENTS

According to Ayurveda, everything in the universe is composed of energy and this energy exists in five different states of density giving rise to five factors or elements (*pancha mahabhuta*), namely:

- ether/space (*akasa*)
- air/motion (*vayu*)
- fire/radiant energy (*teja*)
- water/cohesive factor (*jala*)
- earth/mass (*prithvi*).

These elements are not to be interpreted literally, but rather as metaphors, which help us to understand the universe. They represent five states or qualities of energy that we can recognize as we experience them daily in our physical, mental and emotional lives. According to Ayurveda, everything originally consisted of pure consciousness, non-material energy. From cosmic vibrations the most subtle element, ether, was formed. When it began to move it created the air element. Friction between moving elements gave rise to heat and the fire element. The fire melted and liquefied and created water, some of which in turn solidified, forming earth.

The human body is similarly composed of these five elements, and so the body reflects the greater universe, it is a microcosm of the macrocosm. The five elements exist together everywhere in all things, constantly changing and interacting, in an infinite variety of proportions and each of them has a range of different attributes.

Ether means space that allows for the existence of everything including communication between one part of the body and another, e.g. synaptic space, ultracranial space, abdominal space, as well as self-expression.

Air is gaseous and has airy qualities. It is light, clear, dry and dispersing. It governs all movement, direction and change, stirring all of creation into life. Air is present in the lungs and abdomen for example, and its quality of movement can be seen in all movements in the body, particularly the movements of messages throughout the nervous system.

Fire has the quality of light and heat, and it is dry and upward moving. It governs perception and all transformation in the body. It is responsible for the temperature and colour of the body, for the lustre on the cheeks, the sheen of the hair, the light in the eyes.

Water is liquidity or flowing motion, which gives cohesiveness and holds everything together. It is cool and downward flowing and has no shape of its own. It is present in all the body's fluids, as well as blood, urine, stools, saliva and mucus.

Earth is matter, solidity or stability. It is heavy and hard and gives the body form and substance. It is present in the physical structure of the body, the organs, muscles and bones, teeth and tendons.

Human beings are constantly interacting with the universe and vice versa. We fill space, which gives us a place to live, we breathe the air, drink water, keep ourselves warm with heat and light and consume food provided by the earth. As long as our relationship with the universe is healthy and wholesome, we can be in optimum health. According to Ayurveda, when this harmonious interaction breaks down, it predisposes to dysfunction and disease.

THE *DOSHAS*

There are three primary life forces or humours derived from the five elements known as *doshas*, *Vata*, *Pitta* and *Kapha*, which are responsible for all functions in the body, physical and psychological:

- Ether and Air create the air principle, *Vata*
- Fire and Water yield the fire principle, *Pitta*
- Earth and Water produce the water principle, *Kapha*.

We are all born with our own particular balance of *doshas* which creates our individual constitution and that remains unaltered throughout our lives. The predominant *dosha*, or *doshas*, determine our physique, our mental and emotional tendencies and our predisposition to certain health problems. We generally have a predominance of one or two of the *doshas*. Our constitution (*prakruti*) is largely determined when we are conceived and depends on our parents' constitution, the balance of their *doshas* and their mental and emotional state at the time of conception, and of course *Karma*. The characteristics of our dominant *dosha(s)* will be most apparent in our make up, but naturally it is diluted by those of the other *doshas*. To be alive and well we need all three *doshas* and all five elements. When our *doshas* are in balance, that is they remain in the proportions we were born with, they maintain our health and well-being and when unbalanced we become unwell.

It may be hard for the scientific medical mind to grasp the relevance of the *doshas* in modern medical care or to correlate them with medical concepts it is familiar with. In his book "The One Earth Sourcebook", Alan Tillotson, PhD, addresses this issue to some extent and states that "the concepts behind *Vata*, *Pitta* and *Kapha* describe three elemental processes or energies understood since ancient times as regulatory, destructive (transformation or energy), and creative (growth), respectively.... In time this translates as processes of absorption, transformation and production" (Tillotson et al 2001). He goes on to relate these aspects to the early development of the embryo when cells divide into primary germ layers: ectoderm, mesoderm and endoderm. "The ectoderm develops into our entire nervous system (*Vata*). Our metabolic heart, muscle, bone, uro-genital and vascular (blood and lymph) systems (*Pitta*) arise from the mesoderm. Our nutrient-absorbing digestive tract (*Kapha*) develops from the endoderm." At a cellular level *Vata*, *Pitta* and *Kapha* occur as regulation, energy release and growth respectively. The nucleus embodies *Vata* as the regulatory centre, the cytoplasm containing organelles including the mitochondria, involved in energy production is the province of *Pitta* and the membrane responsible for the transport of nutrients in and out of the cell for growth and development is governed by *Kapha*.

Vata

Vata, a combination of Ether and Air, is the principle of movement. The word *Vata* means wind, from the Sanskrit root "*va*" to blow, direct, move or command (Athique 1998). *Vata* is our life force (*prana*), derived primarily from the breath. It is the energizing force for everything in body and mind, and this is reflected in the circulation of blood and lymph and every impulse of the nervous system. It is the motivating force behind the other two *doshas*, which are incapable of movement without it. For this reason disturbances of *Vata* tend to have more far-reaching implications than those of the other two *doshas* and often affect the mind as well as the entire body.

The qualities of *Vata* are dry, cold, light, irregular, sharp, hard, mobile, subtle, rough and clear. In the body *Vata* controls all movement: the blinking of the eyes, the pulsations of the heart, the movement of air in and out of the lungs, the working of the nervous system, movements involved with digestion and metabolism, elimination of wastes, the circulation of blood and lymph, the movement of nutrients into and wastes out of cells, and the homoeostasis (balance) of the whole body. Mentally and emotionally *Vata* governs the movement of ideas in the mind, inspiration, creativity, spiritual aspiration, mental adaptability, comprehension, fear and anxiety. *Vata* also governs mental balance and well-being.

Vata is air contained in space (ether). It is found in the empty spaces (ether) in the body, like the heart, the thorax, the abdomen, the pelvis, the pores of the bones, the bone marrow, the brain, the bladder, and the subtle channels of the nervous system (Athique 1998). The colon is the site where *Vata* accumulates. The thighs and hips are the main site of musculo-skeletal movement in the body which *Vata* is responsible for. The ears and the skin, the organs of hearing and touch, are governed by *Vata*. *Vata* is excreted from the body via gas and muscular or nervous energy.

Vata's task in the body is to ensure there is enough space for the air to move in and sufficient movement in that space. Air can move freely through the body only when its paths are free from obstacles. Spasm and phlegm for example can obstruct the flow of air through the lungs as in asthma. If there is too much empty space and insufficient movement it can cause stasis, as in emphysema and constipation.

Like the wind, *Vata* predominant children are changeable and irregularity will feature strongly in their physical and emotional make-up. They can be very tall or very short, with a narrow or irregular frame and slight build. They may have crooked teeth, or irregular eyes, perhaps one being larger than the other, or their nose may not be straight. Their weight can change quickly, and when unhappy or stressed they can lose weight easily. Some find it impossible to put on weight, while others become overweight from stress, digestive problems and eating badly. They tend to have prominent bones and joints that often crack. Their appetite is variable, sometimes they are ravenous, other times they have no appetite at all. As a result they tend to eat irregularly, often living on snacks eaten on the hop. They find it hard to sit still and may get up and down from the meal table. However if they do not eat regularly they become hypoglycaemic and can easily feel faint or weak and then feel more anxious.

Vata predominant children tend to feel the cold and may have poor circulation, and any symptoms they have tend to be worse in cold weather. They love warmth and sunshine. Because they are so active and use up so much energy *Vata* children tend to become dried out. They can get dry skin and hair, but the variability that characterizes them means that some parts of the skin may be dry while others are oily. Their skin may become wrinkly when they are still comparatively young. *Vata* children tend to suffer from dry bowels and constipation. With their erratic digestions, they can suffer from wind, bloating and discomfort and tend to be prone to bowel problems like irritable bowel syndrome. *Vata* girls tend to have irregular cycles and often miss periods due to stress, over-activity or being underweight. Their bleeding tends to be light and can be accompanied by cramping pain.

Vata predominant children are active and restless and find it hard to relax. Their sleep tends to be light and easily disturbed with many dreams, and they may suffer from nightmares and insomnia. They can easily get over-stimulated and drive themselves beyond their energy resources. Their stamina tends to be low and they tire easily, but they still push themselves on with their nervous energy until eventually they become exhausted. Vigorous exercise, like running and aerobics, will aggravate their symptoms even though they may temporarily feel better from it. Gentle exercise like yoga or Tai chi is much more suitable and they need to relax.

When in balance *Vata* children are bright, enthusiastic, creative, full of new ideas and initiative, idealistic and visionary. They think fast, talk fast and love being with other people, like travel and change. They are good at initiating things but not necessarily at following through. A clue to their constitution might be had from observing how many unfinished books there are on the bedside table. They are prone to poor memory, lack of concentration, disorganization, fear and anxiety and can suffer from nervous problems like disorientation, panic attacks and mood swings.

Pitta

Pitta is the principle of transformation and heat because *Pitta* is responsible for the chemical and metabolic conversions in the body that create energy and heat. All *Pitta*'s processes involve digestion or cooking, including the "cooking" of thoughts into theories in the mind. It governs our mental digestion, clarity, perception and understanding. *Pitta* comes from the Sanskrit root "*tap*" meaning to heat, cook or transform (Athique 1998). *Pitta* digests nutrients to provide energy for cellular function. Enzymatic and hormonal systems are the main field of *Pitta* activity.

The qualities of *Pitta* are oily, hot, light, subtle, flowing, mobile, sharp, soft, smooth, clear and malodorous. In the body *Pitta* governs appetite, digestion and metabolism of nutrients, thirst, body heat and colour, the lustre of the skin, the shine of the hair and the light in the eyes. Mentally and emotionally *Pitta* governs: mental perception, judgement, discrimination, penetrating thought, willpower, enthusiasm and joy, competition, irritability, anger and courage.

Pitta is composed of Fire and Water and it is the job of *Pitta* to make two normally antagonistic elements cooperate together. All fires in the body, like digestive acids, are contained in water. If there is more fire than water it will, for example, burn the lining of the stomach or intestine and create an ulcer. If there is more water than fire, water drowns out the digestive fire and causes indigestion.

The stomach and small intestine are the main sites of *Pitta*, where the digestive acids with their fiery nature create a storehouse of digestive activity. The blood containing heat, colour and water, is also a *Pitta* site. The eyes are the sense organ that belongs to the element of fire. Other sites include: skin, liver, brain, spleen, sweat and sebaceous glands and the hormonal system. *Pitta* is excreted from the body via bile and acid.

Physically *Pitta* predominant children tend to be medium build and weight, with attractive, well-proportioned figures. Their eyes are medium size, often light in colour and shiny bright. They can be sensitive to sunlight and irritants and easily become inflamed and watery. Their skin tends to be warm to the touch and pale or pink in appearance. It can be sensitive to heat, sunlight and irritants and prone to rashes and pimples. The skin burns easily and there are often moles or freckles. *Pitta* children can blush easily or flush with anger. They sweat easily, even in cold weather and never seem to feel the cold. They are more likely to be intolerant of heat. They may have blond or red hair, which is fine, often straight and oily, and in adulthood turns grey early. Men who go bald early are mostly *Pitta* types as the high level of testosterone that is associated with baldness is a *Pitta* phenomenon.

Pitta predominant children have good appetites and love eating. They hate to miss meals and when hungry can be irritable and hypoglycaemic, with headaches, dizziness, weakness and shaking. Their digestion is good and their bowels efficient, but if they get hot, agitated or angry or eat too many hot, spicy or fried foods, they can suffer from indigestion, heartburn and loose, burning stools. Girls tend to have regular cycles, but may have heavy or long bleeding with bright red blood, preceded by feeling hot and often irritable.

Pitta children are quite methodical and organized. They can be rather obsessive about time and tend to be perfectionists. They often wake up and go to sleep at the same time every day. They sleep well unless they are worried about something such as schoolwork, or an exam the next day. They are highly competitive and their main fear is fear of failure. *Pitta* type children are naturally intelligent and quite fiery. They can be domineering, critical, self-critical, intolerant and do not suffer fools gladly.

Hot weather, getting overheated by, for example vigorous exercise, hot spicy food and red meats, can all increase *Pitta*. When *Pitta* is high it can cause a feeling of increased internal heat, fever and inflammation. Children with an excess of *Pitta* are likely to be irritable, angry, overly critical and achievement orientated, and there is a tendency to be workaholic

in teenage or adulthood. They often have a tendency to inflammation and infection, and skin disorders like herpes, eczema and acne. Bleeding (e.g. heavy periods) and excessive discharges like sweat or urine often occur. High *Pitta* causes yellow colour of the stool, urine, eyes and skin, strong smelling secretions such as sweat and urine, as well as excessive hunger and thirst, burning sensations in the body and difficulty sleeping.

Kapha

Kapha is Earth and Water, the principle of potential energy, of growth and protection. The qualities of *Kapha* are wet, cold, gross, dense, smooth, static, dull, soft, cloudy and heavy. *Kapha* is responsible for the body's nourishment and makes up the bulk of the body's structure, the bones, muscles, tissues and cells as well as the body fluids. It governs the stability and lubrication of the body, moistening mucous membranes and the joints (synovial membranes) and serving to cushion the whole body. It is also responsible for supporting and holding the structures of the body together and on a psychological level provides our emotional support in life. It engenders emotional calm and endurance and enables us to feel love, compassion, devotion, patience and forgiveness. *Kapha* gives us a sense of well-being.

Kapha predominant children tend to be grounded, emotionally and physically strong and resilient. They are placid, kind and thoughtful. They tend to be sweet natured and will often avoid confrontation. They don't like change or the unpredictable aspects of life. They may have a tendency to be lazy, "couch potatoes" who like nothing better than sitting around, relaxing and doing very little. Exerting themselves does often not come naturally although vigorous exercise can make them feel very good and healthy.

Physically *Kapha* predominant children have the biggest and strongest builds of all three types. They tend to have large bones, broad shoulders and big muscles and have a tendency to put on weight easily. Their hair is thick and lustrous, their eyes calm, large and moist, their nails are wide and strong, their lips full and their teeth strong and even. Their appetite is stable though they are often not hungry first thing in the morning when they tend to feel sleepy. They sleep heavily and love to lie in the morning. Their skin is usually cool to the touch, they don't tend to mind extremes of weather, but their symptoms like colds and mucous congestion are often worse in cold damp winter weather.

Kapha keeps the body's earth suspended in its water. The physical body is composed mainly of water and contained within the boundaries of the skin and other tissue linings (earth). Earth alone is immobile and as such it can block organic functions and predispose to disease. Only in solution in water does it function in the body. If the body becomes too solid problems develop, like gallstones and kidney stones, which are concentrations of earth in which the water has dried out too much to permit free flow to continue. When there is too much water and not enough earth in the system, disturbances like oedema can develop. *Kapha* forces water and earth, which would otherwise not interact with one another, to combine properly and remain in balance.

Kapha promotes stasis, which can lead to inertia. Children with excess *Kapha* may feel slow, heavy, lethargic, inactive and have a tendency to accumulate more earth and water, i.e. put on weight and retain water. Emotionally they may feel complacent, greedy, materialistic, acquisitive, or possessive, and mentally passive, slow and dull. There may be a tendency to be stubborn, obstinate and narrow-minded. Excess *Kapha* can predispose to stagnation in the tissues, lymphatic congestion, cellulite, mucous congestion, breathing problems, pallor, feeling cold, sleepiness and low thyroid function. It is associated with low digestive fire, causing a feeling of heaviness in the stomach and nausea after eating, and sluggish bowels.

The primary site of *Kapha* is the stomach. The chest or lungs produce phlegm, as does the throat, head, sinuses, and the nasal passages, which are also *Kapha* sites. The mouth and tongue produce saliva, another *Kapha* fluid. The tongue is the organ of taste, the sense that belongs to the water element. Fat tissue, brain tissue, the joints, lymph, the pleural and pericardial cavities are also the province of *Kapha*. It is excreted from the body via mucus.

Kapha serves as a support and a vehicle for the other two forces, *Vata* and *Pitta*. It acts as a conserving and restraining force on *Vata* and *Pitta* and their active and consuming effect on body and mind, which may otherwise disperse and dissipate vital energy. The subtle energy of *Kapha* is called *ojas*, which is the prime energy reserve in the body responsible for our strength, vitality, immunity and fertility. When *Kapha* is low due to high *Vata* or *Pitta* through stress, poor diet, illness and so on, our immunity as well as our emotional and mental well-being that *Kapha* engenders will be compromised.

Vata and *Kapha* are almost opposite each other in quality. *Kapha* represents all potential states of energy in the body and permits energy to be stored. *Vata* represents all kinetic states of energy in the body and causes stored energy to be released. *Pitta* balances between change and stasis, over-stimulation and inertia. *Vata* and *Kapha* congregate near each other in the body for practical reasons. The heart and lungs are continuously in motion and so require continuous lubrication. Too much motion uses up the lubricant, too much lubricant gums up the works. In the joints the synovial fluid provides lubrication and protection. The brain and spinal cord, whose movement is confined to nerve impulses, swim in cerebrospinal fluid. Mucus protects the lining of the gut enabling the food to pass through it freely.

Vata traits

- A thin frame, erratically proportioned
- Tend to be underweight or lose weight when under stress
- Rough, dry skin which can crack easily
- Eats irregularly and quickly
- Erratic appetite
- Erratic memory, takes things in quickly and forgets easily
- Prone to anxiety, fear, insecurity
- Light sleeper, prone to insomnia
- Active, restless, thinks and does things quickly
- Difficult to sustain energy, concentration, activity
- Changeable mood, intense feelings
- Feels the cold, often dislikes wind. Symptoms worse in cold weather
- Dreams of running, jumping, flying, often fearful.

Pitta traits

- Medium build and weight
- Regular features, well-proportioned body

- Smooth oily skin, often with moles and freckles, which burns easily
- Good, regular appetite, but not prone to gaining weight easily
- Fine shiny hair which falls out easily and goes grey early
- Profuse perspiration, smelly secretions
- Highly intelligent, good memory
- Tendency to be irritable, angry, intolerant and judgemental
- Decisiveness and leadership qualities
- Dislikes intense heat, symptoms often worse in hot weather or if over-heated
- Dream of fire, war, aggression, competition.

Kapha traits

- Large frame, heavy bones
- Big muscles
- Prone to overweight, feeling heavy
- Thick lustrous, oily skin and hair
- Large clear eyes
- Tendency to over sleep
- Tend to be lazy and inactive
- Resistant to change, slow to react
- Loyal and dependable
- Calm, affectionate, forgiving and compassionate
- Slow to learn and slow to forget
- Symptoms worse in cold, damp weather
- Dreams of water, nature, birds and gentle romantic images.

In terms of the cycle of human existence, *Kapha dosha* is responsible for the growth of children to physical maturity, age 0 to 16, *Pitta dosha* is responsible for the maintenance of the body in its maturity, 16–45, and *Vata dosha* is responsible for the decline of the body from 45 to death. These cycles can be extended as we achieve greater longevity (one of the aims of Ayurveda) so that the *Pitta* cycle could continue in some people until age 50–55.

To be healthy, the balance of the *doshas* the individual has at birth needs to be maintained. If the balance is disturbed by diet, the weather or season, lifestyle or state of mind for example, illness of one kind or another eventually results. The disruption may be felt in physical discomfort and pain, or in mental and emotional suffering such as fear and anxiety, anger or jealousy. The current state of

imbalance causing such symptoms to manifest is known as our *vikruti*.

When it comes to treatment, being sensitive, small framed and with a tendency to low weight, *Vata* children generally need smaller doses of medicine and benefit from warming, nourishing and calming herbs. More robust *Pitta* types can be given medium doses and more cooling, and detoxifying herbs, while slow-reacting *Kapha* types may require higher doses of warming, energizing and decongestant herbs over a longer period of time.

THE FIVE SUBTYPES OF THE *DOSHAS*

There are five types of each *dosha* which reside in different places in the body and are responsible for different vital functions. Through them the *doshas* can be understood and treated more specifically.

The five types of *Vata*

The five forms of *Vata* are of prime importance as *Prana* (first type of *Vata*), is the life force, the motivating energy that underlies all activities. The Sanskrit names are formed by adding different suffixes to the root "*an*", which means to breathe or energize (Athique 1998). The forms of *Vata* are also called "*vayu*", another word meaning wind.

Prana Vata

This is the primary air or energy in the body that directs all the other types of *Vata*.

The prefix "*pra*" means inward or towards. It is located in the head, particularly in the brain, and moves inward and downward to the chest and throat, governing inhalation and swallowing. *Prana Vata* governs consciousness, the mind, heart and the senses and gives us inspiration and motivation in life and connects us with our inner self.

Prana Vata brings air and food into the body and enables us to take in impressions, feelings and knowledge. It governs our ability to be receptive to external and internal forms of nourishment, including our inner connection to our life force. When *Prana Vata* is sufficient, it is said that we are immune to all disease. When impaired we become prone to ill health, which can be treated by therapeutic methods such as *Pranayama* (breathing exercises) and aromatherapy, which strengthen it.

Udana Vata

Udana is "upward or outward moving air" ("*ud*" means upward). It resides in the chest and is centred in the throat, and governs exhalation and speech, and various forms of exertion which occur through the outgoing breath. Its action is to move energy from the inside to the outside. *Udana Vata* is said to cause our minds and spirits to ascend. It is responsible for enthusiasm, good memory, strength, motivation and effort, and governs our aspirations and self-expression. It promotes higher values and deeper powers of awareness and when fully developed *Udana Vata* gives us the power to transcend attachment to the outer world. When impaired, *Udana Vata* can cause coughing, sneezing, yawning, belching and vomiting. The practice of yoga promotes the development of *Udana Vata*.

Samana Vata

This means "equalizing air". "*Sama*" means balancing or equalizing as in our word "same". Its function is to balance the inner and outer, the upper and lower parts of the body and their energies, in the process of digestion. Our minds and emotions need to be in balance to be able to absorb nutrients on all levels. It has some ascending action.

Located in the small intestine, *Samana Vata* is the nervous force behind digestion, governing absorption of energy via the digestive system and assimilation of nutrients. When its function is impaired it causes lack of appetite, nervous indigestion, and a range of stress related digestive disorders resulting in poor absorption of nutrients.

Vyana Vata

This means "diffusive or pervasive air". "*Vi*" means to separate. *Vyana Vata* is located in the heart and circulated throughout the body. It governs the circulatory system, the blood supply through the body and specifically to the muscles. Thus it enables the discharge of energy through muscular exertion. Its

action is mainly in the limbs, the prime site of movement in the body. When impaired it can cause poor coordination and difficulty moving, particularly walking.

Vyana Vata has a mainly outward action, which allows us to move and express ourselves in action and to distribute and release energy. Too much *Vyana Vata* can overly diffuse or disperse our energy. It is opposite to *Prana Vata*, which is inward moving.

Apana Vata

This means "downward moving air". "*Apa*" means moving away as *Apana Vata* governs elimination of waste energy. It is located in the lower abdomen and colon, and is responsible for all downward-moving impulses of elimination, including urination, menstruation, defecation, parturition and sex. When impaired it affects these and causes, for example, constipation and diarrhoea. It also governs absorption of water in the large intestine and enables us to take in the full nourishment from the digestion of food, the final stage of which occurs in the large intestine.

Apana Vata supports and controls all other forms of *Vata* and an imbalance of *Apana Vata* is the basis of most *Vata* disorders. So treatment of *Apana Vata* is the first consideration in treatment of *Vata* and this will allow the other *Vatas* to return to normal functioning. *Vata* disorders are the fundamental basis of most diseases and always accompany those of *Pitta* and *Kapha*. For this reason it is always important to consider *Apana* in the treatment of any disease. Keeping all five *Vatas* in balance and properly functioning is the vital key to maintaining health. *Apana Vata* is like the plug on the energy in the body, which can be opened to let waste energy out but if left open will drain *Prana* from the body altogether (Athique 1998). Warding off negativity and not responding to it helps to maintain the proper function of *Apana Vata*.

The five types of *Pitta*

These are sometimes referred to as *agnis* as they all serve to provide or promote fire, digestion, heat and transformation on various levels of body and mind.

Sadhaka Pitta

This means the fire that determines what is truth or reality, from the root "*sadh*" to accomplish or to realize (Athique 1998). It is located in brain and heart and functions through the nervous system and senses and is responsible for intelligence and the attainment of intellectual goals and also spiritual goals. On a material level these include the goals of pleasure, wealth and prestige. When *Sadhaka Pitta* is impaired we suffer from lack of clarity, confusion, delusion.

Sadhaka Pitta governs mental energy, digestion of impressions, ideas or beliefs and our power of discrimination. It has an inward movement, governing the release of energy from our impressions and life experiences to empower the mind. It directs our intelligence within (Athique 1998).

Alochaka Pitta

This is the fire that governs visual perception, located in the eyes, responsible for reception of light from the world around us, for digestion of impressions and vision. Centred in the pupil, *Alochaka Pitta* allows us to see. It has an upward movement that causes us to seek light, clarity and understanding to feed the mind and soul. Clearness in the eyes is a sign of good digestion, efficient liver function, mental clarity and higher intelligence (*Sattva*).

Pachaka Pitta

Located in small intestine, *Pachaka Pitta* governs digestive enzymes that enable digestion. It is also responsible for the regulation of temperature and maintenance of good circulation. When *Pachaka Pitta* is too high it can cause indigestion, hyperacidity and ulcers, and when it is too low, it can cause poor absorption and lack of body heat.

Pachaka Pitta is the main form of support for all other *Pittas*. It is the first consideration when treating *Pitta*, as our primary source of heat is the digestive fire, *agni*. Through discriminating the nutrient from the non-nutrient part of food, *Pachaka Pitta* is responsible for absorption of nutrients as well as the local immunity in the gastrointestinal tract, destroying pathogens entering the body with food.

Brajaka Pitta

Brajaka Pitta is the fire that governs lustre or complexion, and is located in skin. It is responsible for the temperature of the skin as well as maintaining good complexion and skin colour. When aggravated *Brajaka Pitta* causes rashes and discolorations. It governs absorption of warmth, heat and sunlight through the skin and has outward-moving action through which our heat can be diffused through the circulation.

Ranjaka Pitta

Ranjaka means the fire that imparts colour. It is located in liver, spleen, stomach, and small intestine, and gives colour to the blood, bile and stool, as well as other waste materials such as urine and faeces. Its main site is the blood, giving warmth and colour. It has downward moving energy.

The five types of *Kapha*

These protect our organs and tissues from wear and tear caused by the drying effect of *Vata* and the heat of *Pitta*. They help maintain cohesion and strength.

Tarpaka Kapha

Located in the brain and heart in the form of cerebrospinal fluid, *Tarpaka Kapha* gives protection, strength, nourishment and lubrication to the nerves. It cushions the nerves from the effect of stress. It promotes emotional calm and stability, as well as happiness and good memory. Deficiency of *Tarpaka Kapha* can cause discontent, malaise, nervousness and insomnia. It has an inward movement, allowing us to feel the joy of being ourselves. Meditation promotes its secretion.

Bodhaka Kapha

Bodhaka means the form of water that promotes perception. It is located in the mouth and tongue as the saliva that allows us to taste our food as part of the first stage of digestion. *Bodhaka Kapha* also protects the mouth from irritation from harsh/pungent foods and drinks. Deranged sense of taste indicates disturbance of *Bodhaka Kapha* and often precedes

Kapha disorders. *Bodhaka Kapha* has upward moving action. It governs the sense of taste in our life and our refinement of taste as we evolve.

Kledaka Kapha

Kledaka means the water that moistens. It is located in the stomach as the alkaline secretions of the mucous membranes and is responsible for the moistening of food, for the first stage of digestion and protecting the delicate mucous membranes. Impairment of *Kledaka Kapha* manifests as irregular secretion of stomach fluids and excess phlegm.

Sleshaka Kapha

Sleshaka means water that gives lubrication, from the root *"slish"* to be moist or sticky. It is located in joints as synovial fluid, responsible for holding them together and easing movement by preventing friction. Impairment of *Sleshaka Kapha* is involved in arthritis. It has outward action, and gives us the strength and stability necessary for physical movement.

Avalambaka Kapha

Avalambaka means water that gives support. It is located in the heart and lungs, where it provides lubrication. *Avalambaka Kapha* is the main form of *Kapha*, supporting the actions of the other *Kaphas*. It corresponds to basic plasma, *rasa*, which is distributed by lung and heart action, from which all *Kapha* is produced. *Avalambaka Kapha* has a downward action, and gives support. Too much can make us heavy, overweight and prone to pulmonary disorders. Derangement of *Avalambaka Kapha* is behind most accumulations of phlegm in the body. It is the main form of *Kapha* in the treatment of *Kapha* disorders. Clearing the chest of phlegm is the basis for removing phlegm from all the body including water retention.

THE SEVEN TISSUES (*SAPTA DHATU*)

According to Ayurveda the human body is composed of seven *dhatus* (from the root *"dha"* meaning to support) or tissue layers. While the balance of the *doshas* can predispose to ill health, the *dhatus*

can become the sites of disease, in which case they are called *"dushya"*, meaning "that which can be spoiled". For health and strength the seven *dhatus* need to be functioning optimally.

The *dhatus* are formed from digested nutrients, and the five elements derived from these. *Rasa* is the basic plasma of the body from which all other tissues are produced. Each *dhatu* produces the raw material for the next *dhatu* to be produced. This means there is only one *dhatu* in the body that undergoes seven levels of transformation, so problems in any one tissue can easily affect all the rest. Starting from the gross to the subtle the seven *dhatus* are:

1. *Rasa*/plasma – composed primarily of water
2. *Rakta*/blood, specifically haemoglobin – composed of fire and water
3. *Mamsa*/muscle, skeletal and visceral – composed primarily of earth and secondarily of water and fire
4. *Medas*/fat or adipose tissue – composed mainly of water
5. *Asthi*/bone – composed of earth and air
6. *Majja*/marrow and nerve tissue – composed of water and earth
7. *Shukra*/reproductive tissues, male and female – the essence derived from all tissues.

As it is the basic substance of the body, *Kapha* is responsible for all *dhatus* generally, and specifically for five: plasma, muscle, fat, marrow and reproductive tissues. *Pitta* governs blood and *Vata* governs bone.

Rasa/plasma is formed daily from our food, and from it the next tissue, *rakta* (blood) is formed. The process takes 5 days. Each tissue is formed from the one that precedes it and so it takes 35 days to make reproductive tissue.

Rasa means both essence/sap and to circulate. It provides nutrition for the five elements in the body and nourishment to all the tissues. *Rasa* is responsible for tissue hydration and for maintaining electrolyte balance. Psychologically, when *rasa* is sufficient we feel happy and content, with enthusiasm, vitality and compassion for others; our complexion is good, skin and hair are soft and shiny. *Rasa* circulates around the whole body, but the main sites are heart, blood vessels, lymphatic system, skin and mucous membranes. *Plasma* and *Kapha* are closely related, as *Kapha* is contained in plasma.

Excess *rasa* creates an increase of *Kapha* and accumulation of saliva and mucus, which can block channels (*srotas*), and cause loss of appetite and nausea. Deficiency of *rasa* causes dry skin and lips, dehydration, tiredness after slight exertion, intolerance of noise, tremors, palpitations, and aches and pain due to poor nourishment of all the dhatus.

***Rakta*/blood** is composed of fire and water. It is both a fluid and a conveyor of heat because it contains haemoglobin, which carries oxygen for cell respiration. *Rakta* means what is coloured or what is red. It gives us colour literally and figuratively. When *rakta* is sufficient our life energy is good, we have passion for life, faith and love. The skin is warm and radiant, the lips and tongue are a healthy pink and the conjunctiva of the eyes is clear. *Rakta* corresponds to *Pitta*, as *Pitta* is carried in the blood.

Excess *rakta* causes skin problems, boils and abscesses, enlargement of the liver and spleen, hypertension, jaundice, digestive problems, burning sensations, redness or bleeding in the skin, eyes and urine. Deficiency of *rakta* causes pallor, low blood pressure, desire for sour and cold food, dry and dull skin and capillary fragility.

***Mamsa*/muscle** is composed primarily of earth, along with secondary water and fire. It is heavy and makes up much of the bulk of the body. *Mamsa* comes from the root "*man*" meaning to hold firm, as the muscles serve to hold the basic body frame together and give it strength. When *mamsa* is deficient we lack the strength and cohesion that enables us to work hard and exercise. When *mamsa* is sufficient it gives us courage, confidence and endurance with the ability to be open, compassionate, forgiving and happy.

Excess *mamsa* creates swelling or tumours in the muscles, swollen glands, obesity, irritability and aggression. In women it could lead to the development of fibroids, a tendency to miscarriage and low sexual energy. Deficiency of *mamsa* leads to weakness, poor muscle tone and wasting, lack of coordination, fear, insecurity and anxiety.

***Medas*/fat** is mainly composed of water. Its function is lubrication and protection throughout the body but mainly of the muscles and tendons. It helps lubricate the throat to enable a good singing voice, it oils the skin, the hair and the eyes.

Medas promotes feelings of ease, comfort, joy and a sense of well-being and protection. Those who don't feel loved or protected may surround themselves with a layer of fat and become obese.

Excess *medas* leads to obesity, heaviness, tiredness, poor mobility, asthma, low sexual energy, thirst, diabetes, poor muscle development, poor longevity. Emotionally there will be insecurity, fear and possessiveness. Deficiency of *medas* causes cracking joints, tired eyes, enlargement of the spleen, thin limbs and abdomen, dry and brittle hair, nails, teeth and bones, and fatigue.

***Asthi*/bone** is composed of earth, which is the solid part of bone; and air, its porosity. The word *asthi* comes from the root "*stha*", to stand, endure, as its function is to support the body and give it a strong foundation. When *asthi* is sufficient it promotes fortitude, stamina, stability, confidence and certainty. It gives strong bones and flexible movement of the joints as well as strong white teeth. *asthi* is related to *Vata* as *Vata* is contained in the bone tissue. Excess *asthi* creates extra bone tissue, spurs, extra teeth, over-large frame, joint pain, fear, anxiety and poor stamina. Deficiency of *asthi* creates tiredness, joint pain, weak joints, falling hair, teeth and nails, poor formation of bones and teeth, and predisposes to osteoporosis.

***Majja*/marrow and nerve tissue** is composed of a subtle form of water and some earth. *Majja* comes from the root "*maj*" to sink as the bone marrow and nerve tissue is found inside the spinal cord and bones. Its function is to fill the empty spaces in the body, including the nerve channels, bones and brain cavity. It also composes synovial fluid and aids in the lubrication of the eyes, stool and skin as well as the production of red blood cells. On a psychological level *majja* allows adaptation, receptivity, affection and compassion. Healthy *majja* is indicated by clear eyes, strong joints, good powers of speech and tolerance of pain. The mind is sharp and clear and the memory good.

Excess *majja* creates heaviness of the eyes, the limbs, the origins of the joints, deep non-healing sores and infections in the eyes. Deficiency creates weak/porous bones, pain in small joints, dizziness, spots before the eyes, darkness around the eyes, feelings of ungroundedness and poor memory.

Shukra/**reproductive tissue** is the essential tissue form of water that has the power to create new life. *Shukra* means seed and luminous and is also the Sanskrit name for the planet Venus. It includes ovum, sperm and reproductive fluids. When deficient there is a lack of creativity, and sexual debility, impotence or frigidity. When healthy, *shukra* provides strength, energy and vitality for the entire body. It provides resistance to infections and strong immunity, well-formed secondary sex characteristics and a loving and compassionate nature. The reproductive fluid gives light to the eyes and inspiration to the soul.

Excess *shukra* creates excessive sexual desire, often leading to frustration, excess semen, stones in the semen and enlargement of the prostate. Deficiency creates lack of sexual energy and arousal, infertility, insecurity and anxiety.

Ojas is often described as the 8th tissue. It is the subtle essence of all *Kapha* or water in the body and particularly the essence of *shukra dhatu*; it is the ultimate product of nutrition and digestion, as well as the prime energy reserve for the whole body. It gives us immunity, strength, resilience and fertility.

Each *dhatu* is made up of two parts, one stable and the other in formation of the next *dhatu*. The adequate formation of a *dhatu* depends on the previous one being properly formed and the tissue *agni* functioning normally (Table 3.1). If the *dhatu agni* is too low, an excess of the tissue will be produced and its quality will be poor. If the tissue *agni* is too high a deficiency of the *dhatu* will be produced as it is "burnt up".

In this process of tissue formation, secondary tissues (*upadhatus*) are produced, like menstrual fluid from plasma. Waste materials are also produced, like *Kapha* from plasma.

Upadhatus

- Plasma – breast milk and menstrual flow
- Blood – blood vessels and tendons
- Muscles – ligaments and skin
- Fat – the omentum
- Bone – the teeth
- Marrow – the sclerotic fluid in the eyes
- Reproductive tissue – *ojas*.

Table 3.1 Signs of *Dhatu Sara*/healthy quality of the tissues

Rasa-sara	Soft warm skin, oily, uniform in colour, moderate hair which is slightly shiny
Rakta-sara	Red conjunctiva, rosy cheeks, lips, hands, feet, warm skin, happy, good energy but does not tolerate heat
Mamsa-sara	Well-developed muscles, good strength, stamina, well proportioned body shape and good muscle tone
Meda-sara	Big lustrous eyes, thick hair, melodious voice, bulky extremities
Asthi-sara	Strong bones, thick hair, nails, strong teeth, large joints, enduring and forgiving
Majja-sara	Large attractive eyes, bright, intelligent and knowledgeable
Shukra-sara	Handsome, attractive, lustrous eyes and teeth

Table 3.2 Entry of *Vata* into the *dhatus*

Rasa	Dehydration, dry skin, brownish-blackish discoloration, numbness dry cold skin, goose pimples, scleroderma
Rakta	Blood clots, poor circulation, cold hands and feet, anaemia, pulsation, varicose veins, gout
Mamsa	Muscle spasm, tremors, painful stiffness, loss of coordination, wasting, paralysis
Meda	Lack of fat, enlarged spleen (when the fat goes, the spleen is not held in place, sags and gets enlarged), lubrication, loose joints (dislocation), lower back ache, wasting
Asthi	Painful bones, joints, cavities in teeth, cracking joints, osteoporosis, brittle/broken hair, nails, degenerative arthritis
Majja	Bone marrow depression, anaemia, leukaemia, osteoporosis, neuralgical and muscular problems, paralysis, dizziness, coma, psychological problems and anxiety
Shukra	Consumption
Ojas	Lowered immunity, low fertility, weakness

The cycle is completed with the formation of *ojas*, a super fine essence of all *dhatus*.

AYURVEDIC CONCEPT OF DISEASE

When a *dosha* increases and enters into the respective *dhatus* it creates disorders, especially where

Table 3.3   Entry of *Pitta* into the *dhatus*

Rasa	Fever, hives, rash, acne, dermatitis, eczema, bleeding through skin, easy bruising
Rakta	Jaundice, cholecystitis, psoriasis, bleeding through natural openings, chronic eczema/dermatitis, enlarged liver and spleen
Mamsa	Myocytosis, chronic fever, bursitis, ulcers, infection of muscle tissue
Meda	Boils, abscesses, urinary tract infections
Asthi	Inflammatory arthritis, rheumatism, bone abscess, osteomyelitis
Majja	Leukaemia, microcytic or sickle cell anaemia
Shukra	Prostatitis, orchitis, epididymitis, sterility, pelvic infection disorders
Ojas	Hyperpyrexia, low immunity

Table 3.4   Entry of *Kapha* into the *dhatus*

Rasa	Lymphatic congestion, oedema, pale, cold, clammy skin, mild fever, sinus congestion
Rakta	Thickening of blood, increased cholesterol, anaemia, clotting, embolism, hypertension
Mamsa	Myomas, cystic swelling in the muscles, muscular hypertrophy
Meda	Obesity, diabetes, lipomas, enlarged liver, fatty degeneration of the liver
Asthi	Effusion in the joints, swollen joints, *Kapha*-type arthritis, osteoma
Majja	Neurofibromatosis, anaemia, brain tumour
Shukra	Tumours of testicles, enlarged prostate, diabetes, prostatic calculi
Ojas	Low immunity, pneumonia

there is a weakness of one or more *dhatu*. Weakness of the *dhatus* predisposing to disease, can be due to trauma or past injury/*karma* which is hereditary, so we carry the seed potential in the respective tissue. The *dosha* enters with the *agni* first into the *rasa dhatu* then into *rakta*, etc., but if *ojas* is depleted *Vata* can enter in a retrograde fashion (*ojas, majja,* etc.) which is more difficult to cure.

MALAS

Each *dhatu* produces waste products during their process of formation. These are as follows:

- Plasma – *Kapha* (phlegm)
- Blood – *Pitta* (bile)

- Muscles – waste material in the outer cavities, like ear and naval, e.g. ear wax
- Fat – sweat
- Bone – nails and hair
- Marrow – tears and eye secretions
- Reproductive tissue – smegma, waste material secreted by the genitals.

Kapha and *Pitta* in normal amounts not only produce *rasa* and *rakta* but also their excess is excreted as waste materials. So when these two *dhatus* are excessive, *Kapha* and *Pitta* will be over-produced also. Most *Kapha* diseases involve *rasa* and *Pitta* diseases involve *rakta*. *Vata* is closely related to *asthi* and contained within it. Many *Vata* diseases involve the bones, like arthritis and gout. Most deficient states of the *dhatus* present various high *Vata* symptoms. When too little of a *dhatu* is formed, it is unable to nourish the next one which is subsequently depleted also, and so on down the line.

Kapha types tend to have well-developed *dhatus*, but tend towards excess. Their blood and bone (the *Pitta* and *Vata dhatus*) tend to be deficient. Over-development of *Rasa* and production of excess phlegm may block the development of the next tissue, *Rakta*. Over-development of muscle tends to cause under-development of the next tissues, fat and reproductive tissues, over-development of *medas* blocks development of bone, marrow and reproductive tissue. Under-production of a tissue will also block the formation of subsequent tissues. It will fail to nourish more subtle *dhatus* and fail to support the other more gross ones.

There are three primary waste materials (*malas*):

- Faeces (*purisha*)
- Urine (*mutra*)
- Sweat (*sveda*).

Not only do the *malas* ensure elimination of waste products from the body, but they also fulfil other functions. Faeces maintain the tone and temperature of the colon and discharge excess earth and air elements from the body. Urine carries acids from the blood (*Pitta*), as does sweat, and aids blood purification. Sweat aids cooling of the body and moistens the skin and surface hair. It clears excess fat from the body. All three *malas* aid the elimination of excess heat from the body.

Malas can themselves be damaged by excess *doshas* and *dhatus*, which inhibit their eliminative functions, and become sites of disease. If *malas* are not released they accumulate and affect surrounding tissues. Excess faeces cause abdominal pain, distension, constipation, headache, indigestion and dullness. Excess urine causes bladder pain, irritable bladder, water retention and thirst. Excess sweat causes unpleasant body odour and oozing skin disease. Often excess *Pitta* is involved with skin disease like urticaria, eczema, boils and fungal infections. Excess sweating particularly in *Vata* people can cause dehydration, and fatigue.

PREVENTATIVE HEALTH AND TREATMENT

According to Ayurveda, the key to health lies in the understanding of one's basic constitution, (*prakruti*) and how to keep it in balance through diet and lifestyle. Not living according to the needs of our individual constitution will cause the *doshas* to become unbalanced and predispose to ill health. With the knowledge and understanding of how and why we become ill, we can follow a way of life that maximizes our chances of health and fulfilment. The Ayurvedic system provides details of the right foods and drinks for each constitution, whether they should be cold or hot, raw or cooked, which tastes they should have, which herbs and spices should be taken regularly, which is the best form of exercise, which time of year provides optimal conditions and when more care needs to be taken, when is the best time to wake up and go to bed.... Ayurveda is a complete way of life that encompasses guidance for the individual and their relationship to the world without and within them.

When using Ayurveda in practice it is primarily important to assess *prakruti* and *vikruti*, that is the basic constitution and current state of health of each patient. This involves taking a detailed case history and examining the body, paying attention to build, skin and hair type, temperature of the body, digestion and bowel function and temperament,

all of which point to more profound aspects of the patient's condition. Tongue and pulse diagnosis are valuable diagnostic tools used by Ayurvedic practitioners. Once the *doshic* balance, and the state of the *dhatus* and *malas*, etc., has been assessed and the causes of imbalance have been established, treatment and lifestyle advice are relatively straightforward.

The aim of Ayurvedic treatment (*chikitsa*) is to balance the *doshas*, *dhatus* and *malas*. To do this it is important to ensure a healthy digestive fire (*agni*), (see p. 196) eliminate any toxins (*ama*) (see p. 166), clear obstructions in the *srotas*, and balance *prana*, *tejas* and *ojas* (see p. 166). This should be followed by rejuvenation therapy (*rasayana*) to enhance continued good health and vitality.

Before treatment can commence, a sound diagnosis needs to be made. According to Ayurveda this is founded on three basic means of assessment:

- Direct perception (*pratyaksha*)
- Textual authority (*shabdha*)
- Inference (*anumana*).

Direct perception consists of "the eightfold examinations":

- Pulse
- Tongue
- Urine
- Faeces
- Body symmetry
- Eyes
- Voice
- Skin.

A physician will also use "the ten assessments" to help arrive at a diagnosis:

- Constitutional assessment (*prakruti*)
- State of imbalance (*vikruti*)
- Quality of the tissues (*sara*)
- Quality of the body (*sharira sanhana*)
- Body type (*sharira pranama*)
- Daily habits (*satmya*)
- Mental constitution (*manas prakruti*)
- Digestive power (*ahara shakti*)
- Energy levels (*riyayam shakti*)
- Age (*vyas*).

Palliative treatment (*shamana*) (as opposed to *Pancha Karma*) (see p. 167) employs six main techniques to balance the *doshas*, *dhatus* and *malas* and to clear *Ama*:

1. Reducing therapy (*langhana*) for cleaning excesses of *ama/doshas*, etc. (see immune system p. 150).
2. Tonifying (*brimhara*) where there is deficiency using sweet and nourishing tonics (*rasayana*).
3. Drying (*rukshana*) to clear excess fluid using diuretics and astringents.
4. Oleating (*snehana*) to reduce dryness using oils and massage and demulcent herbs.
5. Fomentation or sweating (*svedana*) to dispel coldness, stiffness, and stuck heat by using steam and diaphoretic herbs.
6. Astringent (*stambhana*) therapy to constrict channels (*srotas*) and reduce excess flow of fluids such as diarrhoea or bleeding.

The strategies for treatment that are generally applicable are as follows:

- Treatment of the *dosha*
- Treatment of the *agni*
- Treatment of the *dhatu*
- Treatment of the disease (*ryadhi*)
- Detoxify and clear *Ama* with *Pancha Karma*. Pacify the disease and clear *Ama* with *shamana*
- Treat the *gunas* by increasing *sattva* and reducing *rajas* and *tamas*
- Rejuvenate with tonics.

Through Ayurveda there are a variety of different ways to remedy imbalances of the *doshas* and *dhatus* which all involve enhancing our relationship with the world around us. Ayurveda uses herbal medicines and wholesome foods and addresses every aspect of daily living. The herbs, diet and lifestyle advocated for each individual patient will vary according to their effect on the three *doshas* and the seven *dhatus*. For example, excess *Kapha* can cause catarrh, lethargy, overweight and fluid retention, not to mention a tendency to possessiveness, greed, obstinacy and laziness. A diet consisting of warm, dry, light foods, which reduce *Kapha* would be advised and avoidance of foods with a cold, damp quality such as wheat, milk products and sugar, which would increase *Kapha*, would be recommended. Regular vigorous exercise would be suggested, as well as avoidance of getting up late and taking naps in the day. Activities to stimulate the

mind and body would best suit *Kapha* types who otherwise might be rather unmotivated and passive. Herbal remedies would include warming spices like ginger, cinnamon, cloves and pepper to raise "digestive fire" and cleanse toxins from the body. Bitters such as turmeric and aloe vera may also be prescribed. The specific choice of herbal remedy depends on its "quality" or "energy" which Ayurveda determines according to 20 attributes such as hot, cold, wet, dry, heavy or light, and these arise from the three *gunas*.

THE THREE *GUNAS*

Everything in creation is composed of three prime qualities or "*gunas*", *sattva*, *rajas* and *tamas*, in varying proportions.

Sattva: the quality of love, light, harmony, goodness and virtue. It promotes wisdom and intelligence, perception and clarity as well as joy and contentment. *Sattva* enables spiritual awakening and development of the soul, as well as the awakening of the five senses, enabling us to experience the physical world around us. From *sattva* comes the clarity or inner peace through which we can perceive the truth.

Rajas: the quality of action, mobility, imagination, energy, motivation and turbulence. In the mind *rajas* can create agitation, aggression and competitiveness. In excess it can cause self-motivated or self-seeking action that leads to pain and suffering and attaches us to the material world. Too much *rajas* can dissipate our vital energy and lead to exhaustion.

Tamas: the quality of steadiness, solidity, dullness, heaviness, darkness and inertia that causes sleep, decay, degeneration and death. From *tamas* comes confusion, delusion or ignorance which covers our true nature.

It is mainly on a mental level that the *gunas* have a significant effect. When in balance the *gunas* promote harmony and health. When *rajas* or *tamas* predominate, they can predispose to imbalance and ill health (see also the nervous system, p. 245).

THE 20 ATTRIBUTES

From the three *gunas* come the 20 main attributes, ten pairs of opposites (Table 3.5), the positive and negative aspects of all forces and material objects in the universe:

cold/ hot	(shita/ ushna)	static/ mobile	(sthira/ chala)
wet/ dry	(snigda/ ruksha)	dull/ sharp	(manda/ tikshna)
heavy/ light	(guru/ laghu)	soft/ hard	(mridu/ kathina)
gross/ subtle	(sthula/ sukshma)	smooth/ rough	(slakshna/ khara)
dense/ flowing	(sandra/ drava)	cloudy/ clear	(picchila/ vishada)

In nature and in the body, cold, wet, heavy, gross and dense qualities go together, as do hot, dry, light, subtle and flowing qualities. The former tend to descend and contract and serve to create the body as we see in *Kapha*. The latter ascend and expand and create energy, vitality and mental perception. Foods and herbs all have these qualities and can be used to correct imbalances of these qualities in the body.

Table 3.5   Attributes and the *Gunas*

Gunas	Attributes
Sattva	Neither hot nor cold, neither wet nor dry, light, subtle, mobile, sharp, soft, smooth, clear
Rajas	Hot, a little wet, slightly heavy, gross, mobile, sharp, hard, rough, cloudy
Tamas	Cold, wet, heavy, gross, solid, static, dull, hard, rough, cloudy

Qualities of the elements and the *doshas*

The qualities of *tamas* resemble those of the earth element, the qualities of *rajas* resemble those of fire. Those of *sattva* are like ether.

Generally speaking, like increases like, so a food or herb with cold, wet, heavy qualities will increase those qualities in *Kapha* types. Therapeutically it is opposites that are employed, so that cinnamon with its hot, dry, mobile and clear qualities will help disperse the cold, heavy, solid, static and dull qualities of winter that may otherwise increase *Kapha* symptoms, and lead to ill health.

Doshas	
Vata:	cold, light, dry, subtle, mobile, sharp, hard, rough, clear
Pitta:	hot, a little wet, light, subtle, flowing, mobile, sharp, soft, smooth, clear
Kapha:	cold, wet, heavy, gross, dense, static, dull, soft, smooth, cloudy
Elements	
Ether:	cold, dry, light, subtle, mobile, sharp, soft, smooth, clear
Air:	cold, dry, light, subtle, mobile, sharp, rough, hard, clear
Fire:	hot, dry, light, subtle, mobile, sharp, rough, hard, clear
Water:	cold, wet, heavy, gross, liquid, static, dull, soft, smooth, cloudy
Earth:	cold, dry, heavy, gross, solid, static, dull, hard, rough, cloudy

THE SIX TASTES

Ayurveda also classifies foods and remedies according to six tastes (known as *rasa*), sweet, sour, salty, pungent, bitter and astringent. Understanding the effects on mind and body of each taste and how this relates to the balance of the *doshas*, means that food and herbs can be used as a powerful tool for prevention and treatment of imbalance and disease.

- Sweet, sour and salty substances increase *Kapha* and decrease *Vata*
- Pungent, bitter and astringent tastes decrease *Kapha* and increase *Vata*
- Sweet, bitter and astringent taste decrease *Pitta*
- Pungent, sour and salty substances increase *Pitta* (for more detail see Immune System, p. 150).

THE *SROTAS* CHANNELS OF CIRCULATION

According to Ayurveda, the body contains many channels (*srotas*) through which the basic tissue elements, *doshas* and *malas*, circulate. Excess *doshas* and *malas* can move into *srotas*. *Vata* governs all impulses and energy flow. *Srotas* carry digested food from the digestive tract to the basic tissue elements and provide nutrients for the formation of the seven *dhatus* (see p. 73). The main *srotas* include the gastrointestinal tract, arteries, veins, lymphatic system, respiratory tract, genito-urinary tract as well as fine channels like capillaries and tissue pores.

For proper functioning of a healthy body the *srotas* must be open to allow free circulation of nutrients and other essential substances. If this is impaired/blocked for any reason, the circulating substance accumulates in the channels and the metabolism of the tissue is affected. This gives rise to *ama* (toxins), which then circulate in the body through other channels still functioning.

Srotas which connect us with the outside environment are:
- ***Prana Vaha Srotas:*** Carry wind (*prana*) through the respiratory system (the circulatory system and the digestive system are also involved). *Prana* is absorbed through the lungs and colon and distributed with blood and plasma via the heart.
- ***Anna Vaha Srotas:*** Carry food (*anna*) mainly through the digestive system.
- ***Ambhu or Udaka Vaha Srotas:*** Carry water and regulate water metabolism and includes the urinary tract and the fluid absorbing aspect of the digestive tract.

Srotas which supply the seven dhatus are: *Rasa Vaha Srotas, Rakta Vaha Srotas, Mamsa Vaha Srotas, Medo Vaha Srotas, Asthi Vaha Srotas, Majja Vaha Srotas, Shukra Vaha Srotas.*

Srotas that allow for elimination of wastes (malas) are: *Sveda Vaha Srotas, Purisha Vaha Srotas, Mutra Vaha Srotas.*

Srotas that are specific to the female are: *Artava Vaha Srotas, Stanya Vaha Srotas.*

Srota that is specific for the mind is: *Mano Vaha Srotas.*

For normal, healthy functioning of the body it is essential that these *srotas* channels remain intact and do not get blocked by *ama* which can then predispose to stagnation of the *doshas* or blockage of nutrient flow and eliminative pathways (*malas*) and precipitate symptoms of disease. It is therefore important that these channels be kept clean and competent.

SAMPRAPTI: PROCESS OF DISEASE PATHOGENESIS

According to Ayurveda the cause of disease (*vyadi*) is the impaired equilibrium of the three *doshas*, which then disturbs the digestive fire (*agni*) and leads to the formation of toxins (*ama*), which then affects the nourishment and health of the *dhatus*.

The six stages of disease

A good understanding of the stages of the development of disease is essential for early diagnosis, optimal prognosis and for correct use of preventative and curative measures, so that treatment can be as effective as possible.

All diseases pass through the same six stages of disease and at each level the disease can be halted and addressed if appropriate changes are made to balance the *doshas*. It is useful to ascertain the stage of any disease as it gives a clear indication of the prognosis. The early three stages are represented by vague and ill-defined symptoms, which often lie below the threshold of awareness. Only the three last stages give rise to clear symptoms that are normally associated with illness. If subtle imbalances can be perceived in the first three stages, steps can be taken to remedy the situation and full disease can be prevented.

According to Ayurveda all disturbance of the *doshas* starts with the mind:

- *Avidhya*: ignorance. We take in wrong information and act accordingly.
- *Asatya indrya samartha*: Misappropriate attachment of the senses. We make incorrect judgements, e.g. drinking excess milk even though we have chronic catarrh, believing it to be good for us.
- *Prajnaya paradha*: crimes against wisdom. We don't learn from experience and repeat the same mistakes, e.g. eating sugar even though last time it gave us a hyperglycaemic attack.

Such "crimes against wisdom" lead to:

- Accumulation/*chaya*
- Aggravation/*prakopa*
- Overflow/*prasara*
- Relocation/*sthansan shraya*

- Manifestation/*vyakti*
- Diversification/specification/*bheda*.

1. **Accumulation:** The first stage involves an increase, accumulation and stagnation of the *dosha* in its own site. No signs or symptoms of disease occur yet, just an awareness of the increased *dosha*. For example: increased *Vata* may give a sense of fullness in the abdomen; increased *Pitta* may involve an increased feeling of heat and a slightly acid stomach; if *Kapha* is raised there might be lethargy, heaviness, fluid retention, feeling of cold and liking for substances with opposite qualities, e.g. warming spices, hot drinks and food.
2. **Aggravation:** The *dosha* becomes further excited, provoked by *ahara*/food, *vihar*/activity, *charya*/season/climatic changes (see p. 81) leading to overflow.
3. **Overflow:** From the main site where the *dosha* is produced, the *dosha* overflows and is distributed to other tissues. If *Kapha* is aggravated, *Kledaka Kapha* is affected first. There may be sluggish digestion, lack of appetite, and then as the *dosha* overflows to other sites, there may be a runny nose and mucus. There may be one, two or even three *doshas* involved at the same time. If the aggravated *dosha* is *Vata* but has spread over into specific sites of *Pitta*, then the line of treatment should be as for *Pitta*. If the aggravated *dosha* is *Pitta* and has spread over to specific sites of *Kapha* and vice versa, it should be treated as for the *dosha* of that site.
4. **Relocation:** This represents the prodromal stage of the disease still yet to manifest. The excited *dosha*, having spread to other parts of the body, becomes localized and marks the beginnings of disease relating to those tissues. It interacts with the *dhatus* (see p. 73) in these parts. The sites chosen for the location of the excited *dosha* depend on the strength or weakness of the *dhatus* and this varies from one person to another. At this stage it is still possible to reverse the process with diet and lifestyle changes and the use of herbs.
5. **Manifestation:** The disease is fully manifested by physical symptoms, which occur where the *dosha* has settled, such as a joint in arthritis or the head in migraine.

6. **Diversification/specification:** The stage at which the disease may become subacute, chronic or incurable.

Pathways of disease

There are three pathways of disease classified in Ayurveda:

- the inner path (*antar marga*)
- the outer path (*bahya marga*)
- the middle path (*madhyam marga*).

The inner path is the gastrointestinal tract, running from mouth to anus. It is the pathway that is first disturbed by the *doshas* and the site of the first and second stage of disease, accumulation (*chaya*) and aggravation (*prakopa*). By using herbs to clear *ama* (*ama pachana*) such as Triphala, and methods to balance the *doshas*, the *doshas* can be effectively cleared from the site.

The outer path is the peripheral part of the body and involves the skin, and *rasa* and *rakta dhatus*. Once symptoms appear on the skin, disease has developed into the third stage of disease, overflow (*prasara*). Warm oil massage and steam and fomentation can help to move *ama* back to the inner path to be eliminated.

The middle path involves the vital organs, i.e. the brain, heart, lungs, liver, kidneys and reproductive organs. It also affects muscle, fat, bone, nervous and reproductive tissues (*dhatus*). Once the disturbed *dosha(s)* and *ama* affect the middle path, disease has developed into the fourth and fifth stage, relocation (*stansan – shraya*) and manifestation (*vyakti*), and can progress to the sixth stage, diversification (*bheda*) if not treated. At this stage chronic disease has set in.

Seasonal variations: (*Parinam*)

The three *doshas* are affected by the season by their hot/cold/wet/dry/heavy/light/qualities for example, and are aggravated as a result at certain times, and are alleviated at others.

Kapha is aggravated when qualities similar to it are around and heat is present. When these qualities disappear it calms down. It accumulates in cold, damp, winter weather. The rising heat in the

Late winter/spring	Autumn
Pitta accumulates	*Vata* aggravated
Kapha aggravated	*Pitta* calm
Vata calm	*Kapha* calm
Summer	Winter
Pitta aggravated	*Kapha* accumulates
Vata accumulates	*Vata* and *Pitta* calm
Kapha calm	

spring dilates vessels, *Kapha* melts and becomes aggravated. Then symptoms are likely to come to the fore, such as colds, respiratory infections and hayfever. In the summer the opposite properties to *Kapha* predominate and so symptoms abate.

Pitta accumulates when all the qualities of *Pitta* are there with cold. It is aggravated when these qualities combine with heat in summer. All opposite qualities reduce symptoms and calm *Pitta*.

Vata accumulates when all the qualities of *Vata* are present with heat. When these occur with cold *Vata* is aggravated. All properties opposite to *Vata* will calm symptoms down.

Illness is more likely to occur at the junctions of the seasons, which are times of *Vata* aggravation. Every adaptation to changed circumstances that the body has to make reduces resistance to disease. Ovulation and menstruation are junctions of the menstrual cycle; dawn and dusk are the junctions of day and night; adolescence and menopause are the junctions of life. Seasonal detoxification helps protect against illness developing at such times (see also immune system p. 150).

Foods and herbs taken in a particular season need to be chosen according to their qualities (the three *gunas*, five elements and 20 attributes). In general the substances selected should have the qualities opposite to the season. So if the weather is cold and damp, foods and herbs that are warm and dry and reduce *Kapha*, would be indicated. If diet, lifestyle and routine are not adjusted according to the season to maintain equilibrium of the *doshas*, diseases will develop. The *doshic* fluctuations caused by seasonal variations have considerable significance in the prevention of disease.

Seasonal routines that can be incorporated into our lives need to account for constitutional differences. A healthy person is best adjusting food and

lifestyle to control *Kapha* in late winter and spring, *Pitta* during the summer, and *Vata* during autumn and early winter, while a strongly *Vata*, *Pitta*, or *Kapha* person needs to be aware of balancing their predominant *dosha* all year round.

A *Pitta-Vata* or *Vata-Pitta* person should balance *Vata* in autumn and winter and *Pitta* in spring and summer.

A *Pitta-Kapha* or *Kapha-Pitta* person should balance *Pitta* in spring and summer and *Kapha* in autumn and winter.

A *Kapha-Vata* or *Vata-Kapha* person should balance *Vata* in autumn and early winter and *Kapha* in late winter and spring. Summer will be beneficial to them.

At the junction of winter and spring *Kapha* becomes predominant and this is the best time for all constitutions to clear *Kapha*. A person of *Kapha* constitution will require more strenuous purification than a *Pitta* person, who is best purified with mild purgation. It is best for a *Vata* person to gradually eliminate *Kapha* with medicines rather than emesis, which may increase *Vata*. Between spring and summer both *Pitta* and *Kapha* may profit from purgation, which may or may not be suitable for a *Vata* person, according to their specific condition. According to traditional Ayurveda, *Vata* people respond well to medicated enemas at the joint between autumn and winter.

A *Kapha* person is advised not to slow down digestion by sleeping or being inactive immediately after eating as it increases *Kapha*. *Pitta* people should avoid heat-producing mental or physical activity when digestion is in full swing, as this can irritate *Pitta*. *Vata* people should stay calm and rest during digestion, otherwise high *Vata* will inhibit proper nutrition of *rasa*.

Treating the *dosha* is the first consideration since any disturbance of the *doshas* eventually leads to ill health.

Signs of *Vata* aggravation

Constipation, wind, colic, distension, explosive diarrhoea (aggravated by anxiety), aching pain in the bones, cracking joints, low backache, fatigue, lowered resistance to infection, tinnitus, tingling and numbness, poor circulation, dry skin and hair, brittle nails, pain-cutting/migrating, poor coordination,

Box 3.1   Causes of *Vata* aggravation

Irregular, erratic lifestyle
Irregular eating patterns
Stress, grief, anxiety, fear, shock, loneliness
Change
Too much movement, exercise, running,
jumping, etc.
Flying/travelling
Change of season especially autumn
Dawn and dusk
Suppression of natural urges, e.g. defecation,
eating, urination, passing wind, resting when
tired, sleeping, etc.
Exposure to cold
2–6 am and pm
Over the age of 50
Dry cold weather
Lack of sleep, exhaustion
Bitter, pungent and astringent foods
Dry, light, rough, cold foods
Talking too much
Loud noise

Box 3.2   Causes of *Pitta* aggravation

Heat and damp
Hot weather, summer, getting overheated
Inflammatory situations, anger, jealousy,
arguments, irritation, frustration
10–2 am and pm, midday and midnight
Missing meals
Suppression of emotions
Age 18–50
Overwork, over-commitment, over-competitive
environment
Pungent, sour and salty foods
Caffeine, hot spices
Going to bed late
Too much reading at night
Perfectionism
Bright light

Box 3.3   Causes of *Kapha* aggravation

Sleeping in the daytime, excessive sleep
Lack of exercise, laziness
Cold damp weather, winter
6–10 am and pm
Overeating
Sweet sour and salty foods
Heavy, cold and damp foods

insomnia, restless sleep, tension and anxiety, mental agitation, restlessness. Symptoms are worse at dawn or dusk and between 2–6 am and pm. Symptoms are better in warm weather and aggravated by cold.

Signs of *Pitta* aggravation

Inflammation in stomach and intestines causing heartburn and acidity, inflammatory skin problems (such as eczema and boils), eye problems such as conjunctivitis and blepharitis, heat and burning symptoms, tonsillitis, bronchitis, increased appetite, hypoglycaemia, profuse sweat, yellow discoloration (of the eyes, skin, nails, teeth and urine), fevers, hepatitis, appendicitis, cystitis, dizziness, irritability, anger, aggression, arrogance, perfectionism, over competitiveness, insomnia. Symptoms are worse in heat and between 10–2 am and pm and better in cool weather.

Signs of *Kapha* aggravation

Colds, catarrh, bronchial congestion, hayfever, asthma, low *agni*, slow digestion, slow metabolism,

over weight, lethargy, laziness, poor motivation, foggy mindedness, constipation, poor circulation, excess salivation, possessiveness, acquisitiveness, greed, stubbornness, aversion to change. Symptoms are worse in cold, damp weather and between 6–10 am and pm.

Treatment of the *doshas*

Once the *prakruti* (basic constitution) and the *vikruti* (present state of health) have been established through the various diagnostic methods incorporated into case history-taking, treatment aimed at balancing the *doshas* can begin. The aim is not to balance the *doshas* per se, but to return to the balance of a child's *prakruti*.

Generally speaking if one *dosha* is out of balance treatment should be relatively straightforward. If two *doshas* are out of balance it is more challenging and when three *doshas* are out of balance it can mean that treatment might be more palliative than curative.

When more than one *dosha* is disturbed treatment needs to be aimed at balancing the *dosha* that is causing the most significant symptoms leading to discomfort or distress in the child.

Treatment of *Vata* problems: (*Vata Shamana*)

- Relaxation and rest
- Oleation, i.e. internal and external use of oils particularly sesame oil (see below), followed by application of heat or a warm bath/shower. Oils used for external use include: narayan oil, nilyadi oil, sesame oil, mahanarayan oil, castor oil
- Light purgation using Triphala
- Nasya, i.e. nasal administration of oil, often used for psychological problems, e.g. mahanarayan oil
- Breathing exercises (*pranayama*)
- Herbs: ashwagandha, shatavari, brahmi, bala, gokshura (*Tribulis terrestris*), guduchi, bilva fruit, kushta (*Saussurea cappa*), castor oil plant root (*Ricinus communis*), garlic, particularly aimed at balancing *Apana Vata*
- Formulae: Triphala guggulu, Hingwastaka, Talisadi, Trikulu
- *Rasayana*: ashwagandha, chyawan prash
- Rasayana for digestion: Trikatu.

Treatment of *Pitta* problems: (*Pitta Shamana*)

- Gentle laxatives, such as dandelion root or Triphala to reduce excess *Pachaka Pitta*
- Oleation/massage oils for external use: sunflower oil; coconut oil; kumari/aloe vera oil; bringaraj oil; nilyadi oil; brahmi oil
- Meditation to release suppressed emotions/anger
- Counselling, talking, relaxing in cool areas, e.g. by water
- Soft words/music, uncompetitive activities
- Cold water, milk, goat's milk/meat
- Sweet, bitter and astringent foods and herbs
- Reduction of pungent, sour and salty foods.

Medicines prepared in ghee are good nerve tonics for *Pitta*, as ghee nourishes the brain and nerves. Ghee combines well with bitter herbs enhancing their properties by its *Pitta* reducing properties. They are usually followed by milk.

- Herbs: coriander, cumin, sandalwood (*Santalum album*), aloe vera: (*kumari*), amalaki, turmeric, shatavari, guduchi, punarnava (*Boerhavia diffusa*), manjista, neem
- Formulae: Chandanadi; Pippaliamla; Nimbadi; Pushyanuga
- *Rasayana*: amalaki; guduchi
- Brain *rasayana*: brahmi.

Treatment of *Kapha* problems: (*Kapha Shamana*)

- More exercise, activity
- Reduction of sleep if excessive
- *Vaman*: vomiting/therapeutic or expectorant herbs
- Inhalation of oil/steam, application of heat
- *Nasya* – nasal administration of oils including: eucalyptus oil; nilyadi oil; ginger
- Herbs: punarnava (*Boerhavia diffusa*); haldi (turmeric); ginger; pippali; asafoetida; haritaki; bilva fruit; guduchi
- Formulae: Trikatu; Triphala; Triphala guggulu; Talisadi with lime juice
- *Rasayana* for digestion Trikatu
- *Rasayana* for thyroid problems/overweight Kanchanar guggulu
- Less sweet, sour and salty foods
- More bitter, pungent and astringent herbs and foods
- Hot drinks and foods.

The next consideration in Ayurvedic treatment is the state of the digestive fire (*agni*) (which is discussed in full in the Digestive System (p. 193)).

The therapeutic value of sesame oil

Sesame oil is one of the most important tools of Ayurvedic medicine and something that I use in my practice on an almost daily basis. It is one of the best remedies for balancing *Vata* and since *Vata* derangement is behind imbalances of the other two *doshas*, it deserves pride of place as a remedy. The rich, almost odourless oil expressed from sesame seeds is stable and contains an antioxidant system comprising sesamol and sesamolinal formed from sesamolin, which substantially reduce its oxidation rate (Price and Smith 1999). If properly stored, sesame oil is not likely to go rancid, making it popular as cooking oil in India and China. It is also highly nutritious, rich in vitamins A, B and E as well as the minerals iron, calcium, magnesium, copper, silicic acid and phosphorus. It contains linoleic acid and alpha linoleic acid as well as lecithin, and this may go some way to explaining its benefit to the brain and nervous system. Like olive oil, sesame oil is considered good for lowering harmful cholesterol levels (Patnaik 1993). White seeds produce the most oil, but in India it is said that the best oil for healing is extracted from black sesame seeds.

Sesame oil is immensely popular in India where its use in oil massage (*abhyanga*) is part of everyday life and an important aspect of Ayurveda. It is the favourite oil for massage as its chemical structure gives it a unique ability to penetrate the skin easily, nourishing and detoxifying even the deepest tissue layers. In fact it is said to benefit all the seven tissues (*dhatus*). It is the best oil for balancing *Vata* but can also be used sparingly for *Pitta* and *Kapha*.

People with high *Vata* can be prone to anxiety, nerve and bone disorders, poor circulation, lowered immunity and bowel problems such as wind, constipation and irritable bowel. They tend towards excess dryness both externally and internally. Used regularly, sesame oil is wonderful for reducing stress and tension, nourishing the nervous system and preventing nervous disorders, relieving fatigue and insomnia, and promoting strength and vitality. Those patients who use sesame oil daily have reported feeling stronger, more resilient to stress, with increased energy and better resistance to infection. Its antispasmodic and nervine properties ease pain and muscle spasm, such as sciatica, dysmenorrhoea, colic, backache and joint pain. The antioxidants explain its reputation for slowing the ageing process and increasing longevity. Certainly regular oiling of the skin restores moisture to the skin, keeping it soft, flexible and young-looking. It also lubricates the body internally, particularly the joints and bowels, and eases symptoms of dryness such as irritating coughs, cracking joints and hard stools.

Research into the healing effect of applying sesame oil is beginning to emerge. Those who practise it daily have found that they have less bacterial infection on their skin and that it helps joint problems. This may be related to the linoleic acid that makes up 40% of sesame oil and has antibacterial and anti-inflammatory effects. Sesame oil stimulates antibody production and enhances immunity. It also has anticancer properties and has been shown to inhibit the growth of malignant melanoma (Sharma and Clark 1998).

Daily *abhyanga* is best done in the morning. Rub the oil all over the body and leave it to soak in for 5–15 minutes before taking a warm bath or shower. This allows time for the oil to be absorbed and to nourish and detoxify the tissue layers. The warm water is important as it opens the pores, allowing the oil to permeate further into the body. To ease tension and relieve insomnia, the oil application is best in the evening before bed and should include oiling the soles of the feet. The oil should be room temperature in the summer but needs to be warmed in the winter. Herbal or essential oils can be added to enhance a specific desired effect, e.g. lavender oil for stress and tension, frankincense for arthritic pain, or ginger to increase the circulation.

Oil therapy (*snehana*) using oils internally and externally, is also important in Ayurveda, particularly as a prelude to detoxification (*pancha karma*) (see p. 167). Warm oil is applied in large amounts over the patient's body. According to Ayurveda, applying sesame oil to the skin in this way has a significant detoxifying effect. By stimulating the tissues in the body it helps to prevent toxins from accumulating in the system and to drain into the gut for elimination.

For external use, sesame oil is prepared by heating the oil with one or two drops of water until the water evaporates. Heating the oil has been shown to increase the antioxidant effect. When taken internally, cold-pressed sesame oil is used to moisten dry *Vata* membranes and tissues, and to soften and loosen dry and hardened toxins. It is best taken raw 1–2 tbsp daily.

Caution: *abhyanga* should be avoided immediately after administering enemas, emetics or purgatives, during pregnancy, the first stages of fever or if suffering from indigestion.

References

Athique M 1998 Ayurvedic Anatomy and Physiology. College of Ayurveda, London

Patnaik N 1993 The Garden of Life. Aquarian, Harper Collins, London

Price LP, Smith I 1999 Carrier Oils. Riverhead, Stratford upon Avon

Sharma H, Clark C 1998 Contemporary Ayurveda. Churchill Livingstone, London

Tillotson AK, Tillotson NH, Robert A Jr 2001 The One Earth Herbal Sourcebook. Kensington Publishing Corps, New York

Zysk K 1991 Ascetism and Healing in Ancient India: Medicine in the Buddhist Monastery. OUP, New York

Chapter **4**

Monographs of Ayurvedic herbs commonly used in the treatment of children

CHAPTER CONTENTS

Acorus calamus : Vacha

Family: Araceae
Sanskrit: Vacha
English: Sweet flag, Calamus root
Part used: rhizome
Quality/*Guna*: light/*laghu*, sharp/*tikshna*, flowing/ *sara*
Taste/*Rasa*: bitter/*tikta*, pungent/*katu*
Post digestive/*Vipak*: pungent/ *katu*
Potency/*Veerya*: heating/*ushna*
***Dosha*:** VK- P+
Tissue/*Dhatu*: marrow and nerve, muscle, fat, plasma, reproductive

Constituents

Rhizome bark has 1.5–3.5% volatile oil, including beta-asarone present in variable proportions, eugenol, asarone, caffeine, camphor, camphene, alpha-asarone, alpha-terpineol; sitosterol, galangin.

Action

Nervine, antispasmodic, sedative, analgesic, stomachic, expectorant, decongestant, emetic, laxative, diuretic, thermogenic, antipyretic, anti-inflammatory, antibacterial, antifungal, hypotensive, anticonvulsant, rejuvenative, stimulant, digestive.

Indications

Mental fatigue, poor memory, anxiety, bronchitis, sinusitis, sinus headache, flatulence, arthritis, peptic ulcers, colds, coughs.

Introduction

Acorus calamus actually originated in Europe but has been used extensively for centuries in Ayurvedic medicine, particularly as a rejuvenator of the nervous system, to enhance brain function, relieve headaches and for the treatment of arthritis.

Internal uses

Digestive system

By stimulating *agni*/digestive fire, *Acorus* stimulates appetite and digestion as well as absorption of nutrients. In doing so it helps to clear *ama* from the gut. A decoction of the root is given as a carminative for colic, flatulence and peptic ulcers. By relieving *Kapha* and enkindling *agni*, *Acorus* is considered useful in obesity.

Nervous system

As a nerve stimulant *Acorus* has been used for anxiety, mental fatigue, poor memory, insomnia, nervous debility, depression, epilepsy and other nervous complaints. Asarone and beta-asarone are the constituents credited with the sedative and nervine effects. It is applicable to all conditions of excess *Vata* and has a reputation for being able to enhance awareness and improve memory. Its mechanism is explained by Gogte who states that *Acorus* "alleviates excessive *Kapha* accumulated in the *manovaha srotas* which causes various psychological disorders" (Gogte 2000). In China the powder is blown into the nose of a coma patient to help restore consciousness (Amarasinghe 2003, Williamson 2002). A small piece of root is chewed or the powdered root used as snuff to overcome mental fatigue. In India the powder mixed with ghee is given to newborn babies on the 7th day to enhance brain function and speech development (Amarasinghe 2003, Williamson 2002). It is said to be the best medicine for children having lower intellectual level (Gogte 2000). *Acorus* is one of the main herbs used in India to treat cerebral palsy in children. It is given from the age of two onwards (brahmi and bacopa are given up until then). A poultice of the root is applied to the limbs of paralyzed children (Motley 1994) and the paste applied to painful arthritic joints (Gogte 2000). Research indicates that *Acorus* may affect certain proinflammatory mediators, suggesting a mechanism for its anti-inflammatory effect (Mehrotra et al 2003).

Respiratory system

A decoction of the root is given as a decongestant in catarrh and bronchitis and sinusitis. By clearing *Kapha* and *Vata* from the respiratory tract, *Acorus* is helpful in the treatment of coughs, asthma and laryngitis. For this purpose a piece of the root is often sucked as a lozenge. The powdered root is used as a snuff to relieve nasal congestion, headaches, lethargy and excessive sleepiness (Gogte 2000).

Immune system

The antimicrobial properties of *Acorus* have been put to good use as a herb for fumigation. It inhibits the growth of *Staphylococcus aureus*, *E. coli* and *Shigella*.

Temperature

Acorus is used for alleviating symptoms in fevers such as drowsiness and delirium and as a diaphoretic it can be used for fevers caused by obstruction of sweat.

External uses

Being antiseptic, the juice of the root can be applied to boils, and as an analgesic and anti-inflammatory it can also be applied to arthritic joints, and used as eardrops for earache and tinnitus. In India it is considered very useful for teething problems in children.

Safety profile

Acorus induces vomiting in large doses and is presently classified as an unsafe herb for internal usage by the American FDA. No side effects are known with the therapeutic dose however, although beta-asarone can be carcinogenic in animals. In India the dried root is prepared as a milk decoction to prevent toxicity. It is boiled until the milk evaporates, when it is dried and then powdered.

Dosage and formulations

- Decoction: 1 tsp boiled 4–5 minutes in 11–12 cups of water.
- Milk decoction with powdered ginger (for digestive indications).
- Powder: 100–250 mg intranasally, and for children over 2 for treatment of cerebral palsy up to $\frac{1}{4}$ tsp is given with honey am and pm (Amarasinghe 2003).
- For emesis: 4–5 g fresh powder +10 g rock salt is given with warm water followed by 1 litre warm water.

Research

- Amarasinghe APG 2003 Course lecture notes. Ayurvedic Paediatrics and Gynaecology and Practical Training of Ayurvedic Massage, London
- Gogte VVM 2000 Ayurvedic Pharmacology and Therapeutic Uses of Medicinal Plants. Bharatiya Vidya Bhavan, Mumbai
- Mehrotra S, Mishra KP, Maurya R, et al 2003 Anticellular and immunosuppressive properties of ethanolic extract of *Acorus calamus* rhizome. Int Immunopharmacol 3(1): 53–61
- Motley TJ 1994 The ethnobotany of sweet flag, *Acorus calamus* (Aracae). Economic Botany 48(4): 397
- Williamson E 2002 Major herbs of Ayurveda. Churchill Livingstone, London

Aegle marmelos : Bilva

Sanskrit: *Bilva*
English: Bengal quince, Bael fruit
Family: Rutaceae
Part used: fruit, unripe and ripe, root, seeds, leaves
Quality/*Guna*: light/*laghu*, dry/*ruksha*
Taste/*Rasa*: bitter/*tikta*, astringent/*kashaya*
Post digestive/*Vipak*: pungent/*katu*
Potency/*Veerya*: hot/*ushna*
Dosha: unripe fruit: K- VP+
Ripe fruit: KV- P+ and *agni+*
Tissue/*Dhatu*: plasma, blood, fat, nerve

Constituents

Mucilage, pectin, volatile oil gum and bitters (fruit pulp), alkaloids (roots and leaves), essential oils (leaves and seeds), anthraquinones, coumarins including the active principle marmelocin (fruit and hardwood), tannins (fruit and leaves), triterpenes (roots).

Actions

Unripe fruit: astringent, stomachic, appetizer, digestive stimulant.
Ripe fruit: more laxative, sweet and nutritive properties than the unripe fruit; astringent; haemostatic.
Root: anti-inflammatory, febrifuge, bitter tonic, nervine, cardiac tonic (Gogte 2000).
Leaves: liver stimulant, bitter tonic (Gogte 2000), hypoglycaemic, antimicrobial (Williamson 2002).
Seeds: the essential oil has antibacterial actions.

Indications

Malabsorption, chronic diarrhoea, colic, diabetes, cough, insomnia and bleeding.

Introduction

In India this tree is widely cultivated and is often to be found near temples as it is held as sacred to Lord Shiva. The leaves and wood have been used for pooja (worship). In India the fruit is eaten fresh and is a popular ingredient in drinks, jams and sweets.

Internal uses

Digestive system

Unripe fruit: As an astringent and stimulant, *bilva* is used for chronic weak digestion, low appetite and poor absorption of nutrients as it improves digestive fire and small intestine function. It is considered excellent for those suffering from chronic diarrhoea (Frawley and Lad 2001) and dysentery, as well as for dyspepsia and irritable bowel syndrome. In a randomized double-blind controlled study with patients suffering from irritable bowel syndrome, a combination of *bilva* fruit with bacopa was shown to be effective in 64.9% of the group as opposed to 32.7% of the placebo group (Yadav et al 1989). When used for chronic diarrhoea, the raw unripe fruit has a reputation for working when nothing else has been successful. It is also used for sprue and amoebic dysentery. Half a teaspoonful of powder in a teaspoonful of honey is taken for nausea and vomiting and when ground to a paste and cooked with sugar it is taken for bleeding piles (Gogte 2000).
Ripe fruit: Used as an adjuvant in bacillary dysentery for its ability to heal the intestinal mucosa (Williamson 2002).

Nervous system

Roots: Its nervine properties are useful in treatment of colic, pain, anxiety and insomnia and explain its use in India in the treatment of epilepsy.

Circulatory system

Bilva is considered a tonic for the heart and brain (Williamson 2002). The root is used in cardiac debility and palpitations. The fruit has haemostatic properties and alleviates swelling.

Respiratory system

Because of their bitter and pungent taste the leaves reduce *Kapha* symptoms such as colds and catarrh.

Temperature

The roots are used in decoction for reducing intermittent fevers.

The juice of the leaf has been used for reducing fevers.

Other uses

Leaves: The essential oil has antibacterial and antifungal properties and an aqueous extract has been found to be as effective as insulin at restoring blood glucose levels and body weight to normal (Williamson 2002). Research indicates that *Aegle* has activity against human *coxsackieviruses* (Badam et al 2002) and has an antiproliferative activity on human breast tumour cell lines (Lambertini et al 2004). Other research has demonstrated that extract can protect DNA from radiation-induced damage (*Jagetia* et al 2003).

External uses

The *leaf juice* has been used as an eyewash for conjunctivitis while the leaf powder made into a paste is applied over the eyelids. The *oil* has an antifungal activity (Rana et al 1997) and can be used in creams and ointments for fungal infections including athlete's foot. The *root* bark powder and the *leaf juice* are mixed and used for relieving pain and oedema (Gogte 2000).

Dosage and formulation

- Powder of the fruit: 1–2 g × 3 daily
- Infusion of the leaves 12–20 ml daily
- Juice 10–20 ml daily
- Formulation: Dasmula (ten roots).

Precautions

Unripe fruit is not to be used in acute fevers but can be used in chronic fevers (Frawley and Lad 2001). Large doses can be constipating (Gogte 2000).

Research

- Badam L, Bedekar SS, Sonawane KB, Joshi SP 2002 In vitro antiviral activity of bael (*Aegle marmelos* Corr) upon human coxsackieviruses B1–B6. J Commun Dis 34(2): 88–99
- Frawley D, Lad V 2001 The Yoga of Herbs. Lotus Press, Twin Lakes, Wisconsin
- Gogte VVM 2000 Ayurvedic Pharmacology and Therapeutic Uses of Medicinal Plants. Bharatiya Vidya Bhavan, Mumbai
- Jagetia GC, Venkatesh P, Baliga MS 2003 Evaluation of the radioprotective effect of *Aegle marmelos* (L.) Correa in cultured human peripheral blood lymphocytes exposed to different doses of gamma-radiation: a micronucleus study. Mutagenesis 18(4): 387–393
- Lambertini E, Piva R, Khan MT, et al 2004 Effects of extracts from Bangladeshi medicinal plants on in vitro proliferation of human breast cancer cell lines and expression of estrogen receptor alpha gene. Int J Oncol 24(2): 419–423
- Rana BK, Singh UP, Taneja V 1997 Antifungal activity and kinetics of inhibition by essential oil isolated from leaves of *Aegle marmelos*. J Ethnopharmacol 57(1): 29
- Williamson E 2002 Major Herbs of Ayurveda. Churchill Livingstone, London
- Yadav SK, Jain AK, Tripathi SN, Gupta JP 1989 Irritable bowel syndrome: therapeutic evaluation of indigenous drugs. Indian J Med Res 90: 496

Aloe vera : Kumari

Family: Liliaceae
Sanskrit: *Kumari*
English: Indian aloe, aloe vera
Part use: extract, dried juice of leaves and pulp root
Quality/*Guna*: oily/*snigdha*, sticky/*pichchila*
Taste/*Rasa*: bitter/*tikta*, sweet/*madhur*, pungent/*katu*, astringent/*kashaya*
Post digestive/*Vipak*: sweet/*madhur*
Potency/*Veerya*: cooling/*sheeta*
Dosha: VPK=
Tissue/*Dhatu*: all

Constituents

Polysaccharides, enzymes, vitamins B1, B2, B6, choline, folic acid, essential amino acids, calcium, sodium, chlorine, magnesium, zinc, aloinosides including barbaloin (aloins A and B).

Actions

Alterative, anthelmintic, digestive, laxative, bitter tonic, rejuvenative, purgative, diuretic.

Indications

Intestinal worms, fever, constipation, eye problems, colds, haemorrhoids, coughs, inflammation of skin, chronic ulcers, dysentery, skin rashes, enlarged liver or spleen.

Introduction

Aloe gel has a wide variety of therapeutic uses. It is a rejuvenative for *Pitta* but can be used for all three *doshas*. Legend has it that Cleopatra used it to maintain her beauty and in fact it is excellent for sensitive and allergic skin conditions. It has been a treatment of wounds for over 2000 years. Aloe gel is the clear mucilaginous gel of the inner portion of the leaves, which can be applied to soothe cuts, abrasions and inflammatory skin conditions and when mixed with water it makes the juice. The laxative part of the plant is found in the rind of the leaves and is a bitter, yellow juice. This is not used for children.

Internal uses

Digestive system

Aloe vera juice has a laxative action and can be used to clear toxins and heat from the bowel. It helps control micro-organisms in the gut and acts as a bitter tonic to the liver and the whole of the digestive tract. It enhances the secretion of digestive enzymes, balances acid in the stomach, aids digestion and regulates sugar and fat metabolism. Aloe juice has wonderful demulcent properties, soothing and protecting the lining of the gut. It can be used to treat colitis, peptic ulcers and irritable bowel syndrome. Research has indicated some promise in treating inflammatory bowel disease (Robinson 1998).

Nervous system

Aloe vera has a generally cooling and moistening effect and can be used for problems associated with excess heat and inflammation. It is particularly useful for hot fiery people, who are prone to inflammatory problems and to feelings of anger, irritability and self-criticism. As a nutritive tonic aloe can be combined with shatavari, and as a bitter tonic with gentian (*Gentiana untea*).

Temperature

Aloe vera has cooling properties and can be used to bring down temperatures.

External uses

Externally, aloe gel has remarkable healing powers. It is used for treating burns (Visuthikosol et al 1995) including sunburn, and after radiation therapy (Grindlay and Reynolds 1986, Williams et al 1996). It is also used with success in the treatment of a variety of skin conditions including herpes (Frawley and Lad 2001). In trials, patients with psoriasis demonstrated dramatic results after thrice daily application of aloe vera extract. A total of 82.8% of patients demonstrated significant clearing of psoriatic plaques, compared to 7.7% using a placebo cream (Syed et al 1996). Aloe gel also relieves pain, soothes inflammation (Yagi et al 2002) and has a mildly antibiotic effect (Klein and Penneys 1988). It is applied to haemorrhoids to soothe pain and irritation and speed healing.

Precaution

Do not use when pregnant or in appendicitis and abdominal pain of unknown origin. There are occasionally reports of contact dermatitis from using aloe vera gel (Hunter and Frumkin 1991).

Drug interactions

There is possible interaction with cardiac glycosides.

Research

- Frawley D, Lad V 2001 The Yoga of Herbs (2nd ed) Lotus Press, Twin Lakes, Wisconsin
- Grindlay D, Reynolds T 1986 The Aloe vera phenomenon: a review of the properties and modern uses of the leaf parenchyma gel. J Ethnopharmacol 16(2–3): 117–151
- Hunter D, Frumkin A 1991 Adverse reactions to vitamin E and aloe vera preparations after dermabrasion and chemical peel. Cutis 47(3): 193–196
- Klein AD, Penneys NS 1988 Aloe vera. J Am Acad Dermatol 18(4 Pt 1): 714–720
- Robinson M 1998 Medical therapy of inflammatory bowel disease for the 21st century. Eur J Surg Suppl 582: 90–98
- Syed TA, Ahmad SA, Holt AH, Ahmad SA, Ahmad SH, Afzal M 1996 Management of psoriasis with Aloe Vera extract in a hydrophilic cream: a placebo-controlled, double-blind study. Trop Med Int Health 1(4): 505–509
- Visuthikosol V, Chowchuen B, Sukwanarat Y, Sriurairatana S, Boonpucknavig V 1995 Effect of aloe vera gel to healing of burn wound a clinical and histological study. J Med Assoc Thai 78(8): 403–409
- Williams MS, Burk M, Loprinzi CL, et al 1996 Phase III double-blind evaluation of an aloe vera gel as a prophylactic agent for radiation-induced skin toxicity. Int J Radiat Oncol Biol Phys 36(2): 345–349
- Yagi A, Kabash A, Okamura N, Haraguchi H, Moustafa SM, Khalifa TI 2002 Antioxidant, free radical scavenging and anti-inflammatory effects of aloesin derivatives in Aloe vera. Planta Med 68(11): 957–960

Asparagus racemosus : Shatavari

Family: Liliaceae
Sanskrit: *Shatavari*
English: Wild asparagus
Part used: leaves, root
Quality/*Guna*: heavy/*guru*, unctous/*snigdha*
Taste/*Rasa*: sweet/*madhur*, bitter/*tikta*
Post digestive/*Vipak*: sweet/*madhur*
Potency/*Veerya*: cold/*sheeta*
Dosha: VP- K+
Tissue/*Dhatu*: all tissues

Constituents

Saponins, steroidal glycosides and aglycones, flavonoids including quercetin, rutin and hyperoside, alkaloids, mucilage.

Actions

Galactagogic, antispasmodic, nervine, anti-inflammatory, demulcent, refrigerant, diuretic, general tonic, expectorant, antibacterial, antitumour, antacid.

Indications

General nutritive tonic, gastritis, diarrhoea, dysentery, inflammatory bowel problems, blood purification, dyspepsia, joint pains, anxiety, fever.

Introduction

Shatavari translates "she who possesses a hundred husbands" as this herb is the most important rejuvenative tonic for women in Ayurvedic medicine. As a nourishing herb it is also used for a wide variety of ailments in children. According to David Simon and Deepak Chopra, *shatavari* is nourishing, soothing, cooling, lubricating, useful in conditions when the body and mind are overheated, depleted or out of balance (Chopra and Simon 2000).

Internal uses

Digestive system

The cooling and demulcent properties of *shatavari* are used for soothing dry inflamed mucous membranes throughout the body, for treating problems associated with a disturbance of either *Vata* or *Pitta* giving rise to, for example, heartburn, gastritis, peptic ulcers, colitis, Crohn's disease and irritable bowel syndrome. It relieves hyperacidity as well as diarrhoea and dysentery. In a small trial on eight healthy volunteers, *shatavari* was found to have an equivalent effect to metoclopramide in reducing gastric emptying time (Dalvi et al 1990).

Respiratory system

Shatavari soothes sore throats and dry coughs, and is used generally for treating irritated conditions of the respiratory system.

Immune system

Its immune-stimulating properties combined with its ability to enhance growth and development are particularly applicable to children (Pole 2005). According to Chopra and Simon, *shatavari* has a measurable effect on macrophage function enhancing their ability to fight fungal infections. It enhances the production of natural immune-regulating messenger molecules and protects blood-producing cells in the bone marrow, thus helping the immune system recover more quickly after exposure to toxic chemicals (Chopra and Simon 2000). *Shatavari* also has adaptogenic properties. *Shatavari* has antibacterial activity in vitro against a range of bacteria including *E. coli*, *Shigella* spp., *Salmonella* spp. and *Pseudomonas* (Mandal et al 2000).

As well as being nourishing, *shatavari* is also detoxifying. It is recommended during convalescence and for infections such as herpes and for chronic fevers.

Nervous system

Shatavari is valued in India for its ability to promote clarity of mind and is worth consideration in the treatment of problems such as ADHD in children when used in combination with other brain tonics such as brahmi (*Hydrocotyle asiatica*). It is calming and helps to reduce anxiety and stress.

Reproductive system

Shatavari's main action is on the female reproductive tract. It is considered nourishing and strengthening and it is a successful remedy for problems with fertility, hormonal imbalances and during the menopause (McIntyre 1994). It effectively increases milk production in nursing mothers.

Urinary system

The soothing and cooling properties of *shatavari* can be used for treating irritated conditions of the urinary system.

External uses

Shatavari is used externally to relieve painful swollen joints and muscle tension and is one of the main ingredients of Mahanaryan oil, a well-known oil formulation for the relief of joint and muscle pain. It also reduces development of scar tissue after surgery (Chopra and Simon 2000).

Dosage and formulation

- Infusion: 3–6 oz bid
- Decoction: 2–4 oz bid
- Milk decoction: 2–4 oz bid (with gee pippali, and honey)
- Powder: 3–5 g bid (with honey)
- Mix with equal parts of amalaki and liquorice for heartburn or indigestion.

Research

- Chopra D, Simon D 2000 The Chopra Centre Herbal Handbook. Rider, London
- Dalvi SS, Nadkarni PM, Gupta KC 1990 Effect of *Asparagus racemosus* (Shatavari) on gastric emptying time in normal healthy volunteers. J Postgrad Med 36(2): 91–94
- Mandal SC, Nandy A, Pal M, Saha BP 2000 Evaluation of antibacterial activity of *Asparagus racemosus* willd. root. Phytother Res 14(2): 118–119
- McIntyre A 1994 The Complete Woman's Herbal. Gaia Books Limited, London
- Pole S 2005 An Ayurvedic Herbal. A guide to Ayurvedic Herbs and Formulas. Thesis

Azadirachta indica : Neem

Family: Meliaceae
Sanskrit: Nimba
English: *Neem* tree, Margosa tree, Indian lilac
Part used: flowers, seeds, leaves and bark
Quality/*Guna*: light/*laghu*
Taste/*Rasa*: bitter/*tikra*, astringent/*kashaya*
Post digestive/*Vipak*: pungent/*katu*
Potency/*Veerya*: cold/*sheeta*
Dosha: KP-
Tissue/*Dhatu*: plasma, blood, fat

Constituents

Volatile oil, gum, polysaccharides (fruit pulp); resin: margosin, terpenes, seed: 40% stable oil and sulphur.

Actions

Demulcent, febrifuge, antiseptic, vulnerary, antimicrobial, anthelmintic, insecticidal, alterative, anti-inflammatory, expectorant, bitter tonic, refrigerant, antiemetic.

Introduction

The evergreen neem tree provides one of the best-known blood purifiers and detoxicants among traditional Ayurvedic herbs. It is primarily used for all conditions of excess *Pitta* characterized by heat and burning sensations.

Internal uses

Digestive system

With its bitter taste, *neem* stimulates appetite and digestion as well as the flow of bile from the liver, enhancing liver function. Its hepato-protective activity protects the liver from injury caused by toxins, drugs and viruses. Its astringent, antimicrobial and anti-inflammatory properties contribute to its effect as an antiulcer remedy. *Neem* is often used as a treatment for acidity, heartburn, gastritis, indigestion, nausea and vomiting. It has also been used successfully for eradicating worms.

Nervous system

With its *Pitta*-reducing properties, *neem* is used for anxiety and stress, irritability and it has significant pain-relieving properties.

Circulatory system

A leaf extract has been shown to reduce serum cholesterol levels as well as blood pressure and arrhythmias.

Respiratory system

Neem has decongestant and expectorant action cleaning infection and phlegm from the lungs. It is used in coughs and bronchitis. The seeds are used for tuberculosis.

Immune system

Neem is considered one of the best herbs for a wide range of infections, both chronic and acute. Antibacterial, antifungal and antiparasitic activity has been demonstrated (Fabry et al 1996, 1998) in the leaves and bark. *Neem* has long been used for the prevention and treatment of malaria (Mackinnon et al 1997). As a detoxifying remedy Chopra and Simon recommend *neem* for patients who have been overeating, abusing drugs or alcohol or a prescription drug including antibiotics, steroids or chemotherapy (Chopra and Simon 2000). It is also used for lymphodemitis and inflammatory arthritis.

Skin

As an antimicrobial and detoxicant, *neem* has been used traditionally for a wide range of skin disorders incuding eczema, acne, leucoderma, boils, psoriasis, abscesses and haemorrhoids. It soothes itching and allays inflammation.

Temperature

A decoction of leaves and bark is used to cure fevers, including intermittent fevers of malaria.

External uses

The oil from the seeds is used to treat boils, contagious infections such as scabies, ringworm, head lice, athlete's foot and ulcers, as well as wound healing. It is also used in liniments for inflammatory joint pain and muscle aches. In India *neem* oil is used as nose drops for psoriasis and baldness (Gogte 2000). In some parts of India *neem* twigs are used as toothbrushes providing antimicrobial and astringent effects to tone the gums and prevent infection. *Neem's* ability to inhibit bacterial infection on the surface of the teeth explains its long use in oral hygiene and inclusion in toothpastes to fight tooth decay.

Other uses

The seeds are given in case of delayed and painful childbirth as they cause contractions in the uterus. It is widely used as a component of non-toxic insecticides. *Neem* has been used as a valuable herb for the treatment of diabetes (Sankla et al 1973) and is considered one of the best remedies for obesity. Excreted in breast milk it is used for preventing coughs and skin diseases in infants (Gogte 2000). The leaves are given to a woman after birth as a uterine tonic.

Dosage and formulations

- Powder of leaves mixed with water to form a paste to apply to the skin or neem oil (medicated).
- Daily dose: 10–20 ml juice from leaves or fruit, 2–4 g ($\frac{1}{2}$ tsp) powdered bark, or 5–10 drops oil.

Precautions

Avoid in pregnancy and high *Vata*, depleted and emaciated states. *Neem* may reduce fertility. Toxic effects have been reported.

Drug interactions

Care may need to be used in diabetic patients on insulin.

Research

- Chopra D, Simon D 2000 The Chopra Centre Herbal Handbook. Rider, London
- Fabry W, Okemo PO, Ansorg R 1996 Fungistatic and fungicidal activity of East African medicinal plants. Mycoses 39: 67–70
- Fabry W, Okemo PO, Ansorg R 1998 Antibacterial activity of East African medicinal plants. J Ethnopharmacol 60: 79–84
- Gogte VVM 2000 Ayurvedic Pharmacology and Therapeutic Uses of Medicinal Plants. Bharatiya Vidya Bhavan, Mumbai
- Mackinnon S, Durst T, Arnason JR, et al 1997 Antimalarial activity of tropical *Meliaceae* extracts and Gedunin derivatives. J Nat Prod 60(4): 336
- Sankla R, Singh S, Bhandari CR 1973 Preliminary clinical trials on antidiabetic actions of *Azadirachta indica*. Medicine, Surgery 13: 11

Bacopa monnieri : Brahmi

Family: Scrophulariaceae
Sanskrit: *Brahmi*
English: Thyme-leaved gratiola
Part used: dried whole plant, mainly leaves and stalk
Quality/*Guna*: light/*laghu*, unctuous/*snigdha*
Taste/*Rasa*: bitter/*titka*, astringent/*kashaya*
Post digestive/*Vipak*: pungent/*katu*
Potency/*Veerya*: cooling/*sheeta*
Dosha: VPK =
Tissue/*Dhatu*: all seven, especially plasma, blood, nerve

Constituents

Steroidal saponins; alkaloids: brahmine and herpestine; flavonoids.

Actions

Nervine tonic, diuretic, sedative, cardiac tonic, rejuvenative, antispasmodic, anticonvulsant, antiinflammatory.

Indications

Emotional stress, mental exhaustion, forgetfulness, anxiety, asthma, bronchitis, cough, hoarseness, water retention, rheumatic joint pain.

Introduction

Brahmi derives its name from Brahman meaning pure consciousness, probably because of its ability to calm mental turbulence and aid meditation enabling knowledge of Brahman. [It is often confused with its close relative *gotu kola* (*Centella asiatica*) which is also called Brahmi in Northern India.]

Internal uses

Digestive system

Bacopa has a suppressant action on appetite and so is best combined with warming digestive herbs such as ginger or cardamom (Pole 2005). Its astringent action is useful in diarrhoea due to *Vata* disturbance.

Nervous system

Bacopa is widely used in India and China to enhance brain function and in treatment of mental problems such as epilepsy, anxiety and hysteria. It is reported to have sedative as well as cardiotonic effects due to the presence of hersaponin, one of four saponins isolated from the plant. It has been used traditionally to improve memory and concentration, enhance learning ability and calm mental turbulence. It has a nourishing effect on the nervous system and is prescribed for reducing the effects of stress and nervous exhaustion, depression and in particular for conditions associated with excess *Vata*. A trial of 76 adults suggested that *bacopa* may help decrease the rate of forgetting newly acquired information (Roodenrys et al 2002).

Respiratory system

Bacopa is a popular remedy for treating coughs and colds in children. It can also be used for asthma and hoarseness. A poultice of the entire boiled plant is applied to the chest in bronchitis and chronic cough.

Urinary system

A cooling diuretic, *bacopa* is used for relieving pain of cystitis and irritable bladder.

Temperature

In Sri Lanka *bacopa* is used for relieving fevers.

External uses

A medicated oil containing *bacopa* is applied to inflamed joints to relieve pain and to the head to clear the mind and relieve headaches. The fresh juice of leaves is also applied to inflamed joints to relieve pain.

Dosage and formulation

- Infusion – two cups/day
- Leaf juice 2 tsp
- Alcoholic extract – 30 drops by mouth twice a day
- Powder – 1.25–2.0 g twice a day with warm water
- Forms most of *Brahmi Rasayana*: 10 parts *brahmi*; 2 parts cloves; 1 part cardamom; 1 part pippali
- Combines well with ashwagandha as a nervine and with jatamansi/gotu kola as a sedative (Pole 2005). It is used to prepare a number of important Ayurvedic preparations (Brahmighritam, Brahmirasayanam), which are given to those suffering from anxiety and emotional stress.

Precautions

May cause a rise in blood pressure in large doses.

Research

- Pole S 2005 An Ayurvedic Herbal. A guide to Ayurvedic Herbs and Formulas. Thesis
- Roodenrys S, Booth D, Bulzomi S, Phipps A, Micallef C, Smoker J 2002 Chronic effects of Brahmi (*Bacopa monnieri*) on human memory. Neuropsychopharmacology 27(2): 279–281

Cedrus deodara : Devadaru

Family: Conifereae
Sanskrit: *Devadaru*, deodar, daru, suradaru, Shambhava, Suravha
English: Himalayan cedar
Part used: inner part of the wood and oil used
Quality/*Guna*: light/*laghu*, oily/*snigdha*
Taste/*Rasa*: pungent/*tikta* and bitter/*katu*
Post digestive/*Vipak*: bitter/*katu*
Potency/*Veerya*: hot/*ushna*
***Dosha*:** VK-
Tissue/*Dhatu*: blood, fat, plasma

Constituents

Essential oil (mainly beta-himachalene), hydrocarbons, resin, flavonoids.

Actions

Antimicrobial, insecticidal, anticancer against human epidermal carcinoma of the nasopharynx (Dhar et al 1968).

Indications

Fevers, skin problems, purifying breast milk, urinary disorders, coughs and colds, infectious disease, constipation, worms, headaches and inflammation.

Introduction

This aromatic cedar tree found in India has an Arabic name, Kedron, meaning powerful, of majestic appearance. One of its Sanskrit names is deodar meaning "god's country where tree is grown". This is an excellent plant for all kinds of children's problems, particularly those related to *Vata* and *Kapha*.

Internal uses

Digestive system

With its pungent and bitter tastes *Cedrus* stimulates the appetite and promotes digestion, especially of fats. It is reputed to be one of the best herbs for obesity. The wood is a laxative and anthelmintic, while the oil is more astringent and used for diarrhoea. It calms *Vata* and *Kapha* and so is good for hiccups.

Nervous system

Cedrus has a sedative effect (Gogte 2000) and is topmost in the analgesics for painful conditions like headaches, joint, nerve and muscle pain and sciatica.

Respiratory system

A pungent expectorant, *Cedrus* is used for coughs, colds and catarrh caused by *Kapha*.

Circulatory system

Cedrus is reputed to be cardio-stimulant, a blood purifier, and an inflammatory remedy. It is used to alleviate swelling and is used for mumps (Gogte 2000).

Urinary system

Cedrus has diuretic and antiseptic properties and can be used for urinary disorders.

Temperature

Cedrus is a well-known herb for reducing fevers as it acts as a diaphoretic. It is considered useful in chronic fever caused by *Vata* and *Kapha*.

Immune system

It is a popular Ayurvedic remedy in treatment of children's infectious diseases such as mumps. *Cedrus* has been shown to have an effect on the immune system with an ability to stabilize mast cells. This means that *Cedrus* is well worth consideration in the treatment of chronic allergies. The oil is antiseptic and has been shown to have antifungal properties (Dixit and Dixit 1982). An alcohol extract of *Cedrus* has also demonstrated anticancer properties.

External uses

Cedrus relieves inflammation. The oil has the ability to destroy bacteria from infected wounds (Gogte

2000). It is used in skin disorders, skin ulcers, and arthritis.

Other uses

Cedrus is a popular remedy for women where it acts as a uterine tonic and is used to purify breast milk. Research has indicated that constituents from *Cedrus* have strong antioxidant properties (Tiwari et al 2001).

Dosage and formulation

- Powder: 1–3 g
- Oil 20–40 drops (adult).

Research

- Dhar ML, Dhar MM, Dhawan BN, Mehrotra BN, Ray C 1968 Screening of Indian plants for biological activity, Part 1. Indian J Exp Biol 6: 232
- Dixit A, Dixit SN 1982 A promising anti fungal agent. Indian Perfumer 26(2–4): 216
- Gogte VVM 2000 Ayurvedic Pharmacology and Therapeutic Uses of Medicinal Plants. Bharatiya Vidya Bhavan, Mumbai
- Tiwari AK, Srinivas PV, Kumar SP, Rao JM 2001 Free radical scavenging active components from *Cedrus deodara*. J Agric Food Chem 49(10): 4642–4645

Centella asiatica : Gotu kola

Family: Umbelliferae
Sanskrit: Mandookpani, α-Brahmamandooki
English: Indian pennywort, *gotu kola*
Part used: aerial parts
Quality/*Guna*: light/*laghu*, cooling/*sheeta*
Taste/*Rasa*: sweet/*madhur*, bitter/*tikta*, astringent/*kashaya*
Post digestive/*Vipak*: sweet/*madhur*
Potency/*Veerya*: cold/*sheeta*
Dosha: balances primarily *Pitta* and *Kapha* but also *Vata*
Tissue/*Dhatu*: plasma, blood, nerve

Constituents

Essential oil, fatty oil, beta-sitostenol, tannins, resin alkaloid: hydrocotylin; bitter principle: vellarine; pectic acid, polyphenols, saponins (braminoside, brahmoside), flavonoids.

Actions

Nerve tonic, cardio-tonic, immune stimulant, febrifuge, alterative, diuretic, anthelmintic, vulnerary, rejuvenative, hair tonic, anticonvulsant, anxiolytic, analgesic.

Indications

Skin problems, cuts and wounds, postoperative healing, poor memory, learning problems, childhood infections, urinary problems, insomnia and fever.

Introduction

Another plant named after Brahma, the all-pervading consciousness, because of its central action on the brain. *Gotu kola* is considered a *Sattvic* herb that enhances wisdom and intelligence and is especially useful for children. In Nepal a leaf of *gotu kola* is given to children in a spring ceremony to aid memory and concentration and help them in their school work (Tillotson et al 2001).

Internal uses

Digestive system

Gotu kola is used in the early stages of dysentery in children (Bakhru 1998) with cumin. It can also be used for indigestion, acidity and ulcers as it cools heat and reduces inflammation. Its antibacterial action could contribute to its antiulcer properties.

Nervous system

One of the best tonics for the brain, *gotu kola* reputedly protects against the ageing process and Alzheimer's. It has the ability to improve memory and concentration and is excellent for children with learning difficulties including ADHD and mental problems (Rao et al 1973) autism and Asperger's syndrome. It is also recommended for those who are depleted by stress and anxiety, for relief of insomnia (Ramaswamy et al 1979) and depression, and to calm mental turbulence. As an anticonvulsant it can reduce the duration of epileptic fits.

Circulatory system

Due to its positive effect on microcirculation and capillary permeability (Belcaro et al 1990, Cesarone et al 1994, De Sanctis et al 2001) *Centella* has produced very positive results in the treatment of oedema and venous insufficiency and varicose veins (Cesarone et al 1992). It is also an excellent wound and scar healer and has become increasingly popular for postoperative use (Widgerow et al 2000). It stimulates synthesis of collagen and the production of fibroblasts (Bonte et al 1994, Kim et al 1993, Tenni et al 1988) and helps to protect the skin against radiation. *Gotu kola* is also used to prevent bleeding and other circulatory problems associated with high *Pitta* including anaemia.

Respiratory system

Gotu kola is used for chronic coughs as a decongestant for catarrh.

Immune system

Gotu kola has been demonstrated to be effective against bacteria including *Pseudomonas* and *Streptococcus* spp., as well as against viruses including *herpes simplex* II. It is used to clear toxins from the system and allay inflammation and for this reason it is used in treatment of arthritis and gout.

Skin

A household remedy for skin problems, including boils, acne, ulcers and chronic eczema. As a keratinocyte antiproliferant, it is a promising remedy for psoriasis (Sampson et al 2001). It has also been shown to be active against the *herpes simplex* virus (Yoosook et al 2000). *Gotu kola* has been evaluated with human skin fibroblasts and has been found to increase synthesis of collagen and fibronectin which may provide a mechanism for its well-known actions in wound healing (Tenni et al 1988).

Temperature

Gotu kola clears heat and is good for eruptive fevers.

External uses

The juice of the fresh leaves mixed with turmeric is applied to wounds to speed healing. Prepared in coconut oil it is used to apply to the head to calm the mind, promote sleep, relieve headaches and prevent hair loss. *Gotu kola* oil can also be applied to skin conditions such as eczema and herpes.

Dosage and formulations

- Infusion/decoction: 30–60 ml
- Powder fresh leaves: 1–3 g bid
- Leaf juice: 10–15 ml bid (Chopra and Simon 2000, pp. 94–97).

Drug interactions

None known. May potentiate action of anxiolytic medications.

Research

- Bakhru HK 1998 Herbs that Heal. Orient Paperbacks, Delhi
- Belcaro GV, Grimaldi R, Guidi G 1990 Improvement of capillary permeability in patients with venous hypertension after treatment with TTFCA. Angiology 41(7): 533–540
- Bonte F, Dumas M, Chaudagne C, et al 1994 Influence of asiatic acid, madecassic acid, and asiaticoside on human collagen I synthesis. Planta Med 60(2): 133–135
- Cesarone MR, Laurora G, De Sanctis MT, et al 1992 Activity of *Centella asiatica* in venous insufficiency. Minerva Cardioangiol 40(4): 137–143
- Cesarone MR, Laurora G, De Sanctis MT, et al 1994 The microcirculatory activity of *Centella asiatica* in venous insufficiency. A double-blind study. Minerva Cardioangiol 42(6): 299–304
- Chopra D, Simon D 2000 The Chopra Centre Herbal Handbook. Rider, London
- De Sanctis MT, Belcaro G, Incandela L, et al 2001 Treatment of edema and increased capillary filtration in venous hypertension with total triterpenic fraction of *Centella asiatica*: a clinical, prospective, placebo-controlled, randomized, dose-ranging trial. Angiology 52(2): S55–59
- Kim YN, Park YS, Kim HK, et al 1993 Enhancement of the attachment on microcarriers and tPA production by fibroblast cells in a serum-free medium by the addition of the extracts of *Centella asiatica*. Cytotechnology 13(3): 221–226
- Ramaswamy AS, Periyasamy SM, Basu N 1979 Pharmacological studies on *C. asiatica*. J Res Indian Med 4: 160
- Rao MVR, Srinivasan K, Rao KT 1973 Effect of mandukaparni on general mental ability of mentally retarded children. J Res Indian Med 8: 9
- Sampson JH, Raman A, Karlsen G, et al 2001 In vitro keratinocyte antiproliferant effect of *Centella asiatica* extract and triterpenoid saponins. Phytomedicine 8(3): 230–235

- Tenni R, Zanaboni G, De Agostini MP, et al 1988 Effect of the triterpenoid fraction of *Centella asiatica* on macromolecules of the connective matrix in human skin fibroblast cultures. Ital J Biochem 37(2): 69–77
- Tillotson AK, Tillotson NH, Robert A Jr 2001 The One Earth Herbal Sourcebook. Kensington Publishing Corps, New York
- Widgerow AD, Chait LA, Stals R, et al 2000 New innovations in scar management. Aesthetic Plast Surg 24(3): 227–234
- Yoosook C, Bunyapraphatsara N, Boonyakiat Y, et al 2000 Anti-herpes simplex virus activities of crude water extracts of Thai medicinal plants. Phytomedicine 6(6): 411–419

Coriandrum sativum : Coriander

Family: Umbelliferae
Sanskrit: Dhanya
English: *Coriander*
Part used: seeds, leaves
Quality/*Guna*: light/*laghu*, oily/*snigdha*
Taste/*Rasa*: sweet/*madhur*, bitter/*tikta*, astringent/*kashaya*, pungent/*katu*
Post digestive/*Vipak*: sweet/*madhur*
Potency/*Veerya*: cooling/*sheeta*
Dosha: VPK = especially *Pitta*
Tissue/*Dhatu*: plasma, reproductive

Constituents

Volatile oil (comprising coriandrol, geraniol, borneol, camphor, carvone, and anethole) mostly in the seeds. Also resin, malic acid, alkaloids.

Actions

Carminative, diuretic, decongestant, antispasmodic, diaphoretic.

Indications

Colds, coughs, urinary tract infections, heat and inflammation, digestive problems, fevers, eruptive infections in children.

Introduction

Coriander was mentioned in Sanskrit texts dating back almost 7000 years ago (Foster 1993) and we know that at least 3000 years ago it was an important ingredient in cookery and medicines of the ancient Egyptians. *Coriander* has a cooling effect in the body and is specifically recommended to balance *Pitta*.

Internal uses

Digestive system

Coriander is a good remedy for hot inflammatory conditions, particularly in the digestive tract. It is often used with cumin and fennel. In India they use fresh *coriander* leaf in their food, both to prevent and remedy symptoms such as heartburn, indigestion, wind, colic, diarrhoea and dysentery. They also roast fennel seeds with *coriander* seeds and a little salt and chew them after eating to combat sleepiness after a large meal. Perhaps this is why *coriander* is considered to be nerve and brain strengthening. *Coriander* enhances appetite and improves digestion and absorption of nutrients, and with its relaxant and anti-inflammatory effect in the gut, helps to relieve spasm, griping, gastritis and nervous dyspepsia. The seeds are often combined with laxatives to prevent any griping the latter may cause.

Respiratory system

The seeds can be mixed with turmeric and cumin, and taken in hot teas for colds, flu, coughs and catarrh to aid the body's fight against infection and as a decongestant.

Urinary system

The cooling effects of *coriander* make it an excellent remedy for urinary disorders, particularly those with hot burning symptoms such as cystitis and urethritis. The diuretic effect of *coriander* goes some way to explain its cooling and cleansing effect.

Reproductive system

The relaxant effects of *coriander*, thanks to its high volatile oil content, seen in the digestive tract are also apparent in the uterus, helping to relieve menstrual problems, particularly period pain. In the Arab world women have used *coriander* to lessen the pain of uterine contractions during childbirth.

Immune system

The volatile oils in the seeds have an antibacterial as well as an antifungal action, while the fresh leaves are rich in vitamins A and C, as well as niacin, thiamin, calcium, phosphorus, potassium and iron (Foster 1993). The vitamins have antioxidant properties, helping to prevent damage caused by free radicals.

Temperature

Today in China, as in India, the seeds are used to promote sweating and break a fever and to bring out the rash in eruptive infections like chickenpox and measles (Foster 1993).

External uses

Coriander leaf juice or tea can be taken internally and applied externally to soothe hot, itchy skin rashes such as urticaria and to calm other allergic symptoms such as hayfever and catarrh. In other parts of the world *coriander* has been used for erysipelas (an inflammatory skin condition) and to tone down an over florid complexion.

Other uses

The tea also makes an effective gargle for sore throats and oral thrush. Research indicated that coriander seed oil has strong radical scavenging activity (Ramadan et al 2003).

Dosage and formulation

- Daily dose: 3–6 g ($\frac{1}{2}$ tsp).

Research

- Foster S 1993 Herbal Renaissance. Gibbs-Smith, Salt Lake City, p. 78
- Ramadan MF, Kroh LW, Morsel JT 2003 Radical scavenging activity of black cumin (*Nigella sativa* L.), coriander (*Coriandrum sativum* L.), and niger (*Guizotia abyssinica* Cass.) crude seed oils and oil fractions. J Agric Food Chem 51(24): 6961–6969

Curcuma longa : Turmeric

Family: Zingiberaceae
Sanskrit: Haldi
English: *Turmeric*
Part used: rhizomes
Quality/*Guna*: dry/*ruksha*, light/*laghu*
Taste/*Rasa*: pungent/*katu*, astringent/*tika*
Post digestive/*Vipak*: pungent/*katu*
Potency/*Veerya*: hot/*ushna*
Dosha: VPK=
Tissue/*Dhatu*: plasma, fatty tissue, blood

Constituents

Curcumin, tumerone, and zingiberone, high amounts of a carotene, equivalent to 50 IU of vitamin A per 100 g (Chopra and Simon 2000). Probably the most important component is curcumin, which gives turmeric its intense yellow colour.

Actions

Antioxidant, antibiotic, anti-inflammatory, alterative, digestive, analgesic.

Indications

IBS, digestive problems, skin problems, cuts and wounds, coughs and colds, constipation, anaemia, mucus congestion, fevers, inflammation problems.

Introduction

Turmeric is an amazing healing plant that has not only been valued for its therapeutic properties in Ayurvedic and Chinese medicine for thousands of years, but also has a significant role to play here in the West in prevention and treatment of a wide range of modern day problems. It is an excellent natural antibiotic, and one of the best detoxifying herbs by virtue of its beneficial effect on the liver, a powerful antioxidant with health-promoting effects on the cardiovascular, skeletal and digestive systems. Through its beneficial effect on the ligaments, it is highly valued by those who practise Hatha Yoga. It aids digestion, particularly of protein, it promotes absorption and regulates metabolism.

Internal uses

Digestive system

Turmeric aids digestion, particularly of protein, and promotes absorption of nutrients and regulates metabolism. It also helps to regulate intestinal flora and is worth taking during and after a course of antibiotics and for candida or thrush. *Turmeric* can be given for eradicating worms and for digestive problems such as indigestion, heartburn, wind, bloating, colic and diarrhoea. It has a soothing effect on the mucosa of the gut and boosts stomach defences against excess acid, drugs and other irritating substances ingested and from the effects of stress, thereby reducing the risk of gastritis and ulcers. It is said to lower blood sugar in diabetics. *Turmeric* has beneficial effects in the liver which include stimulating the flow of bile, protecting the liver against damage from toxins and improving the metabolism of fats. It is an excellent spice to add to cooking if concerned about weight. By enhancing liver function *turmeric* helps cleanse the blood of toxins and impurities, which clearly has far-reaching effects in the treatment of a wide spectrum of conditions.

Respiratory system

With its detoxifying effect combined with its immune-enhancing and antimicrobial properties, *turmeric* has long been popular as a remedy for treating respiratory infections such as colds, sore throats, coughs and fevers.

Circulatory system

Turmeric has been shown to lower harmful cholesterol levels, to inhibit blood clotting by blocking prostaglandin production (Srivastava et al 1995) and to help prevent as well as remedy atherosclerosis, thus playing a significant role in the prevention of heart and arterial disease.

Immune system

Turmeric is an excellent natural antibiotic, excellent for treating skin problems such as acne and psoriasis, kidney and bladder problems. It can successfully inhibit infection whether bacterial, viral or fungal. It has powerful antioxidant properties, protecting the body's cells against damage caused by free radicals. It is reported to protect against the development of cancer, and has been used in the treatment of cancer of various kinds, also to enhance the production of several important cancer-fighting cells (Kuttan et al 1987, Nagabhushan and Bhide 1992) to protect the body against environmental toxins and the toxic effects of cigarette smoke, to have a generally immune-enhancing effect in the body and powerful antibacterial properties. In China it is used to treat the early stages of cervical cancer (Kuttan et al 1987). Research has also demonstrated its protective effects against colon and breast cancer.

Curcumin derived from *turmeric* is a powerful, yet safe, anti-inflammatory agent, excellent for treating inflammatory problems such as arthritis, liver and gallbladder problems. It has been found to block the production of certain prostaglandins and to have effects on a par with cortisone and non-steroidal anti-inflammatory drugs but without the side effects (Ghatak and Basu 1972, Srimal and Dhawan 1973). Taking *turmeric* daily has an excellent anti-inflammatory effect, improving morning stiffness, joint swelling and pain with movement experienced by arthritis sufferers.

External uses

Turmeric has antibiotic and anti-inflammatory properties. When powdered it can be mixed with a little water or aloe vera gel, made into a paste and applied to insect bites, spots and pimples, inflamed and infected skin problems including scabies and fungal infestation, and infected wounds. I have found it very successful when treating acne, eczema and psoriasis although care has to be taken with the amount of *turmeric* used because it can colour the skin yellow. It is best once the paste has dried on the skin for a while to wash it off. An alcohol extract of *turmeric* applied externally in skin cancer has been shown to reduce itching, relieve pain and promote healing.

In Ayurvedic beauty care, *turmeric* is mixed with chickpea flour and a little mustard oil and applied to the face to cleanse the skin and keep it smooth and lustrous. Mixed into a paste with honey or aloe vera gel, it has been used traditionally to treat sprains, strains and bruises. A little powder stirred into warm water makes an excellent mouthwash to treat inflamed gums and to relieve toothache. In India they make a tooth powder by mixing it with a pinch of salt and a few drops of mustard oil. It is given to alleviate pain from internal injuries due to falls or accidents.

Dosage and formulations

- *Turmeric* can be eaten regularly and liberally as a culinary spice, added to rice, soups, stews and casseroles and vegetable dishes.
- Daily dose: $\frac{1}{4} - \frac{1}{2}$ tsp of the powder 2 or 3 times daily between meals in hot water or honey, or 2 or 3 cupfuls of the tea between meals.

Precautions

Use with caution during pregnancy as large doses may act as an emmenagogue. Researchers have indicated that regular use of turmeric as a medicine is not advisable for those with duodenal and gastric ulcers or obstruction of the biliary tract or gallstones. Over-use can cause gastrointestinal disturbances in some susceptible people.

Drug interactions

Avoid using large doses concurrently with anticoagulants and non-steroidal anti-inflammatories.

Research

- Chopra D, Simon D 2000 The Chopra Centre Handbook. Rider, London, p. 112
- Ghatak N, Basu N 1972 Sodium curcuminate as an effective anti-inflammatory agent. Indian J Exp Bio 10: 235–236
- Kuttan R, Sudheeran PC, Joseph CD 1987 Turmeric and curcumin as topical agents in cancer therapy. Tumori 73: 29–31

- Nagabhushan M, Bhide SV 1992 Curcumin as an inhibitor of cancer. J Am Coll Nutr Apr; 11(2): 192–198
- Srimal R, Dhawan 1973 Pharmacology of diferuloyl methane (curcumin), a non-steroidal anti-inflammatory agent. J Pharm Pharmacol 25: 447–452
- Srivastava R, Bordia A, Verma SK 1995 Prostaglandins. Leukot Essent Fatty Acids 52: 223–227

Eclipta Alba : Bhringaraj

Family: Compositae
Sanskrit: *Bhringaraj*
English: Trailing eclipta, False daisy
Part used: whole plant, root, leaves, stem and seeds
Quality/*Guna*: light/*laghu*, dry/*ruksha*
Taste/*Rasa*: bitter/*titka*, pungent/*katu*
Post digestive/*Vipak*: pungent/*katu*
Potency/*Veerya*: heating/*ushna*
Dosha: VPK = mainly VP
Tissue/*Dhatu*: plasma, blood, bone, nerve

Constituents

Saponins, alkaloids: ecliptine, wedelic acid, luteolin, triterpene glycosides, flavonoids and isoflavonoids.

Actions

Hepatic deobstruent and tonic, alterative, emetic, purgative, antiseptic, antiviral, rejuvenative, febrifuge, anti-inflammatory, haemostatic, anthelmintic, *rasayana* for *Pitta*.

Indications

Viral hepatic enlargement with biliary stasis, poor hair growth, poor memory, minor cuts, abrasions and burns, skin problems, worms, anaemia, eye problems.

Introduction

Bhringaraj is traditionally used in India to enhance the memory and has a reputation as an anti-ageing agent. It is popular as a remedy for premature greying of the hair and balding, which is attributed to excess *Pitta*. Its bitter taste suggests its cooling properties, which are clearly exhibited by an anti-inflammatory effect and its benefit in a wide range of *Pitta* problems characterized by heat.

Internal uses

Digestive system

Bhringaraj is respected as a remedy for liver problems, including cirrhosis, infectious hepatitis and liver enlargement. There are reports of clinical improvement in the treatment of infective hepatitis (Dixit and Achar 1979). *Bhringaraj* acts as a deobstruent to promote the flow of bile, protecting the liver parenchymal tissue in viral hepatitis and other conditions involving enlargement of the liver. The fresh juice of the leaves is used to improve the appetite and to stimulate digestion.

Nervous system

Bhringaraj is used for insomnia and mental agitation from high *Vata* and *Pitta*. It calms stress and reduces tension. It has also been given for vertigo, dizziness and hearing problems.

Circulatory system

Research found *bhringaraj* to possess myocardial depressant and hypotensive effects (Gupta et al 1976).

Respiratory system

The juice is given with honey to treat upper respiratory congestion in children.

Skin

By benefiting the liver and aiding its detoxifying work, *bhringaraj* makes a good herb for skin problems including urticaria, eczema and psoriasis. It is also helpful in vitiligo. It reduces itching and inflammation and is said to promote a lustrous complexion.

External uses

Bhringaraj hair oil prepared in coconut oil is popular for reversing balding and greying of the hair by nourishing the roots. It is often combined with neem oil for this purpose. The leaf juice is used for its inflammatory properties when applied externally to treat minor cuts, abrasions and burns.

Formulation and dosage

- Fresh leaf juice: 5–10 ml tid
- Leaf powder: 3–5 g bid.

Research

- Dixit SP, Achar MP 1979 Bhringaraj in the treatment of infective hepatitis. Curr Med Pract 23: 6, 237–242

- Gupta SC, Bajaj 1976 UK and Sharma, VM cardiovascular effects of *Eclipta alba*. J Res Med Yoga Homeopathy 113: 91–93

Eletteria cardamomum : *Cardamom*

Family: Zingiberaceae
Sanskrit: Ela
English: *Cardamom*
Part used: seed
Quality/*Guna*: light/*laghu*, dry/*ruksha*
Taste/*Rasa*: pungent/*katu*, sweet/*madhur*
Post digestive/*Vipak*: pungent/*katu*
Potency/*Veerya*: heating/*ushna*
Dosha: VK- (in excess P+)
Tissue/*Dhatu*: plasma, blood, marrow and nerve

Constituents

Essential oils that contain a variety of volatile substances including limonene, cineol, terpineol and terpinene. While there is not a massive amount of scientific data on cardamom, it is known that up to 8% of cardamom seed consists of volatile oil that includes limonene, cineol, terpineol and terpinene (Chopra and Simon 2000).

Actions

Carminative, antispasmodic, decongestant, expectorant, diaphoretic, digestive, circulatory stimulant, nervine.

Indications

Coughs, colds, asthma, weak digestion, poor absorption.

Introduction

In the Middle East they drink an aromatic and spicy brew combining the bitterness of coffee with the sweet, pungent flavour of *cardamom* pods. Not only does *cardamom* enhance the taste of the coffee but also it is reputed to neutralize the over-stimulating effects of caffeine, and in fact can be positively beneficial for the nervous system. In Ayurvedic medicine *cardamom* has long been esteemed for its ability to lift the spirits, reduce pain, restore vitality and induce a calm, meditative state of mind.

Internal uses

Digestive system

Cardamom seeds have a warming and invigorating effect throughout the body, beginning as soon as they reach the stomach. By stimulating *Samana Vayu* and *agni* they stimulate the secretion of digestive juices, improve appetite, enhance digestion and absorption of food, and with their relaxing effect on smooth muscle in the digestive tract they can settle the stomach, especially when it is affected by stress. They can be used for indigestion, colic, wind, and travel sickness. They actually have a balancing effect in the digestive tract for whilst stimulating the flow of digestive juices they can counteract excess acidity in the stomach. In modern Ayurvedic medicine *cardamoms* are a popular remedy for nervous digestive upsets in children, and are often combined with fennel. When simmered in water for a few minutes and taken as a hot tea, they will relieve colic, wind and indigestion, and help to quell nausea and vomiting. They make a good remedy for anorexia and are well worth using to counteract the nausea often experienced while undergoing chemotherapy. A pod can be sucked slowly over an hour or two or a decoction can be sipped through the day. *Cardamoms* are veritably one of the best remedies for gas and they particularly aid the digestion of dairy produce. In India it is common practice to offer *cardamoms* at the end of a meal as a digestive and breath sweetener (Patnaik 1993). They have a mild laxative effect and prevent post-prandial drowsiness.

Nervous system

Today in the West *cardamom* is still highly valued for its ability to relieve tension and anxiety, to dispel lethargy and nervous exhaustion, to lift the spirits and to improve memory and concentration. The essential oil has anti-inflammatory and pain-relieving properties. *Cardamom* is highly effective as an antispasmodic, relieving muscle pain and spasm throughout the body.

Respiratory system

Cardamom seeds chewed slowly can soothe sore throats, clear phlegm and soothe an irritated cough. Their ability to dispel cold and damp may account for their ability to reduce phlegm, which is often a symptom of such climatic conditions. Added to milk products they can actually counteract the mucus-forming properties of milk. Their stimulating expectorant action helps to clear phlegm from the nose and sinuses as well as the chest, making them a good remedy for colds, coughs, asthma and chest infections.

Circulatory system

Their warming and stimulating effects are recommended for those feeling run down and tired, especially in the winter.

Urinary system

The tonic effect of *cardamoms* extends to the kidneys and urinary tract. They are used as a strengthening remedy for a weak bladder, involuntary urination and bedwetting in children, as well as to treat urinary tract infections (Chopra and Simon 2000).

Precautions

Large amounts of *cardamoms* are not recommended to those who suffer from gastro-oesophageal reflux and gallstones. There are no known herb–drug interactions (Skidmore-Roth 2001).

Dosage and formulations

- Daily dose: $\frac{1}{2}$–1 g. Powder in milk decoction.
- Do not buy powdered *cardamom*. Peel pods just before use and crush them when needed.

Research

- Chopra D, Simon D 2000 The Chopra Centre Herbal Handbook. Rider, London, p. 119
- Patnaik N 1993 The Garden of Life. Aquarian, Harper Collins, London, pp. 102–103
- Skidmore-Roth L 2001 Mosby's Handbook of Herbs & Natural supplements. Mosby, St Louis, pp. 168–169

Emblica officinalis (syn. Phyllanthus emblica) : Amalaki

Family: Euphorbiaceae
Sanskrit: *Amalaki*, Emblica myrobalan
English: Indian gooseberry
Part used: dried fruit, ripe fruit, seed, leaves, root, bark, flowers
Quality/*Guna*: light/*laghu*, dry/*ruksha*
Taste/*Rasa*: all except salty
Post digestive/*Vipak*: sweet/*madhur*
Potency/*Veerya*: cooling/*sheeta*
Dosha: VPK = but primarily PV-
Tissue/*Dhatu*: all tissues and increases *ojas*, nutritive tonic, digestive, antacid

Constituents

Ascorbic acid, fatty acids, bioflavonoids, polyphenols, cytokinins, B vitamins, calcium, potassium, iron, tannins, pectin.

Actions

Rejuvenative, antioxidant, hepato protective, *rasayana* for *Pitta*, lowers cholesterol, anti-inflammatory, laxative, hypoglycaemic, cooling, stomachic, tonic, diuretic.

Indications

Gastritis, dyspepsia, acidity, peptic ulcer, general debility, constipation, hypercholesterolaemia, fever, hepatitis, haemorrhoids, skin problems, urinary problems, headaches, bowel problems, chest infections, asthma.

Introduction

The fruit is one of the richest natural sources of vitamin C, containing approximately 20 times the vitamin C content of an orange. *Amalaki* fruit has long been used to treat scurvy. Its antioxidant effects explain its traditional use as one of the best rejuvenative tonics (*rasayana*) in Ayurvedic medicine. It is an ingredient in several important medicinal preparations including Triphala ("three fruits") the well-known bowel tonic and Chayawanprash, a general tonic for people of all ages taken to improve mental and physical well-being, for debility and during convalescence.

Internal uses

Digestive system

With its cooling effects *amalaki* is used for a variety of inflammatory conditions of the GI tract, ulcers, acidity, nausea, vomiting, gastritis, colitis, hepatitis and haemorrhoids. The leaf infusion with fenugreek seeds is given in chronic diarrhoea. Acute bacillary dysentery may be treated with a syrup of *amalaki* and lemon juice. As an ingredient of Triphala, *amalaki* is used as a bowel tonic for chronic constipation and IBS. Its antioxidant properties protect the liver.

Circulatory system

Studies have shown that *amalaki* can produce a decrease in serum LDH (Chopra and Simon 2000) cholesterol levels and reduce fat deposits in the arteries, thus protecting the heart and arteries. In a clinical study normal and hypercholesterolaemic men were given raw *amalaki* fruit for 28 days and both groups demonstrated a decrease in total serum cholesterol levels (Jacob et al 1988). Other studies have indicated that *amalaki* may reduce the risk of blood clots by reducing stickiness of platelets (Sharma et al 1989).

Respiratory system

Amalaki has an antibiotic activity against a wide range of bacteria, and is used traditionally in treatment of lung infections (Chopra and Simon 2000). It is also used in asthma.

Nervous system

Amalaki is a good brain tonic as it improves memory and calms disturbed *Sadhaka Pitta*.

Urinary system

It is used to treat urinary tract infections with success.

Immune system

Amalaki has been shown to slow development and growth of cancer cells (Lambertini et al 2004), probably through its ability to enhance natural cell-mediated cytotoxicity (Williamson 2002). It has antimicrobial properties (Ahmad et al 1998) and is used as an antiviral for colds and flu. Constituents of *amalaki* have been found to be active against a range of organisms including *Staph. aureus, E. coli, L. albicans, Mycobacterium tuberculosis* and *Staph. typhosa* (Khanna and Nag 1973). Research indicates that *amalaki* may have an immunomodulating effect (Sai Ram et al 2002).

Temperature

With its cooling properties, the fruit is commonly used in the treatment of inflammatory problems with a burning sensation anywhere in the body.

Metabolic disorders

Amalaki has been used traditionally for diabetes as it has a reputed hypoglycaemic effect.

External uses

Amalaki is a popular ingredient of hair oils and soaps to prevent hair loss and nourish the hair. It is also used as a remedy for inflammatory eye problems such as conjunctivitis.

The exudation from incisions made into the fruit is used as a collyrium in inflammatory eye conditions. *Emblica* has antioxidant properties, which make it a potentially useful skin care ingredient against oxidative damage (Chaudhuri 2002). *Emblica* also has antifungal activities (Dutta et al 1998).

Other uses

Emblica is active against a variety of snake venoms (Alam and Gomes 2003).

Dosage and formulations

- Infusion: 20–30 ml bid
- Powder: 2–5 g bid
- Chayawan prash: 8–12 g qd or bid. (Because Chayawan prash is a *rasayana* it is recommended that one goes through a period of detoxification before taking it)
- Triphala: *Amalaki* forms $\frac{1}{3}$ of Triphala. $\frac{1}{2}$ tsp in hot water at night.

Precautions

Contraindicated in diarrhoea, dysentery, caution in high *Kapha* and *Ama*.

Research

- Ahmad I, Mehmood Z, Mohammad F 1998 Screening of some Indian medicinal plants for their antimicrobial properties. J Ethnopharmacol 62(2): 183–193
- Alam MI, Gomes A 2003 Snake venom neutralization by Indian medicinal plants (*Vitex negundo* and *Emblica officinalis*) root extracts. J Ethnopharmacol 86(1): 75–80
- Chaudhuri RK 2002 Emblica cascading antioxidant: a novel natural skin care ingredient. Skin Pharmacol Appl Skin Physiol 15(5): 374–380
- Chopra D, Simon D 2000 The Chopra Centre Herbal Handbook. Rider, London
- Dutta BK, Rahman I, Das TK 1998 Antifungal activity of Indian plant extracts. Mycoses 41(11–12): 535–536
- Jacob A, Pondey M, Kapoor S, Saroja R 1988 Effect of the Indian Gooseberry (Amla) on serum cholesterol levels in men aged 35–55 years. Euro J Clin Nutrition 42(11): 939
- Khanna P, Nag TH 1973 Isolation, identification and screening of phyllembliss from *Emblica officinalis* Gaertin. Tissue culture. Indian J Pharm 35(1): 23
- Lambertini E, Piva R, Khan MT, Lampronti I, Bianchi N, Borgatti M, Gambari R 2004 Effects of extracts from Bangladeshi medicinal plants on in vitro proliferation of human breast cancer cell lines and expression of estrogen receptor alpha gene. Int J Oncol 24(2): 419–423
- Sai Ram M, Neetu D, Yogesh B, et al 2002 Cytoprotective and immunomodulating properties

of Amla (*Emblica officinalis*) on lymphocytes: an in-vitro study. J Ethnopharmacol 81(1): 5–10

- Sharma H, Feng Y, Panganamala RV 1989 Maharishi Amrit Kalash (MAK–5) prevents human platelet aggregation. Chica and Terpia Cardiovasolare 8: 227–230

- Williamson E 2002 Major herbs of Ayurveda. Churchill Livingstone, London

Ocimum sanctum : Tulsi

Family: Labiatae
Sanskrit: *Tulsi*
English: Sacred basil, Holy basil
Part used: leaves, seed, root
Quality/*Guna*: light/*laghu*, dry/*ruksha*, sharp/*tikshna*
Taste/*Rasa*: pungent/*katu*, bitter/*tikta*
Post digestive/*Vipak*: pungent/*katu*
Potency/*Veerya*: heating/*ushna*
Dosha: VK- P+
Tissue/*Dhatu*: plasma, blood, marrow and nerves, reproductive

Constituents

Essential oils: including eugenol, carvacrol, linalool, nerol, camphor; triterpenes, sterols, polyphenols and flavonoids; fatty acids: myristic, stearic, palmitic, oleic, linoleic and linolenic.

Actions

Demulcent, antibacterial, antifungal, expectorant, anticatarrhal, antispasmodic, anthelmintic, diaphoretic, febrifuge, nervine, adaptogen, immunostimulant, digestive, laxative.

Indications

Bronchospasm, cough, indigestion, constipation, respiratory tract infections, catarrh, wind, stress-related digestive problems, insomnia, allergies.

Introduction

Holy basil is one of the most sacred plants in India, dedicated to Vishnu and Krishna. With its *Sattvic* qualities it has an uplifting and strengthening effect on mind and body. This is reflected through its immune-enhancing and adaptogenic effects and its beneficial effect on digestion. Its warming properties improve digestion and absorption of nutrients and its diaphoretic and diuretic actions aid the elimination of waste products from the body. The *Kapha* reducing properties of *tulsi* clear lethargy and congestion that dampen the spirits and fog the mind.

Internal uses

Digestive system

In the digestive tract the antispasmodic action helps to relieve spasm and colic, wind and bloating. With its appetizing, digestive, laxative and anthelmintic actions, *tulsi* is used in anorexia, nausea and vomiting, abdominal pain and worms. It also has a mild laxative effect and antiulcer activity, reducing the effect of peptic acid or irritating drugs on the stomach lining and increases the production of protective stomach mucus.

Respiratory system

One of the most important uses of *tulsi* is to clear excess *Kapha* from the respiratory tract. This decongestant action combined with expectorant and antispasmodic actions and the ability to protect against histamine-induced bronchospasm, is helpful in the treatment of asthma and rhinitis. Holy basil has been shown to be active against a range of micro-organisms including *E. coli, Staphylococcus aureus* and *Mycoplasma tuberculosis* as well as against several other species of pathogens including fungi such as *Aspergillus*. It has been traditionally used in the treatment of coughs and colds, fevers, sore throats and flu. It is an excellent remedy for children's fevers, helped by the fact that it is pleasant tasting and the infusion is not difficult to administer to young children.

Nervous system

With its nervine properties, holy basil can be used in anxiety, mild depression, insomnia, and for a variety of stress-related problems such as headaches and irritable bowel syndrome. Its antioxidant actions may account for its adaptogenic effect and its ability to increase resilience to stress.

Immune system

In India *tulsi* is grown in domestic courtyards partly for spiritual purposes but also for the fact that its aroma is said to purify the atmosphere. According to Tillotson the plant gives off ozone, an unstable form of oxygen that helps to break down chemicals and this dispels disease-carrying organisms such as viruses, bacteria and insects (Tillotson et al 2001). Chopra and Simon quote numerous studies that have demonstrated *tulsi*'s anti-inflammatory action, with an ability to inhibit prostaglandin production and one that found *tulsi* to compare with a standard dose of aspirin (Chopra and Simon 2000). Its adaptogenic effect has further applications. Studies show how *tulsi* can protect healthy cells from the toxicity from radiation and chemotherapy and to protect the heart from damage caused by a chemotherapy (Balanehru and Nagarajan 1992, Vrinda and Uma Devi 2001). Trials confirm an anthelmintic activity (Asha et al 2001) and activity against enteric pathogens and candida (Geeta et al 2001).

Urinary system

In the urinary tract *tulsi* relieves dysuria, cystitis and urinary tract infections.

Metabolic system

Another area of substantial research is that of diabetes and *tulsi* has clearly demonstrated its ability to lower blood sugar as well as cholesterol and triglyceride levels (Chopra and Simon 2000). In a study of 40 patients with non-insulin-dependent diabetes mellitus, those taking 2.5 g of dried *tulsi* leaf each morning experienced a definite reduction in their blood glucose levels as well as cholesterol levels (Agrawal et al 1996).

External use

Extracts of *tulsi* can be applied to acne lesions where its antibiotic effect speeds healing. The juice of fresh leaves can be applied to skin conditions ranging from allergic rashes to athlete's foot.

Formulations and dosage

- 1–9 g of dried herb per day
- 5–15 ml daily of 1:5 tincture
- Fresh leaf juice: 15–20 ml with honey tid
- Leaf infusion: 2–3 oz tid
- It is often combined with ginger and black pepper in bronchial asthma. It is given with honey in the treatment of bronchitis and cough
- Daily dose of crushed seeds: 3–5 g ($\frac{1}{2}$ tsp).

The juice of the leaves (1 tsp) along with $\frac{1}{2}$ tsp ginger juice and three grains black pepper are given to cure minor fevers, coughs and indigestion. (For babies $\frac{1}{2}$ tsp juice of fresh basil leaves or an extract prepared from dried leaves or powdered seeds.) The leaf infusion or fresh leaf juice is commonly used in cough, mild upper respiratory infections, bronchospasm, stress-related skin disorders and indigestion.

Precaution

There is a mild antifertility effect in animals but this has not been shown to occur in humans. Some sources recommend avoiding the use of *tulsi* during pregnancy and breastfeeding (Tillotson et al 2001). In severely overheated individuals, *tulsi* can have a mildly *Pitta*-aggravating effect.

Research

- Agrawal P, Rai V, Singh RB 1996 Randomised placebo-controlled, single blind trial of holy basil leaves in patients with noninsulin dependent diabetes mellitus. Int J Clin Pharmacol Ther 34: 406–409
- Asha MK, Prashanth D, Murali B, Padmaja R, Amit A 2001 Anthelmintic activity of essential oil of *Ocimum sanctum* and eugenol. Fitoterapia 72(6): 669–670
- Balanehru S, Nagarajan B 1992 Intervention of adriamycin induced free radical damage. Biochem Int 28: 735–744
- Chopra D, Simon D 2000 The Chopra Centre Herbal Handbook. Rider, London
- Geeta, Vasudevan DM, Kedlaya R, Deepa S, Ballal M 2001 Activity of *Ocimum sanctum* (the

traditional Indian medicinal plant) against the enteric pathogens. Indian J Med Sci 55(8): 434–438, 472

- Tillotson AK, Tillotson NH, Robert A Jr 2001 The One Earth Herbal Sourcebook. Kensington Publishing Corps, New York

- Vrinda B, Uma Devi P 2001 Radiation protection of human lymphocyte chromosomes in vitro by orientin and vicenin. Mutat Res 498(1–2): 39–46

Piper longum : Pippali

Family: Piperaceae
Sanskrit: *Pippali*
English: Long pepper
Part used: root and seeds
Quality/Guna: light/*laghu*, sharp/*tikshna*, oily/*snigdha*
Taste/Rasa: pungent/*katu*
Post digestive/Vipak: sweet/*madhura*
Potency/Veerya: heating/*ushna*
Dosha: VK- P+
Tissue/Dhatu: plasma, blood, fat, nerve, reproductive

Constituents

Volatile oil, alkaloids: piperine, piplartine, lignans, resin, esters.

Actions

Stimulant, carminative, laxative, stomachic, diuretic, febrifuge, tonic, expectorant, anthelmintic, digestive, emollient, antiseptic, emmenagogue, rejuvenative, analgesic, cardiac stimulant.

Indications

Colds, catarrh, coughs, asthma, bronchitis, laryngitis, arthritis, muscle pain, dyspepsia, weak digestion, wind and bloating, worms.

Introduction

A close relative of black pepper, *pippali* has warming and energizing properties and acts as a stimulant and a tonic for those feeling cold and run down in the winter. With ginger and black pepper, *pippali* forms the best-known stimulant formula – Trikatu – for low *agni*, toxins in the GI tract and mucus in the lungs. It can be considered for all problems of excess *Kapha*.

Internal uses

Digestive system

The dried fruits are considered excellent medicine for the digestion. *Pippali* is used for anorexia, dyspepsia, flatulence, constipation, colic and slow digestion. Its antimicrobial properties make it an effective remedy for amoeba and worms, as well as candida. It is prescribed for all conditions associated with excess *Kapha* and low digestive fire. *Pippali* is reported to have a hepato-protective effect, enhancing the liver's ability to break down toxins and to reduce liver damage. *Pippali* stimulates appetite and digestion and enhances absorption of nutrients (Atal et al 1981). The ability of *pippali* to increase absorption has been documented. It has been shown to increase the availability of biologically active compounds by boosting their transport from the stomach into the bloodstream, improving absorption from the small intestine (Barnett 1997). Scientific attention has concentrated particularly on piperine, an alkaloid found in both long and black pepper, which stimulates an enzyme that enhances uptake of amino acids from the GI tract. It has been shown to increase blood concentration of turmeric and vitamins and minerals up to 30% (Tillotson et al 2001). The fact that *pippali* can increase the medicinal effects of herbs means that it has the potential to do this with prescription drugs (Atal et al 1981).

Nervous system

When used in Trikatu, *pippali* promotes energy and vitality. Because *pippali* helps to balance *Vata* it can be used for *Vata* related nervous problems such as tension, anxiety and insomnia.

Circulatory system

Pippali stimulates the circulation and has vasodilatory effects. It has the ability to reduce cholesterol and has also been used for anaemia.

Respiratory system

Pippali's main use is for *Kapha* conditions – for colds, catarrh, bronchial congestion and bronchitis. It has traditionally been used in milk to reduce bronchospasm in the treatment of asthma. It is a good remedy for allergic conditions including hayfever and eczema.

Immune system

Pippali root is used in gout, arthritis and muscle and back pain for its anti-inflammatory effects. Its ability to enhance immunity has been well documented. It activates macrophages and phagocytosis and has been found to be helpful in the treatment of hepatitis. Research has demonstrated its broad-spectrum antibiotic activity against Gram-positive and Gram-negative bacteria (Singh et al 1974) including *Staph. aureus* (Reddy et al 2001). *Pippali* also has antioxidant properties, which may explain its effects as a *rasayana*.

Skin

A rejuvenator of *rasa* and *rakta dhatu*, *pippali* is useful in skin disorders.

Temperature

Pippali fruits are used to bring down fevers and are reputed to be one of the best medicines for typhoid and chronic fevers (Gogte 2000).

External uses

Pippali increases blood flow when used topically so it makes a useful ingredient of liniments for relief of pain and swelling.

Other uses

Alkaloids from *pippali* have been found to have mosquito larvicidal activity equivalent to commonly used organophosphorus insecticides (Lee 2000).

Pippali may have a contraceptive effect as it reduces sperm count, while at the same time it is reputed to be an aphrodisiac. It is used as an antispasmodic for dysmenorrhoea.

Dosage and formulations

- Pippali Rasayana
- Powdered seed and root 0.5–1 g in milk twice daily
- Medicated oil
- Trikatu – $\frac{1}{2}$ tsp in a glass of hot water and honey.

Precautions

Pippali can significantly increase absorption and so care may be needed as it may increase drug absorption. *Pippali* also increases *Pitta* so use cautiously in acidity. Avoid in pregnancy and lactation. No unwanted side effects recorded.

Research

- Atal CK, Zutshi U, Rao PG 1981 Scientific evidence on the role of ayurvedic herbals on bioavailability of drugs. J Ethnopharmacol Sep 4(2): 229–232
- Barnett RA 1997 Tonics. HarperPerennial, HarperCollins, New York
- Gogte VVM 2000 Ayurvedic Pharmacology and Therapeutic Uses of Medicinal Plants. Bharatiya Vidya Bhavan, Mumbai
- Lee SE 2000 Mosquito larvicidal activity of pipernonaline, a piperidine alkaloid derived from long pepper, Piper longum. J Am Mosq Control Assoc 16(3): 245–247
- Reddy P, Srinivas J, Jamil K, et al 2001 Antibacterial activity of isolates from *Piper longum* and *Taxus baccata*. Pharmaceutical Biology 39(3): 236
- Singh RH, Khosa KL, Upadhyaya BB 1974 Antibacterial activity of some Ayurvedic drugs. J Res Indian Med 9(2): 65
- Tillotson AK, Tillotson NH, Robert A Jr 2001 The One Earth Herbal Sourcebook. Kensington Publishing Corps., New York

Rubia cordifolia : Manjista

Family: Rubiaceae
Sanskrit: *Manjista*
English: Indian madder
Part used: root
Quality/Guna: heavy/*guru*, dry/*ruksha*
Taste/Rasa: sweet/*madhura*, bitter/*tikta*, astringent/*kashaya*
Post digestive/Vipak: pungent/*katu*
Potency/Veerya: hot/*ushna*
Dosha: PK- V+
Dhatu: plasma, blood, muscles

Constituents

Red colour due to purpurin, alizarin, iridoids, glucoside-manjistin, purpuroxanthin, anthraquinones, glycosides, triterpenes, beta-sitosterol.

Actions

Alterative, diuretic, emmenagogue, astringent, antipyretic, antitumour, haemostatic.

Indications

Skin problems, diarrhoea, urinary problems, eye conditions, hepatitis, herpes.

Introduction

Manjista is one of the most important detoxifying herbs in the Ayurvedic material medica removing "*ama*" from the blood. It is an effective remedy for inflammatory conditions particularly skin problems. It is one of the main anti-*Pitta* herbs. European madder (*Rubia tinctoria*) has similar properties. Both are called Rubia meaning red as their internal use imparts a red colour to breast milk and urine and a red dye is obtained from the fruit.

Internal uses

Digestive system

Manjista improves appetite (*deepana*) and clears toxins (*pachana*) from the gut. It reduces gut motility and is used in the treatment of diarrhoea with bleeding, Crohn's disease, dysentery, and bleeding ulcers. It is also useful in the treatment of worms.

Nervous system

Manjista is used in nervous disorders particularly those associated with excess *Pitta*.

Circulatory system

Manjista has a long history of use in bleeding disorders. It has been incorporated into prescriptions of Chinese herbs studied for their positive effect on idiopathic thrombocytopenic purpura in children (Tillotson et al 2001) in China. According to Ayurveda, *manjista* stops bleeding by cooling the "heat" predisposing to a bleeding sense tendency and by moving stagnant blood.

Respiratory system

Its antimicrobial and alterative properties enhance resistance to infection. It is used in inflammatory chest problems, tuberculosis and a range of other respiratory infections.

Reproductive system

Manjista is used for all menstrual problems related to disturbance of *Pitta* and *Kapha*, dysmenorrhoea, amenorrhea and clots. It has a reputation for purifying breast milk.

Urinary system

It is used for stones and calculi and urinary tract infections.

Immune system

Manjista has a traditional reputation for breaking accumulations of *Kapha* in bladder, liver and kidneys (Pole 2005). With its anti-inflammatory properties, it is a useful herb for allergic asthma, inflammatory arthritis and autoimmune problems. Studies on constituents of *manjista* confirm its anticancer activity – notably hexapeptides and quinones in particular (Itokawa et al 1993). *Manjista* has also been reported to have hepatoprotective activity, protecting against a variety of liver toxins and to be effective against acute and chronic hepatitis. Several studies have demonstrated that *manjista* has significant antioxidant properties (Shukla et al 1995).

Temperature

Manjista is used to cool heat in the body and relieve fevers. It is traditionally used for chronic pyrexia and puerperal fever (Gogte 2000).

Skin

It is used to clean, cool and clear the blood of all excess *Pitta*, heat, inflammation and toxins/*ama*. It is a popular remedy for the relief of heat and itching in eczema, psoriasis, herpes, scabies and tinea pedis. It is reported to be successful in treatment of vitiligo when given with honey (Gogte 2000).

External uses

A paste prepared from the powder mixed with honey is used for inflammatory skin problems and ulcers and with liquorice for burns and wounds. *Manjista* acts as a vulnerary and speeds healing of trauma to skin and bones.

Dosage and formulations

- Powder 1–3 g
- Decoction 60–120 ml
- Paste
- Medicated ghee.

Precautions

High *Vata* – high doses reported to cause hallucinations (Gogte 2000). Williamson reports no adverse effects have been reported (Williamson 2002).

Research

- Gogte VVM 2000 Ayurvedic Pharmacology and Therapeutic Uses of Medicinal Plants. Bharatiya Vidya Bhavan, Mumbai
- Itokawa H, Ibraheim 22, ya-Fang Q, Tokeya K 1993 Anthraquinones, raphthohydroquinones and naphthohydroquinones dinners from *Rubia cordifolia* and their cytotoxic activity. Chem Pharmaceut Bull 41(10): 1869
- Pole S 2005 An Ayurvedic Herbal. A guide to Ayurvedic Herbs and Formulas. Thesis
- Shukla S, Tripath YB, Sharma M, Shukla VK 1995 Antioxidant property of *Rubica cordifolia* extract and its comparison with vitamin E and parabenzoquinone. Phytother Res 9(6): 440
- Tillotson AK, Tillotson NH, Robert A Jr 2001 The One Earth Herbal Sourcebook. Kensington Publishing Corps, New York
- Williamson E 2002 Major Herbs of Ayurveda. Churchill Livingstone, London

Sida cordifolia : Bala

Family: Malvaceae
Sanskrit: *Bala*
English: Indian country mallow
Part used: root, leaves, seeds, stem
Quality/*Guna*: unctuous/*ruksha*, heavy/*guru*
Taste/*Rasa*: bitter/*tikra*, sweet/*madhura*
Post digestive/*Vipak*: sweet/*madhura*
Potency/*Veerya*: cold/*seetha*
Dosha: VPK = (mainly VP) K+ *ama* in large doses. Increases *ojas*
Tissue/*Dhatu*: all especially nerve

Constituents

Alkaloid: asparagin, ephedrine, phytosterols, mucins, choline, resin acids, linoleic, malvalic and steraulic acid in seeds.

Actions

Cooling, astringent, stomachic, tonic, bitter, febrifuge, demulcent, diuretic, antispasmodic, analgesic, antimicrobial, nervine. It is *rasayana* for all kinds of *Vata* disorders (Frawley and Lad 2001).

Indications

Cystitis, stones, infection, neuralgia, sciatica, infertility, leucorrhoea, rheumatism, dry cough, asthma, tuberculosis, fever, heart disease, convalescence.

Introduction

Bala literally means "what gives strength" owing to its tonic and rejuvenative properties. It is a relative of the European mallow and one of the best nourishing herbs for *Vata* and for all *Vata* problems.

Internal uses

Digestive system

Its soothing and cooling properties can be put to good use in inflammatory gut problems including gastritis, acidity, colitis, irritable bowel syndrome, colic, wind and distension.

Nervous system

With its adaptogenic and strengthening properties, *bala* makes an ideal herb for promoting resilience to stress. Its analgesic properties can be applied to pain as in headaches, shingles, neuralgia, muscle and joint pain. As a *rasayana*, *bala* can be used as a tonic in childhood and old age alike. It is useful for allaying tension and anxiety, for promoting sleep, for nervous exhaustion and any *Vata*-related nervous disorder, including Bell's palsy.

Circulatory system

Bala has a reputation as a heart tonic for relieving arrhythmia, tachycardia, irregular pulse and palpitations.

Respiratory system

As a demulcent and antispasmodic, *bala* can be used for soothing dry coughs, asthma, TB, haemoptysis and bronchitis. Its antimicrobial properties are helpful in chronic respiratory infections related to debility, including chronic bronchitis and bronchiectasis, with emaciation or exhaustion. It is also used during convalescence (Swami Sada Shiva Tirtha 1998).

Urinary system

Bala makes a good soothing remedy for cystitis, irritable bladder, stones, and urinary tract infections, and all problems related to excess *Pitta* and *Vata*.

Immune system

Its nourishing effect on the nervous system and Vata combined with its adaptogenic properties give *bala* an immune-enhancing effect. As an inflammatory *bala* can be used for arthritis. It can be used for chronic infections and conditions such as ME/chronic fatigue syndrome. Traditionally *bala* has been used to increase *ojas* – the vital energy that gives us strength, immunity and preserves against the ageing process.

Temperature

Bala is used to reduce fevers related to a condition of underlying deficiency and weakness. For chronic and intermittent fevers it is often combined with ginger or black pepper (Swami Sada Shiva Tirtha 1998).

External uses

Bala is used as a medicated oil for nerve pain and numbness, muscle tension and spasm, inflammatory problems and eye disorders.

Dosage and formulations

- Balarishta (See Appendix p. 303)
- 3–6 tsp juice
- Powder: 1–3 g
- Decoction milk
- Decoction
- Paste medicated oil.

Precautions

Congestive disorders of high *ama* or *Kapha* (Frawley and Lad 2001).

Research

- Frawley D, Lad V 2001 The Yoga of Herbs Lotus Press, Twin Lakes, Wisconsin
- Swami Sada Shiva Tirtha 1998 The Ayurveda Encyclopedia. Ayurveda Holistic Centre Press, New York

Terminalia belerica : Bibhitaki

Family: Combretaceae
Sanskrit: *Bibhitaki*, Vibhitaki
English: Beleric myrobalan
Part used: fruit
Quality/*Gunas*: light/*laghu*, dry/*ruksha*
Taste/*Rasa*: astringent/*kashaya*, sweet/*madhura*
Post digestive/*Vipak*: sweet/*madhura*
Potency/*Veerya*: heating/*ushna*
Dosha: VPK = (V+ in large doses)
Tissue/*Dhatu*: plasma, muscle, tone

Constituents

Saponins, tannins (17%), glycosides, triterpenoids, mannitol, lignans, beta-sitosterol, polyphenols.

Actions

Laxative, expectorant, bronchodilator, astringent, anthelmintic, lithotropic, eye tonic, tonic, *rasayana* for *Kapha*.

Indications

Asthma, bronchitis, coughs, diarrhoea, colitis, urinary problems, insomnia.

Introduction

Bibhitaki fruit is widely used in rejuvenating formulae for *Kapha* and for symptoms affecting *Kapha* sites, notably the lungs, throat, eyes and hair. It forms one third of the famous three fruit compound, Triphala, with amalaki and haritaki, for chronic bowel problems and general detoxification.

Internal uses

Digestive system

The fresh fruit has stronger laxative properties than the sun-dried, which is more astringent and binding. It is used for haemorrhoids, worms, parasitic infections, chronic diarrhoea and dysentery, as well as constipation as it cleanses the bowels and increases the tone of the bowel muscles (Frawley and Lad 2001). *Bibhitaki* acts on the liver and is considered to be hepato-protective. It has been used traditionally for jaundice and gallstones. It is indicated in inflammatory bowel problems such as colitis and Crohn's disease (Pole 2005) and acts as an antiemetic and antiulcer remedy. Triphala powder has been shown to be effective in healing of ulcers (Williamson 2002).

Nervous system

Bibhitaki is considered a brain tonic and is used for insomnia, often combined with brahmi (Pole 2005). It is helpful for all *Vata* problems.

Circulatory system

Due to its ability to lower cholesterol levels, *bibhitaki* benefits the arteries.

Respiratory system

This is an excellent herb for the respiratory system. With its astringent action, it clears *Kapha* from the lungs, relieving catarrhal congestion, coughs, colds, sore throats, laryngitis, bronchitis and enhancing immunity. Its antihistamine action is useful in the treatment of atopic conditions including eczema, asthma and rhinitis. It has a reputation for improving the voice, presumably due to its decongestant action. It is often combined with long pepper and black pepper for *Kapha* problems, and with ginger for asthma and colds.

Urinary system

Bibhitaki is used for accumulations of *Kapha* in the urinary tract, giving rise to stones and gravel.

Immune system

The lignans have been shown to be effective against malaria and fungal infections (Valsaraj et al 1997). It also is reputed to be antiviral and improve resistance to infection, as its name suggests. Research indicates that *Terminalia* has an inhibitory effect on retroviral reverse transcriptase (Suthienkul et al 1993). *Bibhitaki* means "keeping one free from disease". Triphala has been shown in studies to have an antioxidant action, which may go some way to explain its reputation as a rejuvenative (Rani et al 1997). Its anti-inflammatory action is useful in the treatment of arthritis.

External uses

The high levels of tannins contribute to its vulnerary action, speeding healing of cuts and wounds. *Bibhitaki* also has an antiseptic and anti-inflammatory action on the skin. It is used in oils as a tonic to the hair to promote hair growth and for skin diseases (Gogte 2000). The fruit pulp is applied directly over non-traumatic corneal ulcers (Tillotson et al 2001). *Terminalia* is antimicrobial in vitro (Ahmad et al 1998).

Dosage and formulations

- Powder: 2 g twice daily
- Taken in honey for throat problems can also be mixed with warm water as a gargle.

Drug interactions

None known.

Research

- Ahmad I, Mehmood Z, Mohammad F 1998 Screening of some Indian medicinal plants for their antimicrobial properties. J Ethnopharmacol 62(2): 183–193
- Frawley D, Lad V 2001 The Yoga of Herbs. Lotus Press, Twin Lakes, Wisconsin USA
- Gogte VVM 2000 Ayurvedic Pharmacology and Therapeutic Uses of Medicinal Plants. Bharatiya Vidya Bhavan, Mumbai
- Pole S 2005 An Ayurvedic Herbal. A guide to Ayurvedic Herbs and Formulas. Thesis
- Rani T, Rajani M, Sarkar S, Shishoo CJ 1997 Antioxidant properties of the Ayurvedic formulation Triphala and its constituents. Int J Pharmacol 35(5): 313
- Suthienkul O, Miyazaki O, Chulasiri M, Kositanont U, Oishi K 1993 Retroviral reverse transcriptase inhibitory activity in Thai herbs and spices: screening with Moloney murine leukemia viral enzyme. Southeast Asian J Trop Med Public Health 24(4): 751–755
- Tillotson AK, Tillotson NH, Robert A Jr 2001 The One Earth Herbal Sourcebook. Kensington Publishing Corps, New York
- Valsaraj R, Pushpangadan P, Smitt UW, et al 1997 New anti-HIV, antimalarial and antifungal compounds from Terminalia bellerica. J Nat Prod Jul 60(7): 739–742
- Williamson E 2002 Major Herbs of Ayurveda. Churchill Livingstone, London

Terminalia chebula : Haritaki

Family: Combretaceae
Sanskrit: *Haritaki*, fructus *Chebulic myrobalan*
English: Indian gall nut
Part used: fruit, leaves, stem, bark
Quality/*Guna*: light/*laghu*, dry/*ruksha*
Taste/*Rasa*: all except salty
Post digestive/*Vipak*: sweet/*madhura*
Potency/*Veerya*: hot/*ushna*
***Dosha*:** VPK=
Tissue/*Dhatu*: all

Constituents

Tannins, anthraquinone glycosides, vitamin C, triterpenoid glycosides, gallic acid, chebulic acid, mucilage, sennoside, amino acids, polyphenols, nitrates, ellagic acid.

Actions

Tonic, anti-inflammatory, laxative, astringent, antiseptic, diuretic, alterative, carminative, demulcent, febrifuge, bronchodilator, anthelmintic, cardiotonic, vulnerary, rejuvenating.

Indications

Constipation, diarrhoea, digestive parasites, flatulence, ulcers, wet coughs, eye disorders.

INTRODUCTION

An old Ayurvedic prescription said "As a tonic for promoting strength and preventing the effects of age, *Chebulic myrobalan* should be taken every morning with salt during the rainy season, with sugar in the autumn, with ginger in the first half of winter, with honey in the spring and with treacle in the hot months" (Patnaik 1993). Since the time of Caraka, Ayurvedic physicians have used it in restorative medicines and praised it so highly that by the early 17th century Ben Johnson mentioned it in his play *The Alchemist*. It is known as *haritaki* because it is sacred to Lord Shiva or "Hara".

Internal uses

Digestive system

Haritaki benefits the whole of the digestive tract. It increases digestive fire, acts as a rejuvenative to *Vata* and large intestine and corrects the flow of *Vata* downwards. It increases appetite and improves digestion and absorption. It can be used for gastric disorders, colic and wind, worms, constipation, haemorrhoids, IBS, diarrhoea and vomiting. It can also be used for infections of the gut such as *Shigella* spp., *Salmonella typhi* and for parasites including amoebas as well as for inflammation of the mucous membranes and ulcer. It has an antibacterial effect on *Helicobacter pylori* (Malekzadeh et al 2001). The unripe fruits are more laxative than the ripe ones which are more astringent.

Nervous system

Haritaki is said to promote wisdom, intellect and good sight. According to Vasant Lad it feeds the brain and the nerves (Lad 2002). Probably due to its antioxidant properties *haritaki* is known as an adaptogen, increasing resilience to stress (Fu et al 1992). It is recommended for all *Vata* disorders.

Circulatory system

Haritaki has a reputation as a tonic to the heart and has hypotensive effects. Its antioxidant properties protect the heart and arteries from damage by free radicals. Its ability to reduce serum cholesterol levels and improve the HDL cholesterol ratio (Chopra and Simon 2000) also bears out its reputation.

Respiratory system

A good astringent remedy for catarrh, congestion and *Kapha* type coughs. *Haritaki* sends accumulated *Vata* downwards and helps relieve asthma.

Urinary system

Haritaki is an antiseptic diuretic for cystitis and urinary tract infections.

Immune system

Haritaki has antimicrobial properties and has been shown to be effective against a range of bacterial infections (Phadke and Kulkarni 1989) and viral infections. Its ability to increase resistance to infection probably accounts for its reputation as a rejuvenative and promoter of fearlessness. Research has demonstrated that *haritaki* can inhibit the growth of certain cancer cell lines and therefore may have antitumour activity (Lee et al 1995). In vitro *Terminalia* is active against resistant *Candida albicans* (Bonjar 2004), cytomegaloviruses (Yukawa et al 1996) and has an inhibitory effect on cancer cell growth (Saleem et al 2002).

Temperature

Haritaki is used for *Vata* type fevers and chronic fever.

Skin

It is used for *kushta* (obstinate skin diseases), as well as eruptive infections such as measles.

External uses

The powder is used for cleaning teeth and gums, for stopping bleeding and for infection of the mouth and gums. It has been smoked in pipes for the relief of asthma.

Other uses

It purifies breast milk.

Dosage and formulation

- 3–6 g powder as laxative
- 1 g as rasayana
- Decoction 56–112 ml
- For laxative effect with warm water
- For astringent effect with cold water.

Adverse effects

No adverse effects recorded.

Precautions

Pregnancy, dehydration, emaciation, exhaustion, high *Pitta* (Lad 2002).

Drug interactions

None known.

Research

- Bonjar GH 2004 Inhibition of Clotrimazole-resistant *Candida albicans* by plants used in Iranian folkloric medicine. Fitoterapia 75(1): 74–76
- Chopra D, Simon D 2000 The Chopra Centre Herbal Handbook. Rider, London
- Fu N, Quan L, Huang L, Zhang R, Chen Y 1992 Antioxidant action of extract of *Terminalia chebula* and its preventive effect on DNA breaks in human white cells induced by TPA. Chinese Traditional Herbal Drugs 23(1): 26
- Lad V 2002 Textbook of Ayurveda Fundamental Principles. The Ayurvedic Press, Albuquerque, New Mexico
- Lee SH, Ryu SY, Choi SU, et al 1995 Hydrolysable tannins and related compound having cytotoxic activity from the fruits of *Terminalia chebula*. Arch Pharmacol Res 18(2): 118
- Malekzadeh F, Ehsanifar H, Shahamat M, Levin M, Colwell RR 2001 Antibacterial activity of black myrobalan (*Terminalia chebula* Retz) against *Helicobacter pylori*. Int J Antimicrob Agents 18(1): 85–88
- Patnaik N 1993 The Garden of Life. Aquarian, HarperCollins, London
- Phadke SA, Kulkarni SD 1989 Screening of *in vitro* antibacterial activity of *Terminalia chebula*, *Eclipta alba* and *Ocimum sanctum*. Indian J Med Sci 43(5): 113
- Saleem A, Husheem M, Harkonen P, Pihlaja K 2002 Inhibition of cancer cell growth by crude extract and the phenolics of *Terminalia chebula* retz. fruit. J Ethnopharmacol 81(3): 327–336
- Yukawa TA, Kurokawa M, Sato H, et al 1996 Prophylactic treatment of cytomegalovirus infection with traditional herbs. Antiviral Res 32(2): 63–70

Tinospora cordifolia–caulis : Guduchi

Sanskrit: *Guduchi*/amrit
English: Heart-leaved moonseed/Amrit
Family: Menispermaceae
Part used: stems and leaves
Quality/*Guna*: light/*laghu*, oily/*snigdha*
Taste/*Rasa*: bitter/*tikta*, astringent/*kashaya*
Post digestive/*Vipak*: sweet/*madhura*
Potency/*Veerya*: hot/*ushna*
Dosha: VPK = (primarily P-; with ghee V-)
Tissue/*Dhatu*: plasma, blood, marrow, fat

Constituents

Beta-sitosterol, alkaloids including: berberine and tinosporin, bitters, glycosides, diterpenes.

Actions

Digestive, stimulant/deepana, astringent, rejuvenative, tonic, alterative, diuretic, adaptogen, cholagogue, anti-inflammatory.

Indications

Skin conditions, inflammatory problems, nausea, vomiting, worms, peptic ulcer, fevers, diabetes, liver problems, poor appetite, anaemia, debility.

Introduction

Amrit means the nectar that confers immortality or imperishable and *guduchi* is so called because of its reputation as a rejuvenative, enhancing energy and vitality.

Internal uses

Digestive system

By stimulating the digestion *guduchi* improves appetite and digestion. It is used for heat and inflammation (*Pitta* problems) of the digestive tract including acidity, gastritis, peptic ulcers, nausea and vomiting. Its antifungal properties are helpful in treating *Candida*. Its protective action on the liver explains its traditional use in liver disease and jaundice. It is used for chronic hepatitis, toxic damage to the liver and it aids liver tissue regeneration (Pole 2005). It is used with ghee for constipation.

Nervous system

Guduchi acts as an adaptogen, increasing resistance to stress, both emotional and physical. It increases energy and yet relaxes tension.

Circulatory system

Guduchi is used for problems associated with high *Pitta* including anaemia and bleeding tendency as in bleeding gums and haemorrhoids. It reduces cholesterol and helps to stabilize blood sugar levels.

Respiratory system

By enhancing the immune system *guduchi* can be used for respiratory infections, coughs, colds, flu, sinusitis and for allergies such as hayfever and asthma. It also has decongestant properties.

Urinary system

As a diuretic *guduchi* aids elimination of uric acid from the body and this contributes to its value as a remedy for gout.

Immune system

Guduchi has been valued as a rejuvenative and this may be explained by discovery of its antioxidant properties, as well as antitumour activity. Research has demonstrated that *guduchi* can reduce the side effects of chemotherapy. Many studies have demonstrated its immune-enhancing properties. It enhances antibody production and macrophage function (Kapil et al 1997 cited in Williamson 2002) and improves resistance to infection – fungal, bacterial and parasitic (Rege and Kahanukar 1993). Reports from India show that using *guduchi* prior to surgery meant less postoperative complications including infections (Rege et al 1995). It has an anti-inflammatory action traditionally used for gout (in castor oil) and with ginger for arthritis and is used in the treatment of autoimmune problems such as psoriasis and SLE.

Skin

Guduchi is used for *kushta* (obstinate skin problems) such as eczema and psoriasis.

Temperature

It is used for fever (*jwara*).

External uses

The powder can be mixed with water or aloe vera gel and applied to inflammatory skin problems.

Dosage and formulations

- 1 tsp (1–3 g) powder bid.

Precautions

Excessive doses of berberine inhibit B vitamin assimilation and can cause nausea (Williamson 2002). However, whole plant extract has no reported toxicity.

Research

- Pole S 2005 An Ayurvedic Herbal. A guide to Ayurvedic Herbs & Formulas. Thesis
- Rege NN, Kahanukar SA 1993 Quantitation of microbiological activity of mononuclear phagocytes: an in vitro technique. J Postgrad Med 39: 22–25
- Rege NN, Koti RS, Desai NK 1995 Can we do away with PTBD? HPB Surgery 9: 5–11
- Williamson E 2002 Major Herbs of Ayurveda. Churchill Livingstone, London

Withania somniferum : *Ashwagandha*

Family: Solanaceae
Sanskrit: *Ashwagandha*
English: Winter cherry
Part used: root
Quality/*Guna*: light/*laghu*, oily/*snigdha*
Taste/*Rasa*: sweet/*madhur*, bitter/*tikta*, pungent/*katu*
Post digestive/*Vipak*: sweet/*madhur*
Potency/*Veerya*: hot/*ushna*
Dosha: VK-
Tissue/*Dhatu*: shukra, mamsa, meda, majja

Constituents

Steroid lactones, phytosterols, alkaloids, saponins, iron.

Actions

Sedative, nervine tonic, nutritive, rejuvenative, anti-inflammatory, anticancer, adaptogen, antioxidant.

Indications

Debility, nervous problems, insomnia, lowered immunity, digestive problems, arthritis, skin problems, coughs, asthma, anxiety, fevers, fainting, giddiness and insomnia.

Introduction

Ashwagandha is one of the most important herbs used in Ayurvedic medicine and is fast becoming popular among herbalists here in the West. In India it is held in as high esteem as ginseng in Chinese medicine and has recently been referred to as Indian Ginseng. Its Sanskrit name *ashwagandha* literally means "that which has the smell of a horse", so named because it is said to give the strength and vitality of a horse. It is renowned in India as the best rejuvenative herb, particularly for men, promoting energy and vitality, and has been used for centuries for its restorative properties to remedy conditions of weakness and debility. When the root is taken as a milk decoction and sweetened with honey or raw sugar, it is used to inhibit ageing

and build up strength by catalyzing the anabolic processes in the body. It is often prescribed during convalescence, for weakness and emaciation in children and the elderly and for a wide range of problems associated with old age, such as loss of energy, lack of muscular strength, poor memory, weak eyes, rheumatism, and insomnia. *Ashwagandha* has antioxidant properties limiting damage caused by free radicals, thereby helping to restrain the ageing process.

Internal uses

Nervous system

Ashwagandha is also an exceptional nerve tonic and one of the best remedies for stress. It is the best herb for balancing *Vata* in the body. Along with herbs such as ginseng, liquorice and *Astragalus* it is classified as an adaptogen, helping to modify the harmful effects of stress on mind and body. *Ashwagandha* is considered *Sattvic* in quality, which means it has a highly beneficial effect on mind and body, engendering calmness and clarity of mind, and helping to promote wisdom. With its significant calming and yet strengthening effects, it is excellent for people run down by chronic illness and those suffering from stress, anxiety, overwork, panic attacks, nervous exhaustion and insomnia. It is also well worth using for children with behavioural problems and ADHD. As a painkiller and anti-inflammatory it is used for inflammatory joint problems and can be combined with turmeric.

Respiratory system

Due to its immune-enhancing properties and antimicrobial activity *ashwagandha* is used to increase resistance to respiratory infections. It is also used in the treatment of allergies, rhinitis and asthma due to aggravated *Vata*.

Genitourinary system

Ashwagandha is the best regulator of *Apana Vata*, which governs the lower abdomen. It is excellent for urinary problems, dysmenorrhoea and a variety of gynaecological and menstrual problems associated with excess *Vata*.

Immune system

Ashwagandha, like ginseng, also benefits the immune system and may have a significant role to play in the prevention and management of cancer. Research indicates that *ashwagandha* can inhibit the growth of human tumour cell lines (Jayaprakasam et al 2003), and may also have antitumour effect by acting as an antiradical and protecting against DNA cleavage (Russo et al 2001). Other research has demonstrated that *ashwagandha* may increase the sensitivity of cancer cells to radiation therapy (Devi et al 1996). Its significantly beneficial effects on both the nervous system and immune system mean that this is a remedy that is well worth using in the treatment of autoimmune problems such as multiple sclerosis, psoriasis and rheumatoid arthritis. Research suggests that *ashwagandha* may in part exert its immunostimulating effect by induction of nitric oxide synthase in macrophages (Iuvone et al 2003).

External uses

Prepared as an oil by infusing it in sesame oil, *ashwagandha* can be rubbed into painful arthritic joints, frozen shoulders and used to ease nerve pain such as sciatica, numbness, muscle spasm and back pain. It has a healing effect on the skin and is well worth using for wounds and sores and for dry, itchy skin conditions, including eczema and psoriasis.

Dosage and formulation

- Powder: 5 g in warm water or milk morning and night, sweetened with honey or raw sugar. It can also be taken as a milk decoction or prepared in ghee
- Ashwagandharishta.

Precautions

Although it has traditionally been recommended to pregnant women to strengthen the woman and stabilize the embryo, until further studies are done it is best avoided during pregnancy. Caution with excess *Pitta*.

Research

- Devi PU, Akagi K, Ostapenko V 1996 Withaferin A: a new radiosensitizer from the Indian medicinal plant *Withania somnifera*. Int J Radiat Biol 69: 193–197
- Iuvone T, Esposito G, Capasso F, Izzo AA 2003 Induction of nitric oxide synthase expression by *Withania somnifera* in macrophages. Life Sci 72(14): 1617–1625
- Jayaprakasam B, Zhang Y, Seeram NP, Nair MG 2003 Growth inhibition of human tumor cell lines by withanolides from *Withania somnifera* leaves. Life Sci 74(1): 125–132
- Russo A, Izzo AA, Cardile V, Borrelli F, Vanella A 2001 Indian medicinal plants as antiradicals and DNA cleavage protectors. Phytomedicine 8(2): 125–132

Zingiber officinale : Ginger

Family: Zingiberaceae
Sanskrit: Adrak (fresh), Sunthi (dried)
English: *Ginger*
Part used: rhizomes, leaves
Quality/*Guna*: light/*laghu*, oily/*snigdha*
Taste/*Rasa*: pungent/*katu*
Post digestive/*Vipak*: sweet/*madhur*
Potency/*Virya*: heating/*ushna*
Dosha: KV-
Tissue/*Dhatu*: all

Constituents

1–2% volatile oil – zingerone, gingerol, camphene, borneol, phellandrene, citral.

Actions

Thermogenic, carminative, laxative, digestive, expectorant, analgesic, antispasmodic.
Dried: calminative, diuretic, emollient, appetizer, laxative, stomachic, stimulant, anthelmintic, antimicrobial, decongestant, antioxidant.

Indications

Anorexia, coughs and inflammation, tiredness, nausea, vomiting, asthma, fever, constipation, indigestion, diarrhoea, colic, flatulence, poor circulation.

Introduction

It is the pungent and warming properties of *ginger* that have made it such a valuable medicine. It has a stimulating effect on the heart and circulation, creating a feeling of warmth and well-being and restoring vitality. *Ginger* is an excellent remedy for travel sickness; this was long known by sailors in the East where *ginger* preparations are still taken to keep seasickness at bay during long voyages in stormy seas, and these claims have been vindicated by research (Grontved et al 1988). It also relieves sickness during pregnancy, as well as that related to an upset stomach, over-eating, nervousness and infection.

Internal uses

Digestive system

Ginger is a warming aid to digestion. It invigorates and settles the stomach and intestines, stimulating the appetite and enhancing digestion by encouraging secretion of digestive enzymes. It moves stagnant food and subsequent accumulation of toxins, which has a far-reaching effect throughout the body, increasing general health and vitality and enhancing immunity. It soothes indigestion and calms wind. Its pain-relieving and relaxing effects in the digestive system relieve colic and spasm, abdominal pain, distension and flatulent indigestion, and help relieve griping from diarrhoea and dysentery. It is said to be a good cure for a hangover. It also relieves postoperative nausea (Visalyaputra et al 1998).

Circulatory system

It has a stimulating effect on the heart and circulation, creating a feeling of warmth and well-being and restoring vitality.

Respiratory system

Ginger has a stimulating and expectorant action in the lungs, expelling phlegm and relieving catarrhal coughs and chest infections. Hot *ginger* tea taken at the onset of a sore throat, cold or flu, promotes perspiration, brings down a fever and helps to clear catarrh. In India fresh *ginger* tea is given to children for whooping cough.

Reproductive system

A number of clinical trials report *ginger*'s value in morning sickness (Aikins Murphy 1998). In the uterus it promotes menstruation, and is useful for delayed and scanty periods as well as clots. It relaxes spasm and painful ovulation and periods, and is recommended to invigorate the reproductive system and treat impotence caused by deficiency of vital warmth in the body.

Immune system

The volatile oils are antiseptic (Mascolo et al 1989), activating immunity and dispelling bacterial and viral infections. In the East it has been used for epidemics such as cholera. Fresh *ginger* root is reported to be highly effective in China in treatment of rheumatism, acute bacterial dysentery, malaria and orchitis. A small observational trial supports the use in rheumatism (Srivastava and Mustafa 1992), whilst further research indicates that certain constituents of *ginger* can inhibit prostaglandin synthesis, thus suggesting a possible mechanism of action (Kiuchi et al 1992). *Ginger* has also been shown to have antioxidative (Nakatani 2000) properties, inhibiting free radicals in the body, and thereby further aiding immunity and the circulation.

Temperature

Ginger taken in hot infusion helps to reduce fever.

External uses

Externally, the painkilling properties of chewing fresh *ginger* have been used to relieve toothache. Grated or powdered *ginger* has been used in a paste to cover the scalp to promote hair growth and stop baldness. Dilute *ginger* oil has been used in massage oils and liniments for lumbago, neuralgia and painful joints made worse by cold.

Drug interactions

If given with anticoagulants, *ginger* may enhance bleeding. Use together with caution.

Research

- Aikins Murphy P 1998 Alternative therapies for nausea and vomiting of pregnancy. Obstet Gynecol 91(1): 149–155
- Grontved A, Brask T, Kambskard J 1988 Ginger root against seasickness. A controlled trial on the open sea. Acta Otolaryngol 105(1–2): 45–49
- Kiuchi F, Iwakami S, Shibuya M 1992 Inhibition of prostaglandin and leukotriene biosynthesis by gingerols and diarylheptanoid. Chem Pharm Bull 40(2): 387–391
- Mascolo N, Jain R, Jain SC, Capasso F 1989 Ethnopharmacologic investigation of ginger (*Zingiber officinale*). J Ethnopharmacol 27(1–2): 129–140
- Nakatani N 2000 Phenolic antioxidants from herbs and spices. Biofactors 13(1–4): 141–146
- Srivastava KC, Mustafa T 1992 Ginger (*Zingiber officinale*) in rheumatism and musculoskeletal disorders. Med Hypothesis 39(4): 342–348
- Visalyaputra S, Petchpaisit N, Somcharoen K 1998 The efficacy of ginger root in the prevention of postoperative nausea and vomiting after outpatient gynecological laparoscopy. Anaesthesia 53(5): 506–510

Chapter 5

Common ailments in babies

ADMINISTERING HERBS TO BABIES

There are a variety of ways herbs can be given to babies:

- Infusions and decoctions can be added to bath water, used as hand and foot baths, applied as compresses or used as washes for the skin. Gentle antiseptic herbs such as chamomile, calendula, lavender and rosemary can be prepared in infusions and used as alternatives to baby soaps. (Carle and Isaac 1987, Larrondo et al 1995, Mangena and Muyima 1999). Such herbs have the advantage of enhancing immunity (Amirghofran et al 2000) at the same time as they are absorbed through the skin.

- Babies can be massaged with herbal oils. Any sore or dry areas can be rubbed with lavender oil in a base of sesame or almond oil as an alternative to chemical-based creams. As well as having antibacterial and antiseptic actions (Foster 1997) lavender has an anti-inflammatory action and stimulates tissue repair.

- Weak infusions of herbs can be given internally between feeds (using $\frac{1}{4}$ tsp of herb per cup of boiling water).

- Essential oils can be used in vaporizers and dilute oils can be added to bath water.

- Herbs can be taken by nursing mothers to pass through breast milk to the baby.

- For 10 days or so after the birth, the umbilical cord needs to be cleaned daily as it may get contaminated by urine before it drops off. Antiseptic herbs and oils can be used to dress the cord. Dilute oil of cloves has been widely used in midwifery in the past and is still used today. Distilled witch hazel or rosemary are also applicable and have antiseptic properties (Mangena and Muyima 1999, Iauk et al 2003). Rose water with its antimicrobial and astringent properties, is commonly used. For any redness or inflammation, I have used marshmallow tea, alternated by dilute tincture of calendula, myrrh or echinacea applied on cotton wool. These herbs can also be added to the bath water.

NAPPY RASH

This can usually be avoided if the baby's bottom is washed at nappy changes with dilute herbal infusions of lavender, chamomile or *Calendula*, or with rose water. Since nappy rash can be caused when damp skin is enclosed for long periods with ammonia without enough air to circulate around it, the more the nappy can be left off the better.

To prevent nappy rash

Cream can be rubbed into the nappy area at nappy changes using herbs in a natural base. Chamomile, chickweed (*Stellaria media*), comfrey leaf (*Symphytum off.*) and *Calendula* are healing and demulcent, cooling heat and inflammation and protecting the skin against corrosive effects of urine and stools. Chamomile and *Calendula* have been shown to have an anti-inflammatory effect (Della Loggia et al 1994, Safayhi et al 1994).

Nappy rash tends to occur in more babies with sensitive skins and those who are prone to seborrhoea (indicated by cradle cap or seborrhoeic dermatitis elsewhere on the skin). It may be that nappy rash is the beginning of atopic eczema (see p. 270). Breast-feeding may help to protect against tendency to allergy and to prevent infection associated with nappy rash. Micro-organisms tend to breed better in the alkaline nappy of a bottle-fed baby, than in the more acid stools produced by a breast-fed baby.

Treatment of nappy rash

Should nappy rash develop, it is best treated promptly as it can be very persistent and predispose to secondary infection.

- At each change, the skin can be bathed with dilute herbal infusions or distilled witch hazel, dried thoroughly and applied with calendula, chamomile, chickweed or comfrey leaf cream. If you suspect an infection, calendula and chamomile cream should be beneficial as they have antiseptic properties.

- Egg white and oxygen is an old and effective remedy for nappy rash. Egg white is applied repeatedly to the affected area before putting on a nappy, and in between each application the skin is air dried (a hair dryer is convenient). By doing this, a thick protective layer of albumen is built up, which allows the skin to heal rapidly. I have used this treatment with my own children to good effect. (There may be issues today regarding Salmonella.)

Nappy rash can weaken the skin's defences and predispose to a secondary infection, bacterial, viral or fungal such as thrush.

- *Hypericum* oil is particularly effective for soothing soreness, increasing resilience of the skin to infection and for resolving any secondary viral infection (Miskovsky 2002) such as herpes.

- Essential oil of lavender or chamomile in a base of almond or sesame oil is also excellent.

- For thrush infection, an infusion or cream of chamomile is generally effective (Carle and Isaac 1987).

- Alternatively, I have used a combination of neem, sandalwood and turmeric in a cream base, bathing the skin with an infusion of thyme at nappy changes.

- Yoghurt, calendula cream or powdered golden seal (*Hydrastis canadensis*) can be applied to the skin, after washing it with either dilute cider vinegar or thyme infusion. (See Treatment of Infectious Diseases for more on thrush, p. 262.) Yoghurt has been shown to have an action against *Candida* (Hilton et al 1992), whilst thyme is also known to be antifungal (Pina-Vaz et al 2004).

- If a baby has oral thrush, it may have spread through the system to the anus and caused nappy rash. I have used a couple of drops of diluted *Calendula* tincture with thyme or oregano oil (one drop for each 20 ml tincture) in the mouth, two or three times a day, or a little plain live yoghurt applied round the mouth.

- If the nappy rash is particularly severe, with spots and raised red patches which may develop into red raw areas, or even shallow ulcers, the baby will feel uncomfortable when passing urine or a stool. Chamomile tea can be given between feeds, and soothing comfrey leaf or marshmallow ointment applied, alternated with antiseptic calendula or chamomile cream. The bottom can be washed with infusions of *Calendula*, lavender, rosemary or elderflowers or dilute tincture of myrrh (*Commiphora molmol*) or calendula.

Talcum power is best avoided because it cakes on the skin, holding in the damp and collecting bacteria, and can aggravate nappy rash or introduce a secondary infection.

SEBORRHOEA

Over-production of sebum, causing cradle cap or seborrhoeic dermatitis, with red scaly areas on the face, on or behind the ears, and around the skin creases at the top of the thighs, frequently occurs in small babies. Seborrhoea often settles down of its own accord. There are several things that can be done to help clear it quickly.

Treatment of seborrhoea

- Seborrhoea can be related to an allergy, most commonly to milk products in the cow's milk-based formula of bottle-fed babies. Investigating alternatives may be advised. Women breast-feeding can try avoiding eating all milk products – milk, cheese, cream, yoghurt, ice-cream, etc., for a period of time. They will need to replace calcium and other nutrients derived from milk products until milk is returned to the diet.

- Eating plenty of other calcium-containing foods such as sesame seeds, dried figs, parsley, and watercress, and nettle soup, almond milk, magnesium and vitamin B6 may also help support the immune system of the baby through the breast milk, and help clear the skin.

- Calcium-containing herbs, such as comfrey, horsetail (*Equisetum arvense*), kelp (*Fucus vesiculosus*), marshmallow (*Althea off.*), meadowsweet (*Filipendula ulmaria*), nettles and skullcap (*Scutellaria laterifolia*), used regularly in teas or tinctures are also good for nursing mothers.

- A baby on solid food can be treated directly. Heartsease (*Viola tricolor*) and meadowsweet tea can be made as an infusion and given three times daily.

- Chamomile cream or *hypericum* oil with a little essential oil of lavender, can be applied to the affected areas of the skin two or three times a day until the skin clears.

- A standard dose of burdock decoction (flavoured with peppermint herb and/or liquorice root if desired) can be taken by a nursing mother to help balance the baby's skin function and sebum production.
- Burdock diluted in fennel tea in a ratio of one to three can be given to the baby between feeds.

COLIC

It is not always easy to be sure when a baby has colic. It is indicated when parents have tried everything else to comfort including feeding, changing, cuddling and walking up and down, or the baby cries so much that their face goes red and both legs are drawn up to the stomach as if in pain. Colic tends to occur after a feed, or in the evening when the baby is tired and their digestion does not function so well. It is stressful for the parents when they feel they have tried everything and still the baby seems so distressed.

A baby's digestion is closely connected to their general sense of well-being and security, and this can be affected by those around them. A stressful environment or anxiety on the part of the mother, especially when she is breast-feeding, may aggravate colic further. A baby's colic can also be related to feeding problems, so it is important to check that the baby is latched on properly to the nipple and not gulping air during the feed. This can often happen if milk comes out too quickly at the beginning of a feed (a little could be expressed by hand before feeding), or, if bottle-feeding the hole in the teat may be too small or too big.

It is possible that babies with colic are exhibiting an allergic reaction to food substances coming through the breast milk, or that substances in formula milk are irritating the gut (Kerner 1995) as occurs in lactose intolerance. Many colicky babies have been found to react to cow's milk in breast milk and formula milks. This is more likely in babies born of an atopic family in which problems such as eczema, asthma and hayfever occur. Severe infantile colic is often related to cow's milk protein intolerance (Iacono et al 1991). Other substances coming through breast milk from foods such as wheat, corn and citrus fruits, especially when they occur over-frequently in the mother's diet, can also cause allergic reactions.

Other foods that frequently cause problems in breast milk include:

- alcohol
- beans and lenfils
- tomatoes
- eggs
- vegetables such as:
  - onions
  - leeks
  - garlic
  - green peppers
  - aubergines
  - cucumber
  - courgettes
  - Brassicas
  - (cabbage, cauliflower, brussel sprouts, etc.)
- coffee
- highly spiced foods
- sugar
- chocolate
- too much fruit:
  - oranges
  - grapes
  - green apples
  - plums
  - strawberries
  - gooseberries
  - pineapple

Suspected foods can be omitted from the mother's diet for up to a week while observing any improvement in the baby. The food can be reintroduced after a week and any reaction assessed. When starting a baby on solid foods, any implicated foods are best introduced last and only in small amounts to begin with. Though there is little research available concerning colic, a Cochrane review concluded that an antigen-avoidance diet for mothers during lactation may substantially reduce the child's risk of developing atopic eczema (Kramer 2000) highlighting the importance of this factor. Obviously nursing mothers need to be careful not to compromise their nutrition. Foods omitted from the diet need to be replaced with other foods of comparable nutrient value.

Treatment of colic

- One fluid ounce (30 ml) of weak herbal infusion can be given before each feed to relax the gut and enhance digestion. Useful herbs include: chamomile, caraway, catnip (*Nepeta cataria*), dill (*Anethem graveolens*), fennel (*Foeniculum vulgare*), and lemon balm, which act as carminatives, and marshmallow (*Althea off.*) which is more demulcent. Use $\frac{1}{4}-\frac{1}{2}$ tsp (2–3 ml) of herbs to 4 oz (100 ml) boiling water. After the feed the tea can be given again. In a randomized, placebo-controlled trial of 125 infants, fennel seed oil was found to be significantly superior to placebo in the treatment of colic (Alexandrovich et al 2003).

- A little slippery elm (*Ulmus fulva*) powder mixed with warm water is soothing and nutritive and can be given before a feed in babies over 3 months.

- More concentrated infusions of the above herbs can be added to bath water or used as hand and foot baths.

- Stronger herbal teas can be drunk by the nursing mother, as the antispasmodic volatile oils from these herbs pass through the breast milk to the baby.

- If the mother or baby seem particularly tense, relaxing herbs such as catnip, dill, limeflowers (*Tilia europaea*), chamomile, lemon balm or hops (*Humulus lupulus*) can be added to the herbal tea and bath water for the baby; and skullcap, vervain (*Verbena off.*), passion flower (*Passiflora incarnata*), wild oats (*Avena sativa*), lemon balm or chamomile tea for the mother (see Nervous System, p. 248).

- Essential oils can also be used. Geranium, lavender, chamomile, ginger, fennel or aniseed can be used for their relaxing and antispasmodic properties, diluted (one drop to 1 tsp (5 ml) sesame oil) and added to bath water, used for massage or applied as a warm compress to the baby's abdomen. Often a massage with warm sesame oil followed by a warm bath with herbal infusions or essential oils will relax the baby sufficiently before a feed, and feeding should go more smoothly.

VOMITING

Once a baby is introduced to solids and vomits during or after eating, it may be that the food is indigestible or that there is an intolerance/allergy. If a baby has a runny or blocked nose or a catarrhal cough, swallowed mucus may irritate the stomach and be brought back up after coughing. If the baby seems unwell, off his food, flushed and irritable, or has watery stools, vomiting may be due to infection, i.e. gastroenteritis.

Treatment of vomiting

- Water or herbal teas can be given to replace lost fluids, frequently through the day.
- Reduce any fever with appropriate herbs (see Treatment of Fevers, p. 175).
- To settle the stomach, weak herbal teas of chamomile, catnip, dill, fennel, ginger, lemon balm or meadowsweet, can be given.
- If there are signs of infection, antimicrobial herbs such as echinacea, ginger, elderflowers, chamomile, or thyme can be given.
- If there is accompanying diarrhoea, add agrimony (*Agrimonia eupatorium*) or tormentil (*Potentilla erecta*).
- Drinks or gruel made with slippery elm powder, a pinch of powdered cinnamon or ginger, mixed with warm water or expressed milk, combine antiseptic, carminative and demulcent properties.
- The abdomen or feet can be massaged gently with dilute oils of lemon balm, lavender, spearmint or geranium using a base of sesame oil. Alternatively warm compresses using these oils or the above infusions can be applied to the abdomen.
- Babies on solids are best with no solid foods, just plenty of drink, until the stomach has settled down.

DIARRHOEA

Diarrhoea can occur when a baby is teething, but it can also be related to food intolerance. Even when completely breast-fed, a baby may react to food substances, such as milk, wheat, corn, citrus fruits, coming through the milk. Formula milks can also be to blame. Once a baby starts solid food, food intolerances can become more apparent, so if a baby develops diarrhoea when introduced to new food, it is best removed from the diet and any improvement observed. Culprit foods are best omitted from the diet for several months before they are reintroduced, to allow time for the baby's immature immune system to develop.

Excess fruit, such as citrus fruits, green apples, strawberries and plums, dried fruit, such as apricots, figs or prunes, or fruit juice can also cause diarrhoea.

Gastroenteritis occurs more frequently in bottle-fed babies than those who are breast-fed, as cow's milk formulae tend to produce more putrefactive bacteria in the bowel and do not protect a baby from infection in the same way as breast milk. Water or herbal teas can be given to avoid dehydration. Once the bowels are back to normal, mushy rice and yoghurt, with a little honey and banana is easy to digest and will help re-establish the normal gut flora. Both honey and banana contain the probiotic fructo-oligosaccharide, fermentation of which increases the number of bifidobacteria in the colon (Chow 2002).

Treatment of diarrhoea

- To help settle the stomach, a little fresh lemon juice in warm water can be given to the baby.

- Herbal teas can be given frequently throughout the day made from blackberry leaf (*Rubus fructicosus*) and/or raspberry leaf (*Rubus idaeus*) with a pinch of ginger powder or from chamomile, fennel, spearmint or meadowsweet.

- A drink can be made for babies who are old enough for solids using $\frac{1}{2}$ cup of live yoghurt, $\frac{1}{2}$ cup boiled water, a little grated fresh ginger and a pinch of cardamom. This will help re-establish the normal population of bacteria in the gut and enhance immunity to infection.

- Slippery elm powder with a pinch of ginger or cinnamon powder, made into a drink with a little warm water or milk, is soothing to an irritated gut. Slippery elm (*Ulmus fulva*) contains abundant mucilage that coats inflamed or irritated surfaces in the gastrointestinal tract and protects them from irritation and infection. It has been used for centuries as a nourishing food for recently weaned babies.

CONSTIPATION

Constipation tends to occur more in bottle-fed babies, whose more alkaline stools tend to breed more putrefactive bacteria than those breast-fed. These bacteria can inhibit the beneficial flora that enhance peristalsis, resulting in an irritated gut, and cause a degree of spasm. When constipation occurs in a breast-fed baby it is worth examining the mother's diet for foods that may be irritating the baby's gut. Milk and wheat tend to be the most

common culprits. Suspected foods are best avoided for a week or two and any improvement observed.

In babies on solid food, it is possible that constipation can be caused by a number of factors:

- a low-fibre diet with too much refined food and sugar,
- excess protein from meat and dairy produce,
- insufficient fluid intake,
- poor diet causing a deficiency of vitamins and minerals, particularly vitamin C and magnesium,
- anaemia.

Treatment of constipation

- Increasing fluids between feeds including water from cooked prunes, fig, raisins or apricots is recommended.
- Herbal tea such as chamomile, dill (*Anethum graveolens*), fennel (*Foeniculum vulgare*), ginger, basil, lemon balm and spearmint will all help release tension or spasm in the gut, while marshmallow or slippery elm powder in a little warm water can soothe an irritated gut lining.
- Add a little liquorice water to herbal teas for a more laxative effect if necessary.
- Alternatively, add a little molasses (1 tsp to a cup of tea or hot water) or honey which also has a slightly laxative effect. (Avoid in babies under 10 months.)
- Babies on solid food can be given mashed prunes and apricots, plain natural live yoghurt with a little mashed banana, and garlic can be added to their vegetables.
- Unrefined olive oil in the diet will help re-establish the gut flora.
- Gentle massage of the abdomen with dilute essential oil of ginger, basil, chamomile or rose using sesame oil as a base, can be given in a clockwise direction.
- Hot compresses applied to the abdomen using dilute oils in hot water or stronger herbal infusions (2 × baby's internal dose) can also be effective.

STICKY EYE

This mild infection of the eyes is very common in the first week of life. It is usually due to a foreign substance, perhaps a little amniotic fluid or blood, getting into the eye during the birth.

- A weak infusion (use boiled or distilled water for this) of warm chamomile, *Calendula*, elderflower or marshmallow (*Althea off.*) makes a good wash for both eyes, using clean cotton wool for each eye.
- Eyebright (*Euphrasia officinalis*) eye drops have been found to be effective in a trial for various conjunctival conditions (Stoss et al 2000).
- A little breast milk is also very effective.
- Alternatively a mixture of almond oil and rose water can be used to wipe the eyelid (being careful not to get the oil in the eye).
- A saline solution, made from one teaspoon of sea salt to one cup boiled water, can be effective when used to bathe the eyes.

TEETHING

Some babies tend to dribble a lot when teething, others develop rashes on the face, become irritable, clingy and restless, go off their food or have trouble sleeping, others tend to put anything they can in their mouths to bite on.

> A variety of symptoms can be associated with teething such as fever, cough, breathlessness, vomiting, diarrhoea, conjunctivitis, skin disorders, generalized rashes, thirst, colds and other infections and earache.

The symptoms manifested may provide clues about inherent weaknesses in the baby. Teething acts as a stress phenomenon and a precipitating factor for many illnesses. Nevertheless, it is important to exclude other causes before teething is accepted as a cause. These symptoms may have absolutely nothing to do with teething and should always be checked out as symptoms indicating other illness or imbalance.

Treatment for teething problems

- If there are blisters on the gum overlying an emerging tooth, the baby might gain some relief from something to chew on – either a finger, hopefully not a nipple, a marshmallow root or

liquorice stick or a teething ring cooled in the fridge.
- The gums can also be rubbed to relieve pain.
- An old-fashioned remedy is a teaspoon of honey with a drop of chamomile oil or clove oil.
- Infusions of chamomile, limeflowers, yarrow, fennel or catnip (*Nepeta cataria*) can be given frequently through the day.

Ayurvedic treatment

- Ghee medicated with vacha, musta (*Cyperus rotundus*) and sweet-tasting herbs such as bala, liquorice and shatavari promote easy eruption of teeth.
- The gums can be massaged with powder of amalaki or pippali with honey.
- Formulae containing aloe vera are used for coughs, and for diarrhoea associated with teething.
- For fevers associated with teething a decoction of kiratatikta (*Swertia chiretta*) guduchi, sandalwood (*Santalum album*), ginger, amalaki and musta is traditionally used.

A CRYING BABY

All babies cry; it is their only way to express their needs, but some babies cry more than others. A breast-fed baby may cry more than a bottle-fed baby because breast milk tends to pass through the stomach more quickly, meaning the baby is hungry frequently through the day and night. Most healthy babies stop crying as soon as they are being fed and feel secure, or made comfortable through a change of nappy. Sometimes a baby will still cry, very often in the evenings, if breast milk supply is dwindling, or with "evening colic" (see p. 139).

Parents soon learn to recognize what their baby's cry means – whether hungry, restless, insecure or uncomfortable, tired and irritable, or bored. If it is colic the cry will be more distressed, if the baby is unwell the cry will vary from the normal pattern and could go on intermittently through the day. It could also mean an infection is developing, and once the symptoms manifest properly it can be treated accordingly. Crying could mean teething. Inflamed gums and increased dribbling will confirm this (see p. 139).

It is easier for parents to comfort a crying baby if they know what the trouble is, but what is hardest for most parents is when the baby cries and nothing seems to make a jot of difference. Some babies respond better to noise and fast motion as in a car or pram, rather than quiet and gentle rocking in a cot. Many babies stop crying if they are given attention and this may work better than repeated efforts to relax them into sleep. The anxiety and tension of parents frazzled by hours of walking a baby up and down to lull them to a quiet sleep may have contradictory results once it is picked up by the baby.

Quite naturally a crying baby can profoundly affect the mother's feelings, which can range from anxiety, panic, pure frustration to relief once the crying stops. Both parents may feel very distressed and at the end of their tether. They may benefit from nervine herbs to calm tension and increase resilience to stress (see Nervous System, p. 248). If only for the parents nerves, herbs can be given to calm a crying baby and encourage a restful sleep, particularly the best remedy should the crying indicate the onset of infection.

- Warm herbal baths: Strong infusions of relaxing herbs such as chamomile, catnip (*Nepeta cataria*), cowslip (*Primula vera*), hops (*Humulus lupulus*), lavender, lemon balm and limeflowers (*Tilia europaea*) can be added to bath water.
- Dilute essential oils can be used in bath water; chamomile, geranium, lavender, neroli and rose are all helpful.
- The warmth of the bath is relaxing in itself, and the addition of herbs will help to induce calm, releasing tension in muscles and in the gut, and soothing discomfort related to fevers or skin problems.
- If the baby seems to wake from sleep in a distressed state, catnip is particularly recommended.
- Massage: A sesame oil body massage prior to a bath can be very beneficial (see sesame oil, p. 84).
- Massage of the head, feet or abdomen, can be deeply relaxing and reassuring.
- The above essential oils can be added to a base of sesame oil for message or the oils used in a vaporizer near the bed.
- Herbal teas: Dilute teas of chamomile, catnip, cowslip, hops, lavender, lemon balm and limeflowers can also be given, on a spoon or in a bottle.

AYURVEDIC CARE OF THE NEWBORN

A newborn baby is thoroughly examined and his/her constitution assessed. In babies with *Vata*, *Pitta* and *Kapha* single constitutions, sesame oil, coconut oil and mustard oil are used respectively. It is said that daily massage with the right oils improves the complexion and promotes growth and strength. When the baby starts to crawl, its back and legs are massaged twice daily. Massage at night is said to relieve exhaustion and help the baby to sleep soundly. A drop or two of sesame oil dropped into the ears and the mastoid region daily keeps the area free of irritation and infection (Athavale 2000).

A study of 125 infants, 5–7 weeks old aimed to investigate the effects of massage with various oils or no massage at all on general health. The authors conclude that sesame oil massage significantly improved growth and post-massage sleep (Agarwal et al 2000).

In the Ayurvedic tradition the baby is given warm baths daily medicated with decoctions of herbs such as pippali, and udumbara (*Ficus racemosa*) and aromatic herbs such as sandalwood. In the bedroom dried herbs are tied in bunches and suspended from beams or door frames. Herbs used are normally antimicrobials such as mustard, garlic (Ankri and Mirelman 1999, Rhee et al 2003) kushta (*Saussurea lappa*), and asafoetida (*Ferula asafoetida*). Turmeric is an effective insect repellent (Tawatsin et al 2001) and is hung to dispel mosquitoes and other disease-carrying organisms.

The health of the baby at this stage depends largely on the mother so it is vital that she look after her health first. It is considered important to give an oil massage to the mother immediately after delivery. She should then be given a decoction of *Vata* balancing herbs like dashmula together with pippali, citrak (*Plumbago zeylanica*) and ginger and given jaggery water to drink. This decoction is repeated for the first 3–5 days and helps to purify the blood. She should avoid indigestion, eating in excess and eating incompatible foods, as well as anger, overexertion and sex. A lactating woman is advised to massage regularly with bala oil, (Athavale 2000).

It is important for the mother to have a healthy digestion. If her digestive fire is too high she needs to have plenty of nourishing and cooling foods. If her digestive power is weak she needs to take ghee with medicines that stimulate secretion of digestive enzymes. If she has irregular digestive power she should take medicated ghee as indicated (see *agni* and Digestive System, p. 197).

Recently I was consulted by a couple who had a baby of some months old covered from head to foot with one of the worse cases of eczema I have seen for a while. The baby's skin was severely inflamed, it had been recently infected and was so hot that there was no need to touch his skin to feel the heat radiate off him. His eczema had started when he was 2 weeks old while his mother was breast-feeding him, which she continued to do completely until she introduced solids around 5 months. No remedies that the parents had tried to date made any improvement whatsoever. While interviewing the parents it transpired that the baby's mother also had a history of hot, inflammatory eczema and since pregnancy complained of abnormal heat, which had become so intense that she had a tendency to sweat profusely, to be disturbed at night by the heat and to have great difficulty holding her baby boy as she could not bear the proximity of his equally hot body.

It was clear that treatment was required by both mother and baby and that this was a good example of how the mother's health can affect her breast milk and subsequently the well-being of her baby.

The mother was treated with *Pitta* reducing herbs and diet to reduce her heat and baby and mother got better over the next few months. This certainly vindicates the wisdom of Ayurvedic medicine which holds that the mother's diet and nutrition, amongst other things, can affect the quality of her breast milk and the health of her baby.

Factors affecting breast milk

Diet, nutrition, level of activity, climate, psychological and environmental factors, and any ill health, both during pregnancy and after, can affect the quality of the mother's breast milk and thus the health and well-being of her baby.

More specifically these include:

- Excess of red meat, fish, alcohol, sugar
- Too hot, too cold, too little, too much food
- Stale, fermented, heavy, unbalanced, incompatible, overcooked foods
- Foods that do not suit the mother's constitution
- Salty, sour and pungent food
- Indigestion
- Over or under-activity, tiredness
- Sorrow, anger, anxiety, worry and other psychological disturbances
- Obesity, underweight
- Ill health and disease, fever
- Exertion, working in hot sun, hot weather, insufficient or excessive sleep, sleep in the afternoon
- Suppression of natural urges, e.g. micturition, defecation, sneezing
- Trauma to the breast, breast abscess, infection of the breast.

Should any of these disturb the balance of the mother's constitution or *doshas*, this will in turn disturb the *doshic* balance of the baby. Tension and anxiety, eating too little, too much light food, excess pungent, bitter and astringent foods, cold dry windy weather, insufficient rest, relaxation and sleep and excess activity will increase *Vata dosha* in the breast milk. As a result, the milk can be thin, light (i.e. not oily), a bit frothy, slightly dark in colour, its sweet taste could be tinged with a hint of astringency or bitterness, or the milk could be almost tasteless, due to lack of nutrients, its temperature a little cooler than normal. The baby may have a tendency to be hungry frequently as such milk is likely to be less satisfying than it should be.

Eating excessive pungent, sour or salty foods, a hot climate, fevers, inflammation in the body, getting over-heated, angry or frustrated can cause the milk to be disturbed by *Pitta*. The milk will be of normal consistency perhaps with a yellowish or reddish tinge, a slightly bitter, sour or pungent taste and a strong rather unpleasant smell. Its temperature could be slightly warmer than normal and it may also be rather unsatisfying for the baby who may tend to be hungry frequently.

Eating too much, particularly an abundance of sweet, sour or salty foods, inactivity, lack of exercise, sleeping excessively in the daytime and cold damp, cloudy weather can all cause the milk to be disturbed by *Kapha*. The milk can be heavy, oily, thick and sticky, dense white colour, more sweet tasting

Table 5.1 Characteristics of milk disturbed by *Vata*, *Pitta* or *Kapha*

	Vata	Pitta	Kapha	Ideal
Colour	Darkish	Bluish, yellowish or reddish tinge	Dense white	White
Taste	Sweet with slightly astringent, bitter taste or tasteless	Sweet with slightly bitter, sour or pungent taste	More sweet with slightly salty taste	Natural and sweet
Smell	No smell	Foul smelling like blood	Smell of ghee, oil or animal fat	Natural
Temperature	Normal, slightly cool	Warm	Cool	Warm
Consistency	Thin	Intermediate	Thick, sticky	Mixes easily with water
Foam	Present	Absent	Absent	Absent
Light or heavy	Light	Intermediate	Heavy	Medium
Satiety	Absent	Absent	Heavy	Present
Water test	The milk floats	Produces yellow streaks in the water	It sinks	It mixes easily

(Source: Athavale 2000)

than normal with a slightly salty taste, an oily smell and a slightly cool temperature. It will be more satisfying than milk disturbed by *Vata* or *Pitta* and the baby will tend to be satiated for longer.

It is possible to test breast milk to establish which *dosha* is disturbed. Using a dropper, place one drop of breast milk into a glass of water. Ideally the milk should mix easily with the water. If it is disturbed by *Vata* the milk floats, if by *Pitta* it produces yellow streaks in the water and if by *Kapha* it sinks (Table 5.1).

The effects of *doshic* disturbance of milk on the baby will vary. *Vata* disturbance can have a slightly cooling effect and predisposes to low body weight, trapped wind, bloating, colic, constipation or hunger diarrhoea, retention of urine, breathlessness, insomnia, restlessness, and a tendency to jump easily at the slightest noise. The baby may not be satisfied even after feeding, its growth and weight increase could be slowed as the milk is not as nourishing as it should be. *Pitta* disturbance will have a heating effect, predisposing to low weight, loose stools, indigestion, acidity, vomiting, perianal excoriation,

fevers, hot body, rashes, excessive sweating and thirst, anaemia, yellow tinge to the skin, jaundice, and conjunctivitis. *Kapha* disturbance can have a cooling effect, and predisposes to overweight, wind, abdominal distension, constipation, excessive salivation, vomiting, anorexia, tenesmus, colds, cough, breathlessness, puffiness of face and eyes, itching of the skin, excessive sleep and drowsiness.

The aim of treatment of the mother with such *doshic* disturbances is to purify the breast milk and to balance her *doshas*. In general *Kapha dosha* usually dominates as breasts are situated in the area of the body ruled by *Kapha*. Hence medicines with bitter, pungent, astringent and sweet taste are useful. Mutton soup, vegetable soups and soups of pulses with added ginger, pepper and pippali are recommended by Ayurvedic physicians.

After being massaged with oil, which is followed with a hot bath or shower, the mother is generally given ghee medicated with herbal medicines to purify breast milk, followed by bowel cleansers such as Triphala (a mixture of *Emblica off.*, *Terminalia chebula* and *Terminalia belerica*) or haritaki

(*Terminalia chebula*) with ghee or honey and then sweating is induced.

A well-known herbal formula for purifying breast milk is a decoction of herbs which includes: triphala, ginger, cumin seeds, long pepper, patha (*Cissempelus pareira*), liquorice, cinnamon, *Cedrus deodar*, and mustard can be administered with honey.

Another formulation includes: bibhitaki, citrak (*Plumbago zeylanica*), sandalwood (*Santalum album*), daruharidra (*Berberis aristata*), guduchi, liquorice, turmeric, kutaki (*Picorrhiza kurroa*), kushta (*Saussurea lappa*), musta (*Cyprus rotundus*), nagakesara (*Messua ferra*), patha (*Cissempelus pareira*), vacha, patola (*Trichosanthes*), murva (*Clematis triloba*).

Treatment for *Vata* disturbed milk

- Dashmula decoction three times daily for 3 days

- Decoction or ghee medicated with citrak, acorus, patha, katuki, kushta, ajamoda (*Carum roxburghianum*), bharngi (*Clerondendron serratum*) devadaru, long pepper, ginger and pepper

- Ghee medicated with asafoetida and rock salt

- Oil massage, induction of sweating, mild oily purgatives like castor oil and retention enema with *Vata* balancing herbs are recommended. Such herbs include bala (*Sida cordifolia*), shatavari (*Asparagus racemosus*), and ashwagandha (*Withania somnifera*), *Vata* pacifying herbs can also be applied to the breasts

- Paste of grapes, liquorice and sariva is taken with warm water

- Ghee medicated with bael root

- Decoction of guduchi, ginger and chiretta (*Swertia chiretta*).

The baby can be given ghee medicated with ajamoda (*Carum roxburghianum*), devadaru, long pepper (*Piper longum*) and raw sugar.

Treatment of *Pitta* disturbed milk

Give a decoction of either

- Triphala, musta (*Cyprus rotundus*), and chiretta (*Swertia chiretta*)

- Shatavari, patola leaves (*Trichosanthes kirilowii*), neem, sariva (*Hemidesmus indicus*), padmaka (*Prunus cirasoidus*), guduchi, and sandalwood

- Sariva decoction. Cold pastes or sprays of *Pitta* calming herbs such as those listed above, can be applied to the whole body and locally to the breasts.

Treatment of *Kapha* disturbed milk

Emetics such as *Acorus calamus*, mustard and long pepper are given to clear *Kapha*. Herbs such as devadaru, musta, patha (*Cissempelus pareira*), ginger and haritaki are all recommended.

Warm paste of bael root (*Aegle marmelos*) and liquorice can be applied to the breast, allowed to dry and then washed off before feeding. Neem, long pepper and ginger with honey and ghee may also be helpful.

TONICS FOR INFANTS

The growth and development of the brain occurs rapidly in infants and for this reason in India infants are given brain tonics from birth. These are administered in the morning until the baby is a year old, by allowing the baby to lick a small amount from the mother's finger.

- Paste of brahmi and shankapushpi (*Convolulus pluricaulis*) with ghee and honey.
- Brahmi, mandukaparni, Triphala, citraka, vacha (*Acorus calamus*), shatavari with honey and ghee.
- Manjishta, triphala, brahmi and bala in equal quantities licked with honey and ghee.
- Vacha, liquorice, saindhava (rock salt), haritaki (*Terminalia chebula*), ginger (*Zingiber officinales*), ajamoda (*Carum roxburghianum*), kushta (*Saussurea lappa*), pippali (*Piper longum*) and cumin seeds, powdered and mixed with ghee are licked to improve speech.

Tonics can also be given according to the constitution. Oil massage and ashwagandharishta are recommended for a *Vata* child, ghee and amalaki for a *Pitta* child and honey, pippali or haritaki for a *Kapha* child.

A general tonic for a breast-fed baby is prepared from honey medicated with vacha, jatamansi (*Nardostachys jatamansi*), shatavari, apamarga

(*Achyranthes aspera*), sariva (*Hemidesmus indica*), brahmi, pippali, turmeric, kushta and sindhava (rock salt). A tonic for mixed feeding is prepared from ghee medicated with vacha, liquorice, pippali, citrak and Triphala and tonic for a baby on all solid food is prepared from a ghee medicated with dashmula, tagara (*Valeriana wallichi*), pepper, liquorice, grapes and brahmi.

References

Agarwal KN, Gupta A, Pushkarna R, Bhargava SK, Faridi MM, Prabhu MK 2000 Effects of massage and use of oil on growth, blood flow & sleep pattern in infants. Indian J Med Res 112: 212–217

Alexandrovich I, Rakovitskaya O, Kolmo E, Sidorova T, Shushunov S 2003 The effect of fennel (*Foeniculum vulgare*) seed oil emulsion in infantile colic: a randomized, placebo-controlled study. Altern Ther Health Med 9(4): 58–61

Amirghofran Z, Azadbakht M, Karimi MH 2000 Evaluation of the immunomodulatory effects of five herbal plants. J Ethnopharmacol 72(1–2): 167–172

Ankri S, Mirelman D 1999 Antimicrobial properties of allicin from garlic. Microbes Infect 1(2): 125–129

Athavale VB 2000 Bala Veda Pediatrics & Ayurveda. Chaukhamba Sanskrit Pratishthan, Delhi

Carle R, Isaac O 1987 Die Kamille – Wirkung & Wirksamkeit. Zeitschrift für Phytotherapice 8: 67–77

Chow J 2002 Probiotics and prebiotics: A brief overview. J Ren Nutr 12(2): 76–86

Della Loggia R, Tubaro A, Sosa S 1994 The role of triterpenoid in the topical anti-inflammatory activity of *Calendula officinalis* flowers. Planta Med 60(6): 516–520

Foster S 1997 Herbal Renaissance. Gibb Smith, Salt Lake City, p. 116

Hilton E, Isenberg HD, Alperstein P, France K, Borenstein MT 1992 Ingestion of yogurt containing *Lactobacillus acidophilus* as prophylaxis for candidal vaginitis. Ann Intern Med 116(5): 353–357

Iacono G, Carroccio A, Montalto G, et al 1991 Severe infantile colic and food intolerance: a long-term prospective study. J Pediatr Gastroenterol Nutr 12(3): 332–335

Iauk L, Lo Bue AM, Milazzo I, Rapisarda A, Blandino G 2003 Antibacterial activity of medicinal plant extracts against periodontopathic bacteria. Phytother Res 17(6): 599–604

Kerner JA Jr 1995 Formula allergy and intolerance. Gastroenterol Clin North Am 24(1): 1–25

Kramer MS 2000 Maternal antigen avoidance during lactation for preventing atopic disease in infants of women at high risk. Cochrane Database Syst Rev (2): CD000132

Larrondo JV, Agut M, Calvo-Torras MA 1995 Antimicrobial activity of essences from labiates. Microbios 82(332): 171–172

Mangena T, Muyima NY 1999 Comparative evaluation of the antimicrobial activities of essential oils of *Artemisia afra*, *Pteronia incana* and *Rosmarinus officinalis* on selected bacteria and yeast strains. Lett Appl Microbiol 28(4): 291–296

Miskovsky P 2002 Hypericin – a new antiviral and antitumor photosensitizer: mechanism of action and interaction with biological macromolecules. Curr Drug Targets 3(1): 55–84

Pina-Vaz C, Goncalves Rodrigues A, Pinto E, et al 2004 Antifungal activity of thymus oils and their major compounds. J Eur Acad Dermatol Venereol 18(1): 73–78

Rhee MS, Lee SY, Dougherty RH, Kang DH 2003 Antimicrobial effects of mustard flour and acetic acid against *Escherichia coli* O157:H7, *Listeria monocytogenes*, and *Salmonella enterica* serovar *Typhimurium*. Appl Environ Microbiol 69(5): 2959–2963

Safayhi H, Sabieraj J, Sailer ER, Ammon HP 1994 Chamazulene: an antioxidant-type inhibitor of leuktriene B4 formation. Planta Med 60(5): 410–413

Stoss M, Michels C, Peter E, Beutke R, Gorter RW 2000 Prospective cohort trial of Euphrasia single-dose eye drops in conjunctivitis. J Altern Complement Med 6(6): 499–508

Tawatsin A, Wratten SD, Scott RR, et al 2001 Repellency of volatile oils from plants against three mosquito vectors. J Vector Ecol Jun; 26(1): 76–82

Chapter 6

The immune system

SUPPORTING THE IMMUNE SYSTEM

The body is inherently endowed with a unique ability to protect and heal itself from injury and disease. Among the intricate mechanisms our bodies possess to prevent the entry of pathogenic micro-organisms are antiseptic tears in the eyes, antiseptic saliva in the mouth, sticky mucus and hairs to trap organisms in the nose and sneezing which expels them forcibly. There is mucus and the mucociliary escalator preventing invasion by micro-organisms into the lungs, and coughing which expels them forcibly. There are acids in the stomach and flora in the intestines to check unwanted organisms, which the bowels expel with any accompanying toxins. The bladder flushes out organisms and toxins through urine. The vagina is acid and destroys organisms and finally there is skin, which is waterproof and protects underlying tissues by secreting sebum and antiseptic oils. These homoeostatic mechanisms can be enhanced or compromised by everyday living. A healthy lifestyle is one that obviously protects the body's immune efforts.

The role of medicine is to assist the efforts of the body to heal itself, as a child's innate vital force endeavours to maintain homoeostasis and health. If too many pathogenic influences – poor diet, lack of fresh air, a new or virulent infection, for instance – overburden the homoeostatic mechanism temporarily, then "sickness" results. Unwanted organisms and toxins, which are generally dealt with by the body's immune and eliminative system, begin to accumulate in the body. However, the healing energy or vital force of the body rallies its defences and directs its force towards throwing them off. To do this, energy is withdrawn from normal daily processes, such as digestion and assimilation, and directed towards cleansing and eliminating the waste products through the natural channels – bowels, kidneys, skin and lungs – and the stimulation of the immune system. The various signs, symptoms, "illnesses" and conditions are not so much signs of disease as evidence of the body carrying out its own self-cleansing process.

It is possible to enhance the efficiency of this healing process in many ways. Firstly it is important that children avoid eating heavy food and

that "remedies" to suppress the action of the vital force are not prescribed unnecessarily. It is inadvisable, for example, to give medicines indiscriminately to stop vomiting or diarrhoea, or to bring down a mild fever, as these are the very mechanisms children possess for warding off disease quickly. Such symptoms could be interpreted as signs of *health* not disease. Each child's case obviously has to be judged on its own merits, for if either vomiting or diarrhoea persist for too long or the fever is rising quickly, some treatment may be required. However, suppression of the efforts of the vital force may only serve to push the illness further into the body or into a more chronic state. As the defensive system is weakened by such suppression, it is less able to ward off subsequent threats to health and thereby predisposed to further illness.

It is common for babies and children to suffer from frequent colds, coughs, catarrh and ear infections. The mucus produced results from irritation of the sensitive linings of the nose, throat and chest by infection, environmental chemicals or allergens. The excess mucus acts protectively to dilute the irritants and minimize the damage to the mucous membranes. Anticatarrhal medicines or astringent nose drops are directly antagonistic to the inherent healing action of the body, and its strength is thereby depleted, its efforts to eliminate the irritants reduced. The outcome of this can be the development of chronic catarrh and/or frequent respiratory infections. As simple symptoms are suppressed and healing energy is depleted, so the nature of the subsequent illness may change to that of a more serious or chronic nature. A case of infantile eczema may be "cured" by hydrocortisone cream but it may be linked to the development of asthma later in childhood.

The complexity of the immune system is being increasingly understood, as are the many health problems related to immunity. These not only constitute the common colds, flu's and allergies that children are prone to, but also more serious immune-related problems such as psoriasis, asthma, Epstein–Barr virus, chronic fatigue syndrome and arthritis. Herbs have been used for millennia to enhance resistance to disease and the fight against invading micro-organisms in infection. Our understanding of how these herbs actually interact in the body is also growing. Many herbs are known as "immunoregulators" and have the ability not only to stimulate an underactive immune system but also to prevent it from over-reacting to invaders or substances that it misinter-prets as pathogens in allergic and autoimmune disease.

The link between health and diet and stress has been made very clearly and is something that every modern therapist is aware of and addresses through their practice, as fundamental to preven-tion and recovery. Naturally a positive outlook, fun, laughter, serenity, being in conducive sur-roundings, and clean air, can all boost immunity. Love, displays of affection and touch are vitally important to the well-being of children. Touch and communication will not only let the child know they are loved, but also give a sense of security and the resilience to cope with difficult situations that may arise. It is clear that affectionate touch and massage are deeply relaxing and that they can sig-nificantly reduce stress levels. Touch has been shown to increase immunity, accelerate growth in infants and reduce aggressive tendencies. A review of massage therapy for children found that massage resulted in "lower anxiety and stress hormones and improved clinical course" in a number of medical problems (Field 1995). A child who is emotionally distressed is more likely to fall prey to infection and to have a greater tendency to develop food and chemical intolerances. Negative thoughts and feelings have been shown through skin tests to affect local immunity in the skin, while calming thoughts and meditation have been shown to increase the skin's immunity and the activity of white blood cells in the blood. Gentle massage and a bath with some relaxing essential oils such as laven-der or chamomile before putting children to bed, will have far-reaching effects, not only helping to ensure a good sleep and recovery from the stresses of the day, but also enhancing immunity and helping to prevent disease.

Exercise is also important for the maintenance of health and immunity, and parents need to encour-age their children to take daily exercise. Obviously it is important to strengthen muscles but also to promote circulation of blood and lymph and to ensure the removal of wastes and toxins from cells and tissues, including the bowels.

THE ROLE OF DIET

It is said that the choice of diet made can influence long-term health prospects more than any other action parents may take. Clearly the right foods are essential to provide a child with energy and nutrients to build a strong and healthy body, but food can also play more subtle parts in a child's overall well-being. Certain foods are harder to digest and may be slow to provide energy; some can cause a child to feel tired, heavy and lethargic, while others can make children irritable, over-stimulated, jumpy and hyperactive.

Raw materials for the immune system

Proteins

Proteins are vital not only to growth and repair, but also for immunity, providing raw materials for the formation of antibodies. Meat, poultry, fish, eggs and soya beans provide complete proteins. There are three vegetable sources of protein: grains; nuts and seeds; beans and pulses. Two out of these three need to be combined in the same meal to provide all the essential amino acids to make a complete protein.

Essential fatty acids

These are fats that cannot be made by the body and have to be taken in the diet. Essential fatty acids (EFAs) are vital to a healthy immune system, and yet the average diet is still very low in these and high in harmful fats despite increasing health awareness. EFAs are crucial to the normal func-tioning of lymphocytes and their production of antibodies, to a healthy skin, blood, and kidneys, to the formation of cell membranes, as well as to the normal functioning of the brain and nervous sys-tem. Research has demonstrated that children with a history of recurrent respiratory infections fare better when taking supplements of essential fatty acids. A double-blind trial was carried out on 20 children who were given 596 mg linoleic acid and 855 mg alpha-linoleic acid daily for 4 months and followed up for another 2 months. The number of respiratory infections in the children given essen-tial fatty acids was reduced (Greenfiles 1997).

There are two main groups of EFAs: omega-6 (the principal types being linoleic acid (LA) and arachidonic acid), and omega-3 (the main one being linolenic acid (LNA)). Generally we need omega-3 and omega-6 oils in a ratio of 2:1.

Food sources include:

- **Omega-6:** Safflower seeds, sunflower seeds, pumpkin seeds, corn oil, evening primrose oil, sunflower oil, safflower oil, grains, vegetables, dried beans, sprouted seeds and beans.
- **Omega-3:** Linseed oil, soya beans, soya oil, walnuts, walnut oil, wheatgerm, wheatgerm oil, fresh oily fish (sardines, tuna, wild salmon, herring, mackerel), cod liver oil, dried beans, sprouted beans, spinach and cabbage, wheat.

All oil sources of EFAs need to be cold-pressed, fresh, and unrefined; most commercial oils are heat-extracted, and heat damages the essential fatty acids, as does sunlight. They are also chemically refined, bleached and hydrogenated, which destroys most of their nutritional value. Canning, processing and cooking can all destroy essential fatty acids. Once taken in through the diet, EFAs have to be converted into other forms through metabolism before they can be used. The enzymes involved in their metabolism require other nutrients vitamins A, C, E and B6 and minerals zinc, copper, magnesium, and selenium, to process them into prostaglandins.

Vitamins, minerals and trace elements

A variety of vitamins, minerals and trace elements are essential to the immune system as well as EFA metabolism.

Vitamin A has an antioxidant action. It is crucial to the production of T and B white blood cells, responsible for antibody production. Deficiency can compromise antibody formation and reduce resistance. A serious deficiency can cause atrophy of the lymphatic tissue in the thymus gland and spleen, severely reducing immunity.

The most important of the B vitamins is vitamin B6, but they are all necessary for the health of the mucous membranes as a first line of defence against micro-organisms, and are crucial in the production of T and B white blood cells and the formation of antibodies. Vitamin B6 needs zinc in order to be fully effective.

Vitamin C has an antioxidant action and it helps to protect against virus infections. It stimulates macrophages, and encourages antibody response and the production of T-killer cells. Vitamin C can also reduce the allergic response, as well as the immunosuppressive effects of stress, through its effect on the adrenal glands.

Vitamin E enhances the production of antibodies and the activity of macrophages, and strengthens resistance, particularly to viruses. It works synergistically with selenium. Like vitamins A and C, it is an antioxidant, reducing cell damage caused when oxygen combines with other substances, and it helps prevent damage to the lungs caused by pollution in the atmosphere. Antioxidants are vital for the immune system, helping protect the white blood cells from destroying themselves in the battle against infection.

Copper is necessary for a child's resistance to infection, but in excess can actually suppress the immune system.

Iron is also important. T cells and B cells require oxygen, and haemoglobin to carry it in the bloodstream. However, excess iron can actually reduce resistance, since micro-organisms require iron to multiply.

The metabolism of EFAs into prostaglandins requires magnesium, which when balanced with calcium, is also responsible for normal muscular relaxation. The overuse of artificial fertilizers and phosphorus in preserved foods means magnesium tends to be deficient in diets where there is a predominance of refined or junk foods.

The average diet also tends to be deficient in both selenium and zinc, both vital to the immune system, because poor soil and the overuse of artificial fertilizers produces foods low in these substances. Zinc deficiency can occur among young children who derive much of their nutrition from milk and cheese.

The best way to ensure that children have sufficient of these nutrients is through a diet that is high in fresh, organically grown foods, with as much fresh fruit and vegetables as possible, but that is low in saturated fats. Childrens' diets should provide whole grains, nuts, seeds, beans and pulses, oily fish and cold-pressed vegetable oils. Refined foods, packaged, canned, and frozen foods, excess sugar and salt, fatty meats, dairy produce, cakes, biscuits and sweets should be largely avoided. Many of these are actually classed as "antinutrients", that is they have either very little nutritional value or they disturb EFA metabolism and therefore adversely affect immunity.

Foods to be avoided

- Excessive sugar can compromise the metabolism of EFAs and deplete B vitamins and minerals, particularly magnesium and copper.
- Excess salt, found particularly in processed foods, can upset the sodium/magnesium/potassium balance in the body, and lead to a loss of magnesium and potassium.
- Excessive saturated fats and refined oils can interfere with the body's ability to use EFAs; partially hydrogenated vegetable oils are particularly implicated.
- Preserved, processed foods and soda drinks often contain large amounts of phosphates, which interfere with the absorption of nutrients such as magnesium and calcium from the digestive tract.
- Pesticide residues in food inhibit the body's use of vitamin B6 and increase the body's need for antioxidants.
- When oils are heated, especially oil kept hot all day or used repeatedly to deep-fry fish, chicken and chips, free radicals are created causing damage to cell membranes and EFAs. Antioxidants help prevent such damage, and their defence system involves a number of nutrients including vitamins A, C, B and E and zinc, copper, sulphur and magnesium. Heated oils, pesticides in food, and environmental pollutants all increase the body's requirements of these nutrients, and diverts them from being available to the immune system.

To avoid the possible health risks of food additives and pesticides, parents need to be encouraged to buy fresh organic foods, and if buying manufactured foods to read labels. If parents feel they cannot afford all organic foods, they can be advised to wash everything thoroughly with water and cider vinegar ($\frac{1}{4}$ cup per gallon of water). Vinegar is said to accelerate the breakdown of some pesticides. They can also remove the outer leaves of green vegetables, like cabbage and lettuce, which contain more chemical residues than the inner leaves. Root vegetables can be scrubbed or peeled, and any fruit that has been waxed (such as apples, citrus fruits, peppers, tomatoes) needs to be peeled also.

AYURVEDA AND IMMUNITY

Immunity is known in Ayurveda as *vyadhi kshamatva*. The importance of good digestion is often overlooked when considering immunity and is something that features predominantly in the Ayurvedic system. If the "digestive fire" is good, the food eaten will be digested and assimilated well and the residue of wastes remaining to be eliminated from the body will be minimal. If however, the digestive fire is low, much of what is eaten will remain in the gut as partially digested or undigested food, which begins to ferment and produce toxins. These can permeate the body and in turn lower resistance to a range of health problems, including coughs and colds and flu bugs that children are so prone to in winter. Bearing this in mind among the first steps to enhance immunity are to improve digestion and assimilation and to detoxify the system (see Digestive System, p. 193).

Dietary recommendations

According to Ayurveda one should take the appropriate food for one's constitution, which should be modified according to the season. Ideally food is best eaten in clean and pleasant surroundings for optimal digestion. It is important to be relaxed, and to taste and enjoy one's food. The food should be warm, pleasant, clean, fresh, well-cooked, easy to digest and consist of all the six tastes. Children should eat plenty of foods that promote growth and development, i.e. *Kapha* foods.

In terms of quantity, it is recommended that a child should eat enough food to fill the stomach a third full, and drink water during meals till the total liquid intake is equal to another third. The remaining third of the stomach should remain empty to allow space for the digestive juices to flow, for the stomach contents to churn and mix well with the digestive enzymes, and for free movement of gas. If too much food is eaten it overloads the digestive power and digestion is diminished, as it is when food is eaten too frequently, at irregular times or with too much water. It is best not to drink water before meals as it dilutes the digestive juices. Similarly it is advisable not to drink water after eating oily foods or a large amount of food as the water reduces digestive power.

The six tastes

Ayurveda classifies foods and herbs according to six tastes, sweet, sour, salty, pungent, bitter and astringent. Like the *doshas*, the six tastes are derived from the five great elements (Box 6.1). In fact each substance in nature is composed of all five elements although one or two may predominate. So when we experience a food as sour for example, it means it is mainly sour but contains other secondary tastes. Understanding the effects of each taste on mind and body and the balance of *Vata*, *Pitta* and *Kapha*, means that foods and herbs can be more specifically chosen according to the needs of the individual child. This classification can make them more effective tools for prevention and treatment of imbalance and disease, and has been of enormous value to me in formulating prescriptions and giving dietary advice in my practice.

Rasa is the Sanskrit word which means both taste and emotion. This suggests that taste and emotion correspond with one another. An emotion tends to produce in the body its corresponding taste, just as eating foods or herbs of a specific taste tends to create its corresponding emotion. How much of each *dosha* your body produces depends primarily on which tastes you consume.

- Sweet, sour and salty substances increase *Kapha* and decrease *Vata*
- Pungent, bitter and astringent tastes decrease *Kapha* and increase *Vata*
- Sweet, bitter and astringent tastes decrease *Pitta*
- Pungent, sour and salty tastes increase *Pitta*.

Sweet

Composed mainly of elements Earth and Water, the sweet taste has the effect of increasing *Kapha* and decreasing *Pitta* and *Vata*. Its qualities (*gunas*) are cooling, heavy and unctuous. It reduces *agni*/digestive fire. Sweet-tasting foods are nourishing and soothing to body and mind. They relieve hunger and thirst and produce a feeling of satiety in body and mind after digestion. They promote growth and development of all tissues. Sweet-tasting foods are said to enhance strength and vitality and prolong life. They have a lubricating effect on the skin and hair and nourish the sense organs. Over-indulgence in sweet foods is said to lead to

Box 6.1 The six tastes	
Elements	**Tastes**
Ether and Air	Bitter/*Tikta*
Air and Fire	Pungent/*Katu*
Fire and Water	Salty/*Lavana*
Water and Earth	Sweet/*Madhura*
Earth and Fire	Sour/*Amla*
Earth and Air	Astringent/*Kashaya*

lethargy, overweight, heaviness, colds, coughs, complacency, and a tendency to constipation, increasing the naturally inert complacency of *Kapha*, cooling the anger of *Pitta* and comforting the anxiety of *Vata* (Athique M 1998).

Sour

Composed mainly of Earth and Fire, the sour taste increases *Pitta* and *Kapha* and decreases *Vata*. Its qualities (*gunas*) are heating, heavy and unctuous. Sour-tasting foods and herbs have a refreshing effect, stimulating the mind, encouraging elimination of wastes and increasing the flow of saliva and other digestive juices. They increase appetite, improve digestion and regulate peristalsis. They build up all tissues except the reproductive tissues (Athique M 1998). After digestion sour tasting foods are said to increase the desire for more, either food or general acquisitiveness. Sour promotes the evaluation of things in order to determine their desirability. Over-indulgence in evaluation is said to lead to envy or jealousy, which may manifest as depreciation of the thing desired, as in the Sour Grapes syndrome. This can increase *Kapha*'s aquisitiveness, if envy of another's success incites one to obtain more for oneself. *Pitta* can increase if jealousy changes into anger or resentment and envy helps reduce *Vata* by focusing the mind and motivating consistent action.

Salty

Composed mainly of Water and Fire, salty tasting foods and herbs increase *Kapha* and *Pitta* and decrease *Vata*. Their qualities are heavy, heating and unctuous. Salty is called "all tastes", *sarva rasa* in Sanskrit, because it can enhance all flavours in food while at the same time increasing appetite for food. The salty taste aids elimination of wastes, thereby having a detoxifying effect. While in small amounts it promotes appetite and digestion, in large amounts it aggravates *Pitta* symptoms such as indigestion, heat and rashes. It also is said to weaken muscles and can cause premature ageing. Excess salty foods increase water retention.

The salty taste is associated with zest for life, which enhances all appetites. Over-indulgence is said to lead to hedonism, which distracts the mind. Small amounts increase the mind's desire for intensity of experience. Over-use is said to make the mind weak, increasing complacency as long as one is able to indulge, which increases *Kapha*. It increases the fieriness of *Pitta's* anger whenever there is an obstruction to gratification and decreases *Vata* by allaying fears (Athique M 1998).

Pungent

Composed mainly of Fire and Air, the pungent taste increases *Pitta* and *Vata*, and decreases *Kapha*. Its qualities (*gunas*) are heating, light and dry. Pungent foods and herbs flush secretions from the body and reduce *Kapha*-like secretions such as mucus, semen, milk and fat. They stimulate the flow of digestive juices, improving appetite, digestion and absorption. Pungent herbs and foods help to destroy bacteria and parasites, and their heating effect cause the eyes to water and the nose to run, and increase circulation and sweating. They stimulate the mind and senses and help to reduce obesity, remove obstructions and open the channels (Frawley D 2000). Pungency is associated with extroversion, the tendency to excitement and stimulation and particularly the craving for intensity, too much of which can lead to irritability, impatience and anger. Pungency relieves *Kapha* by increasing motivation and temporarily relieves *Vata* by enhancing self-expression. In the long run it increases *Vata* by dispersing energy, leaving one depleted and exhausted. Strongly pungent medicines are contraindicated in children and conditions associated with high *Pitta*.

Bitter

Composed mainly of Air and Ether, the bitter taste increases *Vata* and decreases *Pitta* and *Kapha*. Its qualities (*gunas*) are cooling, light and dry.

Bitter-tasting foods and herbs in small amounts are said to return all tastes to normal and decrease food craving and are considered the best of all six tastes. Bitter tastes increase appetite and improve digestion and have a detoxifying effect in the digestive tract, helpful in the treatment of skin disease and fevers. They also help to reduce weight and aid elimination of excess water from the body. The bitter taste is associated with dissatisfaction, which promotes a desire to change. Swallowing a bitter pill means dispelling delusion and facing reality. By stimulating a desire for change, bitter taste can reduce the complacency of *Kapha*, but overuse increases *Vata* as dissatisfaction and continuous change can increase insecurity and anxiety.

Astringent

Composed mainly of Air and Earth, the astringent taste increases *Vata* and decreases *Pitta* and *Kapha*. Its qualities are cooling, light and dry. Astringent-tasting foods and herbs tone, dry and constrict all parts of the body, reducing secretions. Their styptic properties promote healing of wounds, and reduce bleeding. They help to reduce excess water by their drying effect. Excess astringent-tasting foods and herbs inhibit excretion of faeces, urine and sweat and cause accumulation of toxins in the body (see *Vata* diseases, p. 178). Astringency is associated with introversion, shrinking away from excitement and stimulation. Too much introversion can increase insecurity, anxiety and fear, that characterizes *Vata* types.

When taste is experienced in the mouth it is transmitted to the brain, which determines the type of substances that have been ingested and the digestive enzymes needed for optimal digestion. By the time the food reaches the gut the digestive organs should be prepared. For this reason it is important that children taste the food they are eating properly, and this is best ensured by sitting down to eat at the table, and doing nothing else that would distract them, such as watching TV.

According to Ayurveda there are three different effects of food and herbs:

- *Rasa* or Taste. The effect foods and herbs have before digestion, determined by taste buds while food is in the mouth.

- *Virya* or Energy, experienced during digestion. Hot food increases the body's ability to digest, freeing energy for other metabolic tasks. Cold food requires extra energy for its digestion. The gut obtains this from the rest of the body, which must reduce its other activities as a result. This may explain why certain foods tend to make one lethargic after eating.
- *Vipaka* or Post Digestive Effect, occurs after digestion when the nutrients are assimilated deep within the tissues (Box 6.2).

Sour, Salty and Pungent are always hot.
Sweet, Bitter and Astringent are always cold.

A substance may have a heating taste with a cold energy, which means that when it enters the body it increases digestive power but during digestion it does not aggravate *Pitta*. A substance may have a cooling taste and hot energy, reducing appetite when eaten but increasing digestive juice flow while digestion is going on. A good example of this is the bitter taste.

Cooling tastes (sweet, bitter and astringent) have a cold and contracting effect on the emotions. They decrease our desire to eat more. Heating tastes have a hot and expansive effect, increasing our desire to eat more. Cooked onions for example are sweet in taste, hot in energy and sweet in post digestive effect. They satisfy hunger with their sweet taste and promote anabolism with their sweet post digestive effect, but their hot energy does not permit *Kapha* to be disturbed by their sweetness (Athique M 1998).

Salty is the most important taste to control *Vata* as it is heavy, oily, heating and improves digestion. Sour comes next, then sweet. Bitter is the best taste to control *Pitta* as it is cooling and drying. Then sweet, then astringent. Pungent is the best taste for controlling *Kapha* because it is heating, light and dry and flushes secretions from the body. Bitter comes next, then astringent.

A child with a *Pitta* constitution is advised to drink water after meals as otherwise he may suffer from burning in the stomach and *Pitta* disorders like eye diseases, headache and piles. Eating hot food and drinks in excess increases *Pitta*. Taking excess cold food and drinks gives rise to *Kapha* and *Vata* diseases such as anorexia, colicky pain, hiccup, headache, laziness and increased stools (Tables 6.1–6.3).

Daily activities

The daily activities of a child will clearly have an effect on their general health. In Ayurveda there are clear guidelines for a healthy lifestyle that addresses almost every aspect of daily living and this is the basis of preventative medicine. This is known as *dinacharya* or daily routine (Athavale 2000).

Rising

Parents should teach children how to pray or meditate regularly on rising. A regular bowel movement on rising is ideal for maintaining health. The face can be washed with a decoction of amalaki. The hands should be washed regularly, before praying, eating and when they are dirty.

Teeth and gums

According to Ayurveda, teeth are a by-product of bone. In India neem and liquorice stems are chewed and used as a toothbrush. A universal toothpaste is made from sesame oil mixed with fine powder of ginger (*Zingiber officinale*), pepper, pippali (*Piper longum*), cardamom, triphala, khadira (*Acacia catechu*) and rock salt. Ground almond shell is also used to make tooth powder in India. The gums can be massaged daily with triphala powder mixed with sesame oil to nourish bone tissue (*asthi dhatu*). Cavities in the teeth and receding gums are signs of *Vata* aggravation in the skeletal system, and often related to a deficiency of calcium, magnesium and zinc. To prevent these problems it is recommended that children chew a handful of

Box 6.2	Effects of foods and herbs	
Taste	**Energy**	**Post Digestive**
Sweet	Cold	Sweet
Sour	Hot	Sour
Salty	Hot	Sweet
Pungent	Hot	Pungent
Bitter	Cold	Pungent
Astringent	Cold	Pungent

Table 6.1 *Vata* reducing diet

	Decrease		Increase	
Fruits	Dried fruits		Sweet fruits	Apricots
	Cranberries		Avocado	Bananas
	Persimmon		Berries	Cherries
	Watermelon		Coconut	Figs (fresh)
	Pears		Grapefruit	Grapes
	Pomegranate		Lemons	Mango
	Apples		Melons (sweet)	Peaches
			Papaya	Pineapples
Vegetables	Brussels sprouts	Cabbage	Beets	Okra (cooked)
	Cauliflower	Leafy greens	Cucumber	Potato (sweet)
	Celery	Lettuce	Green beans	Courgette
	Eggplant	Mushrooms	Onion (cooked)	Asparagus
	Onions (raw)	Parsley	Radishes	
	Peas	Peppers	Cooked vegetables	
	Potatoes	Spinach	Carrots	
	Sprouts	Tomatoes	Garlic	
	Raw vegetables	Broccoli		
Grains	Barley	Buckwheat	Oats (cooked)	
	Corn	Millet	Rice	
	Oats (dry)	Rye	Wheat	
Animal foods	Lamb		Beef	
	Pork		Chicken or turkey	
	Rabbit		(white meat)	
	Venison		Eggs (fried or scrambled)	
			Seafood	

Others
Legumes: None except mung beans, tofu, black and red lentils
Nuts: All are OK in small quantities
Seeds: All are OK (in moderation)
Sweetening agents: All are OK except white sugar and aspartame
Condiments: All spices are good, except excess cayenne, dry ginger and cinnamon
Dairy: All dairy products are OK (in moderation)
Oils: All cold pressed oils are good, particularly sesame

calcium-rich black sesame seeds every morning, then brush the teeth without toothpaste so that the residue of the sesame seeds is rubbed against the teeth, polishing and cleaning them. To prevent receding gums, tooth infection and cavities, the gums can be massaged daily with sesame oil. Take a mouthful of sesame oil and swish it from side to side for 2–3 minutes then spit out the oil, then gently massage the gums with the index finger (Lad 1999). Chewing food well stimulates the gums and helps to keep them healthy. Eating four figs every day is said to strengthen teeth and gums alike.

Drinking cold water

Pitta constitution children should take cool water first thing in the morning. When taken in through the nose, using a netty pot, water is said to improve eyesight and is good for the sinuses.

Eyes

Anu taila in the nose and sesame oil in the ears is said to be good for the eyes. Adequate sleep is important. Taking $\frac{1}{4} - \frac{1}{2}$ tsp of Triphala regularly at night with honey and ghee is a good eye tonic.

Table 6.2 *Pitta* reducing diet

	Decrease		Increase	
Fruits	Sour fruits	Apricots	Sweet fruits	Apples
	Berries	Bananas	Avocado	Coconut
	Cherries	Cranberries	Figs	Grapes (dark)
	Grapefruit	Grapes (green)	Mango	Melons
	Lemons	Oranges (sour)	Oranges (sweet)	Pears
	Plums (sour)	Papaya	Pineapples (sweet)	Plums (sweet)
	Peaches	Pineapples (sour)	Pomegranate	Prunes
	Persimmon		Raisins	
Vegetables	Pungent		Sweet and bitter	Brussels sprouts
	vegetables		vegetables	Cucumber
	Carrots		Cabbage	Celery
	Garlic		Cauliflower	Leafy greens
	Peppers (hot)		Green beans	Mushrooms
	Spinach		Lettuce	Peas
	Beets		Okra	Peppers (green)
	Eggplant		Parsley	Sprouts
	Onions		Potatoes	Asparagus
	Radishes		Broccoli	
	Tomatoes		Zucchini	
Grains	Millet	Oats (dry)	Rice (basmati)	Rice (white)
	Rice (brown)	Rye	Wheat	Oats (cooked)
	Buckwheat	Corn	Barley	
Animal foods	Beef		Chicken or turkey (white meat)	
	Lamb		Rabbit	
	Seafood		Eggs (white)	
	Eggs (yolk)		Shrimp (small amount)	
	Pork		Venison	
Dairy oils	Buttermilk	Cheese	Butter (unsalted)	Cottage cheese
	Sour cream	Yoghurt	Ghee	Milk
	Almond	Corn	Coconut	Olive
	Safflower	Sesame	Sunflower	Soy

Others
Legumes: All OK except lentils
Nuts: No except coconut
Seeds: No except sunflower and pumpkin
Sweetening agents: All OK except molasses and honey and aspartame
Condiments: No spices except coriander, fresh ginger, cardamom, fennel, turmeric and a small amount of black pepper

Milk with shatavari is recommended for the eyes. Looking at or touching auspicious objects is said to be good for the mind.

Ears

Sesame or coconut oil can be dropped into the ears daily.

Nose

Two drops of anu taila oil are recommended, administered to the nose each morning. Children with *Pitta* constitution or a tendency to nosebleeds can use ghee mixed with a little saffron. For a dry nose that tends to block easily, sesame oil medicated with bala can be used as nose drops.

Table 6.3   *Kapha* reducing diet

	Decrease		Increase	
Fruits	Sweet and sour fruits	Avocado	Apples	Apricots
	Figs (fresh)	Coconut	Berries	Cherries
	Grapes	Grapefruit	Cranberries	Figs (dry)
	Melons	Lemons	Mango	Peaches
	Bananas	Oranges	Pears	Persimmon
	Pineapples	Papaya	Pomegranate	Prunes
		Plums	Raisins	
Vegetables	Sweet and juicy vegetables		Pungent and bitter vegetables	Sprouts
	Courgettes		Brussels sprouts	Asparagus
	Potatoes (sweet)		Carrots	Broccoli
	Cucumber		Celery	Cabbage
	Tomatoes		Garlic	Cauliflower
			Lettuce	Eggplant
			Okra	Leafy greens
			Parsley	Mushrooms
			Peppers	Onions
			Radishes	Peas
			Beets	Potatoes (white)
				Spinach
Grains	Rice (white)	Rice (brown)	Millet	Oats (dry)
	Oats (cooked)		Rice (basmati)	Small amount of rye
	Wheat		Barley	Corn
Animal foods	Beef		Chicken or turkey (dark meat)	
	Lamb		Eggs (not fried – scrambled)	
	Pork		Rabbit	
	Seafood		Shrimp	
			Venison	

Others
Legumes: All are good except kidney beans, soy beans, black lentils and mung beans
Nuts: None
Seeds: No except sunflower and pumpkin
Sweetening agents: No sweeteners except raw honey
Condiments: All spices are good except salt
Dairy: None except ghee and goat milk
Oils: None except almond, corn or sunflower in small amounts

Bhastrika, i.e. forceful expiration from each nostril with the mouth closed, keeps the air passages clean and helps prevent respiratory infections.

Voice

Sucking cloves is recommended for the voice. Two drops of anu taila oil in the throat and gargling with sesame oil medicated with clove or rose is also recommended. Cold drinks and ice cream should be avoided.

Gargling

After brushing the teeth, the mouth should be rinsed and the child should gargle with water. Sesame oil is particularly recommended if the gums are sensitive to sour foods.

Oil massage

Massage of the body with sesame oil for 15 minutes every day improves the complexion of the skin and condition of the hair, tones muscles and blood vessels and exerts a soothing action on the skin and nervous system. If short of time, oil can be used to drop in the ear and massage the neck, head, spine and soles. Sesame oil massage is said to improve vision, enhance the five senses, induce restful sleep and is reputed to delay ageing. Oil massage of the soles is reputed to be good for the eyes. It can be done in all seasons except summer.

Exercise

Exercise should be taken regularly in the morning till the child perspires or feels the need to mouth breathe. Vigorous exercise should be taken in winter and spring. Yoga is good for the spine and organs of digestion, respiration, etc. and is advised for older children, to help keep the mind strong.

Bathing

A bath should be taken regularly, at least once a day. A healthy child should use warm water for the body and cold water for the head, and scrub the skin with a paste of devadaru (*Cedrus deodar*) amalaki (*Emblica off.*). Warm water medicated with holy basil leaves is good for *Vata* constitution. Children with *Pitta* constitution can use cold water with sandalwood or manjista (*Rubia cordifolia*). *Kapha* children are best with hot water medicated with kadambari (*Anthocephalus indicus*) or pepper.

After the bath is the recommended time for prayer.

Diet

Children should eat sweet, nourishing and strengthening foods such as fresh cow's milk, butter and ghee. As well as modifying diet according to the constitution it should also be varied according to the child's state of health and the season (see p. 151). Heavy foods are best avoided at night. After lunch the child should take a short walk and sleep in the afternoon. In the evening the child should stroll in the open air, play outdoor games to refresh mind and body. Before bed the child should pray or meditate again.

Sleep

Absence of worries, oil massage, instilling drops into the ear, a bath, a good dinner and a comfortable bed in a soothing environment should ensure a good night's sleep.

Rasayanas

Tonic herbs, which are renowned for their ability to improve the quality of the tissues, should be started in early infancy. They include: ashwagandha, bibhitaki, pippali, shatavari, gotu kola, amalaki, haritaki, liquorice, guduchi, bala, gokshura (*Tribulus terrestris*), punarnava (*Boerhavia diffusa*) and Chayawan prash (the most important ingredient of which is amalaki).

Rasayanas can be physical as well as more subtle. Good conduct, pursuit of one's studies, true knowledge and meditation act as rasayanas.

HERBS FOR THE IMMUNE SYSTEM

The immune system is composed of many different parts working together to protect the body. It has built-in regulators that tell it when to turn on and off. It consists of the lymph system organs, white blood cells, and specialized cells and chemicals including antibodies. Should pathogenic micro-organisms overcome our homoeostatic mechanisms and invade the body, the immune system rallies its defences to deal with it by general (non-specific immunity) and specific means (cellular immunity). Macrophages work with cytokine chemicals in general immunity while lymphocytes and antibodies destroy specific antigens. The thymus gland aids the production of and stores T cells to attack cells infected by bacteria, fungi and viruses. It is also responsible for secreting hormones that regulate immune activity. The thymus gland is important to the establishment of children's immunity and for this reason is larger in children than in adults. It requires adequate dietary zinc in order to function efficiently. There are certain herbs that are capable of enhancing the function of the thymus gland including echinacea, ginseng (*Panax ginseng* and *Eleuthrococcus senticosus*), neem leaf, and liquorice (Tillotson et al 2001).

The spleen, liver, tonsils, adenoids and wall of the intestine also contain lymphatic tissue. The latter is responsible for maintaining lymphocytes capable of responding to all the antigens that enter the body through food entering the digestive tract. Common childhood infections such as rubella and chickenpox cause lymphatic swelling and tenderness as the immune system rallies its defences.

Cellular immunity

When specific immune responses (cellular immunity) are called into action, molecules on the surface of infecting organisms (antigens) stimulate lymphocytes and produce antibodies to destroy the antigens. These have a memory so that antigens are recognized should infection reoccur, ensuring the body is able to respond effectively to the organisms before an infection develops next time.

B cells and T cells are the major lymphocytes responsible for antibody formation. T cells mature in the thymus gland and comprise 60–70% of blood lymphocytes. Certain herbs are able to enhance antibody response, including echinacea, golden seal (*Hydrastis canadensis*), ginseng, guduchi and punarnava (*Boerhavia diffusa*) (Tillotson et al 2001).

There are three types of T cells. Killer T cells attack infected or damaged cells with cell poison and release chemicals that attract phagocytes and interferon, which inhibits viral infection. Several herbs are capable of increasing natural killer (NK) cell activity including liquorice, garlic, ginseng, mistletoe (*Viscum album*) ganodema and shitake mushrooms (Tillotson et al 2001). Shitake mushrooms have been shown to exhibit antifungal activity and exerted an inhibitory activity on HIV-1 reverse transcriptase and leukaemia cells (Ngai and Ng 2003).

Other T-helper cells communicate with B cells to help the killer cells. They secrete interleukin 2, which stimulates further production of T cells stimulating their defence mechanisms, while T-suppressor cells control the action of other lymphocytes and stop this action from getting out of hand, calling a halt to the defences once the infection is resolved. If suppressor cells are low, infection and inflammation can persist. Garlic, ginseng, astragalus (*Astragalus membranaceous*) and liquorice have been shown to regulate T-cell activity.

B cells produce antibodies to bind to specific antigens. These antibodies mature in bone marrow and are distributed to other lymph tissue – spleen, tonsils, GI tract, etc. and make up 10–20%

of blood lymphocytes. Some then transform into plasma cells which make the antibodies for the bloodstream: IgG, IgA, IgE, IgM, etc. IgA is an antibody found in mucosal secretions in the upper respiratory and digestive tract. Liquorice, carotene – vitamin A, and schizandra (*Schizandra chinensis*) berry all increase IgA supply. IgG is the most prevalent antibody in blood serum. Increasing IgG in early stages of infection can speed resolution of infection. Echinacea and golden seal increase IgG and IgM. In vitro research suggests that codonopsis (*Codonopsis dangshen*) may stimulate Ig production by B cells (Shan et al 1999). Other B cells transform into B-memory cells, which provide further immunity against recurrences. Liquorice, ginseng, ashwagandha, astragalus, and carthamnus flower (*Carthamus tinctorius*) have been shown to modulate B-cell activity (Tillotson et al 2001).

In chronic inflammation and allergy, IgG needs to be reduced and both liquorice and guduchi decrease IgG. IgE found in respiratory and intestinal mucosa, binds to mast cells and basophils and stimulates secretion of chemicals such as histamine. Herbs that reduce and inhibit IgE-mediated allergic reactions, include echinacea, garlic, golden seal, feverfew (*Tanacetum parthenium*) turmeric and chamomile. An extract of seven plants including *Emblica off.*, *Terminalia chebula*, *T. bellerica*, *Albizia lebbeck*, *Piper nigrum*, *Zingiber officinale* and *P. longum* has been shown to have an antihistamine and antiallergic effect in vitro (Amit et al 2003). Many herbs have been demonstrated to act on the reticuloendothelial system, increasing numbers and activity of phagocytes. These include ginseng, guduchi, codonopsis, cat's claw (*Uncaria tormentosa*), ashwagandha, liquorice, garlic, astragalus, echinacea and olive leaf (*Olea europea*).

Neutrophils are phagocytes that live in bone marrow and aid in prevention and treatment of bacterial infections, fungal and parasitic infections and cancer. Garlic, guduchi, black cumin (*Nigella sativa*), ginseng and mistletoe increase neutrophil activity. Eosinophils and basophils secrete chemicals that break down antigen–antibody complexes related to allergy. Boswellia gum (*Boswellia serrata*), feverfew and turmeric root all affect eosinophil function. Mast cells are activated when antigens bind to their surface IgE receptors causing allergic reactions and they release histamine and other chemicals that increase vascular permeability. It is important to calm mast cell action to resolve chronic allergies. The following herbs stabilize mast cell activity: liquorice root, ginkgo leaf (*Ginkgo biloba*), lavender oil, katuki (*Picrorrhiza kurroa*), devadaru (*Cedrus deodar*), *Andrographis panniculata*, vasaca leaf (*Adhatoda vasica*). Celery seed (*Apium graveolens*), arjuna bark (*Terminalia arjuna*), echinacea, ginkgo leaf, flaxseed (*Linum usitatissimum*), peppermint leaf and grapes all contain luteolin which inhibits histamine and leukotriene release.

Non-specific immunity

Cytokines are immune system messenger molecules which are responsible for attacking viruses, anti-inflammatory effects, activation of immune cells and blood cell formation. Mistletoe (*Viscum album*) has been shown to stimulate a number of pro-inflammatory cytokines (Gorter et al 2003). astragalus, echinacea, *Panax ginseng* and garlic also affect cytokines.

Interferon is secreted by cells when attacked by a virus, signalling killer T cells to increase their activity and intervene with viral replication. Ginseng, garlic, ashwagandha, mistletoe and liquorice all enhance interferon activity.

Interleukins are proteins that stimulate white blood cell activity. Interleukin 1 helps produce fever, interleukin 2 (T-cell growth factor) stimulates T-cell production and has an effect on nerve cells and conduction of nerve impulses. Ginseng, ashwagandha, nigella, astragalus, garlic, bupleurum root (*Bupleurum chinense*) and cat's claw bark all moderate production of interleukins (Tillotson et al 2001).

When out of balance, the immune system can be either overactive or underactive. If overactive the body becomes vulnerable to inflammation and tissue destruction. If deficient and underactive, resistance is lowered and one becomes susceptible to infection. T-cell deficiency increases susceptibility to yeast infections, bacterial sepsis and Epstein–Barr infections (Tillotson et al 2001). B-cell deficiency includes susceptibility to staphylococcal and streptococcal infections. Since babies are born with very little of their own immunity, only that inherited from their mother which lasts for the first year (passive immunity), breast-feeding is important as it provides many of the raw materials needed for immunity. In order to produce specific antibodies to specific infecting micro-organisms, an initial infection is necessary. This is one of the reasons children up to the age of 8–10 years tend to develop infections frequently.

Once bacteria and viruses have been eliminated by the body's defences, the debris needs to be cleared by the liver. All foods and toxins absorbed via the intestines are also taken to the liver where white blood cells (natural immunity cells like Kupffer cells) destroy unwanted matter, dead cells, hormones, toxins, drugs, pesticides and food additives, by enzymatic reactions in the liver. Efficient functioning of the liver is therefore vital to the maintenance of a healthy immune system. If it is struggling under too great a burden of toxins, the liver will not be able to respond effectively in response to an infection when necessary. There are several herbs which have been well documented for their ability to support liver function including milk thistle (*Cardus marianus*), dandelion (*Taraxacum off.*) and rosemary (*Rosmarinus off.*).

Self-heal (*Prunella vulgaris*), although largely neglected by Western herbalists, is an important herb in Chinese medicine. The bitters have a stimulating action on the liver and gallbladder, and self-heal is prescribed for symptoms of jaundice and liver problems. It is also recommended for gout. Self-heal is used for headaches, particularly when related to tension and photophobia. Research has indicated that *Prunella* has a potent antiviral action, including activity against HIV (Zheng 1990, Yamasaki et al 1993). This combined with an immunomodulatory effect of the polysaccharides (Markova et al 1997) makes *Prunella* well worth bearing in mind when considering immunity especially since it grows as a weed in temperate climates. Rosmarinic acid contributes to antioxidant effects of *Prunella* (Lamaison et al 1991), whilst trials suggest it has antimutagenic effects, indicating possible use as an anticancer herb (Lee and Lin 1988). Self-heal can also be taken for swollen glands, mumps, glandular fever and mastitis. As an astringent, it can be taken for diarrhoea and colitis.

Spices such as ginger, cinnamon, cardamom, coriander, clove, black pepper and asafoetida are some of the best remedies for the digestion and for raising immunity and these can be taken in food and as tasty hot teas. The pungent effects of ginger, for example, warm and strengthen the digestion, stimulate the flow of digestive juices and invigorate the whole system. The volatile oils are highly antiseptic (Mascolo et al 1989), activating immunity and dispelling bacterial and viral infections. Similarly cinnamon is warming and strengthening, invigorating the digestion and detoxifying the body. The volatile oil in cinnamon is one of the strongest natural antiseptics known. Its antimicrobial properties make it an excellent medicine to prevent and resolve a whole range of infections. A hot cup of cinnamon tea, with its expectorant and decongestant actions, is often used in the relief of coughs and colds, flu and catarrh. Cinnamaldehyde found in cinnamon essential oil has strong antibacterial activity (Chang et al 2001), whilst cinnamon essential oil has also been found to have antifungal effects (Ranasinghe et al 2002).

Some of the most significant immune enhancers that are used by modern herbalists include echinacea (*Echinacea angustifolia*), golden seal (*Hydrastis canadensis*), liquorice (*Glycyrrhiza glabra*), garlic (*Allium sativum*), guduchi (*Tinospora cordifolia*) and astragalus (*Astragalus membranaceus*).

Without doubt the most popular immune-boosting herb in this country today is echinacea. This amazing herb can improve the immune system in many ways including increasing activity of T cells, interferon and natural killer cells and raising properdin levels (Kim et al 2002, Barrett 2003). Properdin activates the alternative complement pathway, which is responsible for increasing non-specific host defence mechanisms like neutralization of viruses, destruction of bacteria and increasing the migration of white blood cells to the areas of infection. There has been some discussion that echinacea may work best as a preventative if it is not taken continuously, but there is little evidence to back this up. Echinacea has been shown to be one of the best alternatives to antibiotics, useful for all chronic and acute bacterial and viral infections. For good effect it should be taken every 2 hours during acute infections.

There is recent evidence that sheds some light on how echinacea can affect the immune system. The study involved 48 healthy women who received one of six treatments for 4 weeks:

- An extract of *E. purpurea*
- *E. purpurea* + *E. angustifolia*
- Ultrarefined *E. purpurea* + *E. angustifolia*
- *E. purpurea* + *E. angustifolia* + larch arabinogalactan, another immune-booster
- Larch arabinogalactan
- Placebo.

Complement properdin, a mark of immune function, was measured initially and at the end of the trial. After 4 weeks of treatment, those taking *E. purpurea* + *E. angustifolia* as well as those taking *E. purpurea* + *E. angustifolia* + *larch* arabinogalactan showed significant increases in complement properdin − 21 and 18%, respectively. These treatment groups also showed improvements in overall physical and emotional health. Larch arabinogalactan (*Larix occidentalis* extract) on its own did not increase complement properdin but, the authors admit, the duration of the study may have been too short for any significant change brought on by this herb to be noticeable. These findings suggest that, with or without larch arabinogalactan, echinacea appears to boost that part of the immune system ultimately responsible for killing viruses and bacteria (Kim et al 2002).

The antibiotic activity of golden seal's alkaloids against a wide range of infecting organisms, including *Staphylococcus* spp., *Streptococcus* spp., *Diplococcal pneumonia*, are well documented (Hwang et al 2003, Scazzocchio et al 2001). Golden seal also has remarkable immunostimulatory activity, increasing blood supply to the spleen and thereby promoting optimal activity of the spleen and the release of immune-potentiating compounds. One of the alkaloids, berberine, is a potent activator of macrophages (Kang et al 2002). It should be noted that only sustainable sources of golden seal should be used.

Liquorice is another great immune enhancer. Honoured for thousands of years as a treatment for inflammatory conditions, modern studies have documented that liquorice has steroid-like actions (Shibata 2000). It enhances immunity by stimulating formation and efficiency of white blood cells and antibodies. It is effective against candida and several types of bacteria including the *Staph.* spp. It has antiviral effects and contains a compound that enhances interferon production (Pompei et al

1979, Shinada et al 1986). This in turn increases antiviral activity, as interferon binds to cell surfaces and stimulates the synthesis of proteins that impair the ability of viruses, including herpes, to survive. It contains phyto-oestrogens, sugars and flavonoids. The most investigated component is glycyrrhizic acid, which seems to be responsible for many of liquorice's anti-inflammatory properties. In the stomach glycyrrhizic acid is converted into glycyrrhetic acid, which inhibits the enzyme that metabolizes the natural steroid cortisol, resulting in higher circulating levels of this steroid with its anti-inflammatory effects. Components of liquorice act as powerful antioxidants. Liquorice is particularly useful for treating respiratory tract infections such as pharyngitis, bronchitis and pneumonia. Numerous studies have demonstrated it to be beneficial to the liver and to support the adrenal glands, providing protection from the effects of stress.

Astragalus taken regularly as a preventative also boosts resistance to colds, flu and other viruses. Chinese research supports the fact it has an immune-enhancing action (Sun et al 1983). It has antiviral and antibacterial properties, stimulates production of interferon and enhances the production of T cells. *Astragalus membranaceus* extract is effective in enhancing human immunofunction and antitumour activity. It could be applied in clinical practice for immuno modulation and tumour treatment (Wang et al 2002). Astragalus has a broad anti-inflammatory effect in human amnion and may be considered a promising agent to protect preterm labour (Shon and Nam 2003).

Preliminary research suggests that chamomile, calendula, burdock, red clover (*Trifolium pratense*), marshmallow (*Althaea off.*) all have immune-boosting properties similar to echinacea. They all have a long history of use by herbalists in treatments of immune-related properties. Burdock, for example, has been used around the world to inhibit and slow the growth of cancerous tumours. Aromatic herbs including thyme, lavender, bergamot (*Citrus bergamotia*), rosemary, tea tree (*Melalenca alterifolia*), eucalyptus, cardamom, cinnamon, ginger, black pepper, sage (*Salvia off.*) and lemon balm (*Melissa off.*) all contain immune-stimulating compounds, notably the volatile oils. Other herbs indicated to inhibit tumour growth are gotu kola, kelp (*Fucus*

vesiculosus) and dandelion. Olive leaves (*Olea europea*) have been shown in vitro to be active against *E. coli* and *C. albicans* (Markin et al 2003).

The root of the Peruvian rain forest herb "una de gato" or cat's claw (*Uncaria tomentosa*), which got its name because of its claw-like stems, has been used by the Peruvian Indians for centuries for immune problems. It is now a popular remedy here for treating immune problems, acute infections, rheumatoid arthritis, gastric ulcers, colitis, Crohn's disease, herpes, candida, and leaky bowel syndrome associated with allergies. It has been shown to significantly enhance proliferation of human B and T lymphocytes (Wurm et al 1998). Cat's claw is particularly applicable for prevention of coughs and colds and also for treating urinary tract problems associated with lowered immunity.

Elderberries (*Sambucus nigra*) have attracted attention lately for their immune-enhancing properties and their ability to increase antibody response to infection. For centuries they have been popular as a flu remedy. Lately they have been found to contain compounds, lignans and flavonoids, that help to prevent flu viruses from penetrating the cell membranes. With their bitter and pungent tastes, they have a detoxifying effect and help resolve heat and inflammation. They are used in the treatment of respiratory tract infections including sore throats and sinus infections. Elderberry syrup (Box 6.3) is a palatable way to administer this to children and may be preferable to taste buds than bitter golden seal or tongue numbing echinacea.

The humble garlic bulb, much maligned for its malodorous effects, has been revered throughout

---

Box 6.3   Recipe for Elderberry syrup

Two cups of elderberries
500 ml water
$\frac{1}{4}$ cup of honey
$\frac{1}{4}$ cup of lemon juice
  Cook the berries in the water for a few minutes until they are soft and blend with the honey and lemon juice. Pour the puree into a clean bottle and store in the fridge. Take a tablespoonful in hot water once or twice a day as a preventative of infections.

history. It is one of the best antimicrobial herbs in the *Materia Medica*. It is an excellent detoxificant, it stimulates digestion, and is an effective expectorant and decongestant for coughs, colds and catarrh. Its antibiotic activity was noted by Louis Pasteur in 1858 and garlic was employed by Albert Schweitzer in Africa for the treatment of amoebic dysentery. Modern research from numerous studies has shown garlic to significantly enhance various aspects of the immune system and to have antimicrobial activity against many types of bacteria, virus, worms and fungi, including *Candida albicans*. It has even proved itself effective against infections that have become immune to antibiotics (Weber et al 1992).

The best and of course most economical way to take garlic is to eat it regularly. It is best raw as cooking destroys a large percentage of its medicinal properties. This is a recipe for a Greek dip known as Skordalia which my children were given regularly when they were young and which fortunately they loved (Box 6.4).

Citrus/grapefruit seed (*Citrus paradisi*) extract is known to be an effective antimicrobial remedy. It contains constituents which include flavonoids, citric acid and vitamin C. Laboratory tests have demonstrated its effect on a variety of different pathogenic bacteria and fungi in 10–500 parts per million and 500–2000 parts per million, respectively. Tests carried out by Kerry Bone showed that a 0.5% concentration of citrus seed extract was effective against a wide range of bacteria including

Escherichia coli, Salmonella typhi, Staphylococcus aureus and *Streptococcus pyrogens, Enterococcus faecalis, Corynebacterium* spp., *Proteus, Bacillus, Mycobacterium* spp., *Pasteurella multocida*; also against fungi including: *Aspergillus flavus, Aspergillus niger, Penicillium* spp., *Fusarium* spp., *Trychophyton interdigital, Candida albicans* and micro-organisms: *Pseudomonas* and *Coliform*. A study was carried out on a group with atopic eczema, whose faecal microflora had raised counts of haemolytic coliforms and *Staphylococcus, Candida* spp. and pathogenic *Clostridium* spp. as well as raised levels of lactic acid-producing bacteria. When a dose of 150 mg/four drops of citrus seed extract was given three times daily, counts of *Candida, Goetrichum* and haemolytic *E. coli* as well as *Staph. aur.* were reduced (Bone 1996).

Ginseng is another remarkable herb, famous for its ability to boost energy and immunity and to increase resilience to stress, both physical and mental/emotional. *Panax ginseng* is recommended to children for convalescence, when run down by illness or stress, increasing white blood cell count and aiding the liver and spleen in their immunological work. It is not to be taken in the acute phase of disease or if there is inflammation. Siberian ginseng (*Eleutherococcus senticosus*), a similar well-known adaptogen also increases resistance to both physical and emotional stress and improves immunity.

Guduchi (*Tinospora cordifolia*) is known in Sanskrit as Amrit nectar, which means immortality. This herb has demonstrated its ability to enhance antibody and cellular immunity. Many studies have evaluated the effects of guduchi on the immune system and showed that it can enhance antibody production and improve macrophage function (Kapil and Sharma 1997). It does not appear to have direct antibiotic activity but to stimulate the body's immune defence system to function more effectively against bacterial, fungal and parasitic infections (Thatte et al 1992). It is used traditionally to treat a wide range of infections but it also acts as an adaptogen which enables the body to cope better with physical and mental stress. It is considered rejuvenative as well as detoxifying. It is often a component of formulae to treat chronic skin problems such as eczema.

Amalaki (*Emblica officinalis*) and shatavari (*Asparagus racemosus*) are other immune-enhancing

---

Box 6.4   Skordalia

Two potatoes, peeled
Four large garlic cloves, peeled
Juice of one lemon
$\frac{2}{3}$ cup of water
$\frac{2}{3}$ cup of olive oil
Six black peppercorns
Salt to taste
   Cook the potatoes in water until soft. Drain. Puree all the ingredients together. This is a tasty immune-enhancing dip to eat with crackers or raw vegetables or to stir into soups and casseroles.

herbs traditionally used to nourish *ojas* (see Introduction to Ayurveda, p. 63). When *ojas* is abundant and circulating freely, all cells and tissues in the body function optimally and support all processes in the body. Depletion of *ojas* makes us vulnerable to infection and ill health. Studies have shown that amalaki has antibiotic activity against a wide range of bacteria explaining its traditional role in the treatment of lung infections (see also p. 114) (Ahmad et al 1998). The immune-modulating properties of shatavari have been well documented. It has been shown to have a measurable effect on macrophage function and to enhance their ability to destroy the *Candida albicans* fungus (Rege and Dahanukar 1993). Shatavari has also been shown to aid immune system recovery after exposure to toxic chemicals (see also p. 164) (Thatte and Dahanukar 1988, Rege et al 1989).

Turmeric has long been used as a natural antibiotic. Studies from around the world have confirmed that turmeric can inhibit the growth of bacteria, yeast and viruses and has antitumour properties (see also p. 108).

Ashwagandha (*Withania somnifera*) has been shown to have a measurable effect on the immune system. It is classified as an adaptogen, helping to modify the harmful effects of stress, both physical and mental. Known as Indian ginseng, ashwagandha is an effective antioxidant and has a traditional use as a rejuvenative after illness and as an energy and nerve tonic. Research has shown that ashwagandha protects the immune system from the effects of toxic chemicals (Ziauddin et al 1996). This immune-protecting property has been researched for its ability to reduce the side effects of radiation and chemotherapy in the treatment of cancer. One of the classic uses of ashwagandha is to calm mental turbulence and as a brain tonic. It is certainly very helpful in the treatment of a range of stress-related disorders, including tiredness and lowered resistance.

ENHANCING IMMUNITY THROUGH DETOXIFICATION

One of the main tenets of Ayurveda is that proper digestion is a requirement for optimum health, and incomplete or disordered digestion can be a major contributor to the development of many diseases. The problem is not only that ingestion of foods and nutritional substances is of insufficient benefit when breakdown and assimilation are inadequate, but also that incompletely digested food molecules can be absorbed into the body, leading to the development of food allergies. In addition partially digested or undigested foods can ferment and produce toxins/*ama* that are then absorbed into the bloodstream and can wreak havoc with our immune systems. Our bodies are systems that take in, transform and release energy. If the system becomes overloaded beyond its capacity to transform or release energy, the body's balance is destabilized despite homoeostatic mechanisms to restore balance, and ill health results.

Ayurvedic detoxification and "rejuvenation" is the primary approach to maintaining positive health. Detoxification of the body and "rejuvenation" (nourishment of the tissues) are not confined only to treatment of disease but also to enhancing resistance.

To understand the cause and treatment of this accumulation of toxins and its subsequent damage, from an Ayurvedic perspective, it is important to clarify the concepts of *agni* and *ama*. *Agni* or digestive fire transforms and metabolizes nourishment from the environment. When *agni* is strong this nourishment is digested into its fundamental five elements and then these are absorbed eventually to become our cells and tissues (see *dhatus*, p. 75). When healthy, any of the digested food that is not useful to the body is eliminated via the three pathways of elimination (*malas*): urine, faeces and sweat (see *malas*, p. 76).

When *agni* is not functioning properly, toxins (*ama*) can accumulate from the incompletely metabolized food materials. The accumulation of *ama* in the body's cells and channels (*srotas*) disrupts the flow of nourishment to the cells and tissues. *Ama* is described as heavy, thick, cold and sticky, while *agni* is light, clear, hot and pure. *Ama* not only predisposes to disease but also blocks the action of *agni* and therefore the further digestion, absorption and assimilation of nutrients. If *ama* has accumulated over a period of time it compromises both proper mental and physiological functioning, giving rise to mental and physical fatigue, general aches and pains, poor digestion, body odour, bad breath and malaise. The condition of the tongue reflects the presence of *ama* in the system and there is often an unpleasant white coating, particularly noticeable in the morning.

Ama is usually associated with one of the three *doshas*. (It is possible to have *Vata*, *Pitta* or *Kapha* imbalances either with or without *ama*.) If there is toxicity in the body, it is hard to balance the *doshas* until *ama* has been removed and eliminated from the system. *Ama* conditions, known as *Sama*, vary according to the *doshas*:

● *Sama Kapha* is indicated by indigestion and mucus congestion
● *Sama Pitta* by indigestion, hyperacidity and diarrhoea, fever or skin conditions
● *Sama Vata* occurs with tiredness, abdominal distension, gas and constipation.

Once the *ama* has been removed, more specific measures for balancing the *doshas* and nourishing the cells and tissues can be effective. So the first stage of treatment with Ayurveda normally involves some detoxification.

Methods of detoxification

There are two levels of detoxification treatment

● Preliminary detoxification, which involves enhancing digestion and elimination called "palliation therapy"
● Secondly and more deep acting is the thorough cleansing of the *srotas*, known as "purification therapy", or *Pancha Karma*.

Pancha in Sanskrit means five and *karma* means actions, referring to the five actions that are considered the most powerful purifying and rejuvenating procedures in Ayurveda. These five actions are:

● purgation
● emesis
● nasal instillation
● enemas
● blood letting.

Palliation therapy is a slower and gentler method of detoxification and best suited to children, and does not require the stronger purification methods of *Pancha Karma*. Instigated from time to time or over a period of time, palliation can be as effective as *Pancha Karma* and is what

I incorporate into my practice. *Pancha Karma* necessitates in-patient care in special therapy centres. There are some existing in the UK but otherwise this is only available in India and Sri Lanka.

Shamana – "Palliation Therapy"

According to Ayurveda there are seven aspects of *shamana* designed to pacify aggravated *doshas* and clear *ama*.

1. *Agni deepana*, raising the digestive fire using pungent heating herbs
2. *Ama pachana*, clearing *ama*
3. *Kshud nigraha*, fasting from food
4. *Trut nigraha*, fasting from water
5. *Vyayama*, exercise including yoga
6. *Atapa*, lightening or drying the body by sitting in the sun and warming the body to raise metabolism
7. *Maruta*, lightening and drying the body by sitting in fresh air and doing breathing exercises (pranayama).

Traditionally, a few days of detoxification are recommended at the change of seasons. Since the changing seasons predispose to accumulations of a specific *dosha*, recommending cleansing at seasonal transitions can be very helpful for reducing or eliminating accumulations of either *Vata*, *Pitta* or *Kapha*.

Herbs for detoxification

Of the six tastes (see p. 79) pungent and bitter tastes are the best for cleansing *ama*. By increasing digestive fire with warming and pungent herbs *ama* is "burnt" away, and this is known as "*agni deepana*" (raising digestive fire) and *ama pachana* (clearing *ama*). Sweet, salty and sour tastes increase *ama*, as they are said to feed toxins. Astringent has a neutral effect; although it can dry up *ama*, it can hold it in the body by its contracting action.

Agni deepana

The best pungent herbs for raising digestive fire include cayenne, cinnamon, black pepper, ginger, long pepper, asafoetida (*Ferula asafoetida*), and mustard, and these are ideal for *Sama Kapha* but may aggravate excess *Pitta*. Warming herbs and spices such as cardamom, turmeric, cumin, coriander, basil and fennel, are also good regulators of *agni* and *ama*, and can be used more generally.

Well-known formulae for *agni deepana* include:

- Trikatu: (black pepper, long pepper and ginger). This has stimulant, expectorant properties and is specific for low *agni* and high *ama*. It reduces *Kapha* and *Vata* and increases *Pitta*. It can be helpful for *Sama Pitta* conditions in combination with bitter herbs.
- Trikulu: (clove, cinnamon, cardamom) digestive and cleansing for *Vata* and *Kapha*.
- Hingwastaka: (salt, asafoetida, trikatu, ajmoda (*Carum roxburghianum*), black cumin (*Nigella sativa*), cumin). This is one of the best remedies for *Vata*.
- Lavanbhaskar: (five salts compound (see Appendix p. 302)). This is recommended for *Vata*. It has laxative properties.
- Manibadhra: (rock salt, cumin, pippali, ginger, ajwan (*Trachyspermum animi*)).
- Talisadi: (talisha (*Abies webbiana*), trikatu, bamboo manna (*Bambusa bambos*), cardamom, cinnamon, raw sugar). This has expectorant, stimulant, and anti-*Kapha* properties and is good for colds and flu, taken with lime juice or honey. It increases *agni* in *Vata* and *Kapha* conditions.
- Sitopaladi: (rock candy, bamboo manna, long pepper, cardamom, cinnamon). This is an expectorant, which reduces *Kapha* and *Vata* and can be taken for coughs, colds, catarrh, loss of appetite, and debility.
- Trisugandhi: (cinnamon, cinnamon leaf, cardamom). A diaphoretic and stimulant, recommended for indigestion, poor appetite, wind, distension, to improve digestion and increase *Agni*.
- Lavangadi: (cloves, camphor, cardamom, cinnamon, nutmeg, vetivert, ginger, cumin, bamboo manna, jatamansi (*Nardostachys jatamansi*), long pepper, sandalwood, cubeb (*Piper cubeba*), raw sugar). This reduces *Vata* and *Kapha*, and increases *agni* and *Pitta*. It is recommended for poor appetite, colds, coughs, gas, colic, diarrhoea, nausea and vomiting.

Ama pachana

Bitter-tasting herbs "scrape" *ama* from the tissues (*ama pachana*) and can be used to relieve fevers or infections caused by it with their cooling effects. They are excellent where there is heat, inflammation, fermentation and toxins in the blood, and for any *ama* condition related to eating excess sweet or fatty food. They are best for *Sama Pitta* and *Sama Kapha* conditions and can be used in small amounts for long-standing *Sama Vata* conditions.

The best-known Ayurvedic bitters include katuka (*Picrorrhiza kurroa*) (CITES listed, only from sustainable sources), neem, aloe, turmeric, and guduchi. Western bitters include dandelion root, burdock, gentian (*Gentiana lutea*) and dock root (*Rumex crispus*).

Other remedies for *ama pachana* include:

- Triphala
- Haritaki and sugar/castor oil (good for *Vata*)
- Amalaki (good for *Pitta*)
- Guduchi and ginger
- Coriander
- Castor oil and ginger powder
- Triphala guggulu (good for *Kapha*)
- Aloe vera juice.

Cleansing the bowels is another pathway of detoxification that can be combined with a light, detoxifying diet. Gentle laxatives can be used for constipation or irregular bowel habits. Laxative herbs are contraindicated if there is diarrhoea, debility or emaciation, even if the tongue is coated or there are other signs of *ama*. There are other herbs and formulae that can cleanse the bowel without being laxative.

The best-known and most effective such Ayurvedic formula for cleansing the bowel is Triphala. It can be used generally as it helps balance all three *doshas* and combines all six tastes. It clears *ama* and raises digestive fire, improves metabolism and nourishes the tissues.

Aloe vera juice, taken with warming spices like ginger, black pepper and turmeric, is another excellent bowel cleanser. It is particularly good for *Sama Pitta* and *Sama Kapha*.

Bitter purgatives like rhubarb or senna (*Cassia senna*) should be combined with warming spices such as ginger to protect the digestive fire and to clear *ama*. Soothing bulk laxatives like flaxseed and psyllium are not recommended in *ama* conditions as they can further clog up the system. With their sweet taste they are said to feed rather than clear *ama*.

A healthy diet is one of the most important tools for reducing *Ama* accumulation, and it is advisable for children to follow an *ama*-reducing programme for a few days. This involves eating foods that are freshly prepared, nutritious and appetizing, and minimizing tinned, devitalized, junk or stale foods. Foods that are light and easy to digest are best, such as rice, vegetable soups and lentils, also grains such as barley and basmati rice, with plenty of freshly steamed or lightly sautéed vegetables or freshly juiced fruits and vegetables which are easier to digest than raw, hard foods. Seeds can be eaten in small amounts, however refined carbohydrates such as white flour and sugar, fried foods and dairy products should be reduced to a minimum. Also, fermented foods and drinks, including vinegar, chutneys, pickles and cheese should be minimized. Cold foods and drinks, oily, heavy, and salty foods, including nuts, should be avoided completely. White meat, turkey or chicken and fish are preferable to red meats. Ginger tea is an excellent way to raise the digestive fire and clear *Ama* from the digestive tract. It is best given in the morning before breakfast and again before lunch. It can also be sipped throughout the day. Hot water and a squeeze of lime make a good alternative and may be preferable for some children's palates.

Kshud nigraha: fasting

For growing children complete fasting from all food is not recommended, although reduction of foods when unwell is very natural for children who will normally be unwilling to eat.

- *Vata* predominant children can fast on such occasions on hot liquid soups

- *Pitta* predominant children can fast on fruit juices such as grape/pomegranate
- *Kapha* predominant children will recover more quickly if they simply drink water or herbal teas.

Seasonal variations: *Parinam*

The three *doshas* change according to the season (Table 6.4) and are aggravated at certain times, accumulate and are alleviated at others (see also p. 81).

The ideal times to undergo detoxification for a *Vata* person would be at the end of summer before autumn sets in, as this is at the crossover time just before *Vata* is aggravated. For a *Pitta* person the ideal time would be late spring, just before the summer when *Pitta* becomes aggravated and for a *Kapha* person at the end of winter before spring begins. These are the recommended times to undergo gentle cleansing and restore balance to the body. There is some consensus between East and West regarding cleansing toxins in spring, for it has long been a tradition in Britain to do a spring detox using cleansing herbs like dandelion, nettles and cleavers (*Galium aparine*), and eating plenty of fresh fruit and vegetables including plenty of greens. During the spring, the rising heat and stimulation of growth, brings to the surface internal toxins that have been accumulated through the winter. This is the best time to eliminate them in order to avoid illness through the summer. Once cleansed the body is better able to heal itself even without medication and if medication is given it has a better chance of reaching its target sites. This should mean greater efficacy with fewer side effects. In the process of detoxification as toxins are released, headaches or other symptoms such as pimples, bowel changes or malaise, may be experienced temporarily.

Table 6.4 Seasonal variations

Spring	Summer	Autumn	Winter
Vata calm	*Vata* accumulates	*Vata* aggravated	*Vata* calm
Pitta accumulates	*Pitta* aggravated	*Pitta* calm	*Pitta* calm
Kapha aggravated	*Kapha* calm	*Kapha* calm	*Kapha* accumulates

References

Ahmad I, Mehmood Z, Mohammod F 1998 Screening of some Indian medicinal plants for their antimicrobial properties. J Ethnopharmacol 62: 183–193

Amit A, Saxena VS, Pratibha N, et al 2003 Mast cell stabilization, lipoxygenase inhibition, hyaluronidase inhibition, antihistaminic and antispasmodic activities of Aller-7, a novel botanical formulation for allergic rhinitis. Drugs Exp Clin Res 29(3): 107–115

Athavale VB 2000 Bala Veda Pediatrics & Ayurveda. Chaukhamba Sanskrit Pratishthan, Delhi

Athique M 1998 Ayurvedic Anatomy and Physiology. College of Ayurveda, London

Barrett B 2003 Medicinal properties of Echinacea: a critical review. Phytomedicine Jan; 10(1): 66–86

Bone K, Morgan M 1996 Clinical Applications of Ayurvedic and Chinese Herbs: Monographs for the Western Herbal Practitioner. Warwick, Australia: Phytotherapy Press

Chang ST, Chen PF, Chang SC 2001 Antibacterial activity of leaf essential oils and their constituents from Cinnamomum osmophloeum. J Ethnopharmacol 77(1): 123–127

Field T 1995 Massage therapy for infants and children. J Dev Behav Pediatr 16(2): 105–111

Frawley D 2000 Ayurvedic Healing. Passage Press, Salt Lake City

Gorter RW, Joller P, Stoss M 2003 Cytokine release of a keratinocyte model after incubation with two different Viscum album L extracts. Am J Ther 10(1): 40–47

Greenfiles 1997 Vol. 11 No. 1, (Spring) quoting J Internat Med Res 1996, 24, 325–330

Hwang BY, Roberts SK, Chadwick LR, Wu CD, Kinghorn AD 2003 Antimicrobial constituents from golden seal (the Rhizomes of Hydrastis canadensis) against selected oral pathogens. Planta Med Jul; 69(7): 623–627

Kang BY, Chung SW, Cho D, Kim TS 2002 Involvement of p38 mitogen-activated protein kinase in the induction of interleukin-12 p40 production in mouse macrophages by berberine, a benzodioxoloquinolizine alkaloid. Biochem Pharmacol May 15; 63(10): 1901–1910

Kapil A, Sharma S 1997 Immunopotentiating compounds from Tinospora cordifolia. J Ethnopharmacol 58: 15–20

Kim LS, Waters RF, Burkholder PM 2002 Immunological activity of Larch arabinogalactan and Echinacea: a preliminary, randomized, double-blind, placebo-controlled trial. Altern Med Rev Apr; 7(2): 138–149

Lad V 1999 The Complete Book of Ayurvedic Home Remedies. Judy Piatkus Limited, London

Lamaison JL, Petitjean-Freytet C, Carnat A 1991 Medicinal Lamiaceae with antioxidant properties, a potential source of rosmarinic acid. Pharm Acta Helv 66(7): 185–188

Lee H, Lin JY 1988 Antimutagenic activity of extracts from anticancer drugs in Chinese medicine. Mutat Res 204(2): 229–234

Markin D, Duek L, Berdicevsky I 2003 In vitro antimicrobial activity of olive leaves. Mycoses 46(3–4): 132–136

Markova H, Sousek J, Ulrichova J 1997 Prunella vulgaris L. – a rediscovered medicinal plant. Ceska Slov Farm 46(2): 58–63

Mascolo N, Jain R, Jain SC, Capasso F 1989 Ethnopharmacologic investigation of ginger (Zingiber officinale) J Ethnopharmacol 27(1–2): 129–140

Ngai PH, Ng TB 2003 Lentin, a novel and potent antifungal protein from shitake mushroom with inhibitory effects on activity of human immunodeficiency virus-1 reverse transcriptase and proliferation of leukemia cells. Life Sci 73(26): 3363–3374

Pompei R, Flore O, Marccialis MA, Pani A, Loddo B 1979 Glycyrrhizic acid inhibits virus growth and inactivates virus particles. Nature Oct 25; 281(5733): 689–690

Ranasinghe L, Jayawardena B, Abeywickrama K 2002 Fungicidal activity of essential oils of Cinnamomum zelanicum (L.) and Syzygium aromaticum (L.) Merr et L.M. Perry against crown rot and anthracrose pathogens isolated from banana. Lett Appl Microbiol 35(3): 208–211

Rege NN, Dahanukar SA 1993 Quantitation of microbicidal activity of mononuclear phagocytes: an in vitro technique. J Postgrad Med 39: 22–25

Rege NN, Nazareth HM, Bapat RD 1989 Modulation of immunosuppression in obstructive jaundice by Tinospora cordifolia. Indian J Med Res 90: 478–483

Sand J, Walton R, Rountree B 1994 Smart Medicine for a Healthier Child. Avery Publishing Group, New York

Scazzocchio F, Cometa MF, Tomassini L, Palmery M 2001 Antibacterial activity of Hydrastis canadensis extract and its major isolated alkaloids. Planta Med Aug; 67(6): 561–564

Shan BE, Yoshida Y, Sugiura T, et al 1999 Stimulating activity of Chinese medicinal herbs on human lymphocytes in vitro. Int J Immunopharmacol 21(3): 149–159

Shibata S 2000 A drug over the millennia: pharmacognosy, chemistry, and pharmacology of licorice. Yakugaku Zasshi Oct; 120(10): 849–862

Shinada M, Azuma M, Kawai H, et al 1986 Enhancement of interferon-gamma production in glycyrrhizin-treated human peripheral lymphocytes in response to concanavalin A and to surface antigen of hepatitis B virus. Proc Soc Exp Biol Med Feb; 181(2): 205–210

Shon YH, Nam KS 2003 Protective effect of Astragali radix extract on interleukin 1beta-induced inflammation in human amnion. Phytother Res 17(9): 1016–1020

Sun Y, Hersh EM, Talpaz M, et al 1983 Immune restoration and/or augmentation of local graft versus host reaction by traditional Chinese medicinal herbs. Cancer Jul 1; 52(1): 70–73

Thatte UM, Dahanukar SA 1988 Comparative study of immunomodulating activity of Indian medicinal plants, lithium carbonate and glucan. Methods Find Exp Clin Pharmacol 10: 639–644

Thatte UM, Kulkarni MR, Dahanukar SA 1992 Immunotherapeutic modification of *Escherichia coli* peritonitis and bacteremia by *Tinospora cordifolia*. J Postgrad Med 38: 13–15

Tillotson AK, Tillotson NH, Robert A Jr 2001 The One Earth Herbal Sourcebook. Kensington Publishing Corps, New York

Wang RT, Shan BE, Li QX 2002 Extracorporeal experimental study on immunomodulatory activity of *Astragalus membranaceus* extract. Zhongguo Zhong Xi Yi Jie He Za Zhi 22(6): 453–456

Weber ND, Andersen DO, North JA et al 1992 In vitro virucidal effects of *Allium sativum* (garlic) extract and compounds. Planta Med 58(5): 417–423

Wurm M, Kacani L, Laus G, et al 1998 Pentacyclic oxindole alkaloids from *Uncaria tomentosa* induce human endothelial cells to release a lymphocyte-proliferation-regulating factor. Planta Med 64(8): 701–704

Yamasaki K, Otake T, Mori H, et al 1993 Screening test of crude drug extract on anti-HIV activity. Yakugaku Zasshi 113(11): 818–824

Zheng M 1990 Experimental study of 472 herbs with antiviral action against the herpes simplex virus. Zhong Xi Yi Jie He Za Zhi 10(1): 6, 39–41

Ziauddin M, Phansalkar N, Patki P 1996 Studies on the immunomodulatory effects of Ashwagandha. J Ethnopharmacol 50: 69–76

Chapter **7**

Fevers, infections and allergies

UNDERSTANDING FEVERS

Fever is the natural accompaniment of many infections. It is a vital response to invading pathogens and a symptom of the body's fight against infection. Although the popular response to a child's fever is to suppress it immediately, this may not always be best for the child. Fever is not a disease and may even be a friend.

Symptoms of an infection manifest once certain micro-organisms have an opportunity to multiply in the body and as they are broken down by the immune response, pyrogens are released which raise the setting of the body's internal thermostat. As a result the metabolism of the body is increased and this has the effect of enabling the infecting organisms to be combated more quickly and efficiently by the body. In fact, fever itself has a natural antibiotic and antiviral effect. To illustrate this point we know that a protein known as interferon is released during a viral infection to overcome infection and this is more effective when the child has a fever than when the temperature remains normal. Once the infection is successfully resolved and the fever is no longer required by the body, the thermostat will reset itself.

Of most concern when a baby or young child has a persistently raised temperature is the possibility of a febrile convulsion. Although most children are unlikely to experience convulsions even with a high fever, some children are more susceptible. The younger the child and the higher the fever, the more likely the convulsion, hence the need for tepid sponging combined with febrifuge herbs during a fever, especially when fevers occur in babies. *Roseola infantum* with its red rash of spots and high fever is more commonly associated with convulsions than other infectious diseases. The other concern when treating children's fevers is to keep the child as comfortable as possible. Fevers are usually accompanied by variable degrees of discomfort which may be distressing to the child. It is important to find a balance between keeping a child comfortable enough to rest and recover and suppressing the fever and thus prolonging the illness.

It is worth considering at this point why some children succumb to an infection while others close to them do not. While bacteria and viruses have largely taken the blame for the onset of infection,

they are perceived by the herbalist as the precipitating factors in disease, not the real underlying cause. What also requires consideration therefore is the general state of resistance in the child, which will determine either whether they fall prey to minor infections such as colds, flu and chest infections, or eruptive infections like chicken-pox and measles, and if they do, how efficient they are at resolving the disease with a minimum of complications.

A child's response to invading micro-organisms relates to a number of factors: the general constitution of the child, inherited familial tendencies, diet and lifestyle, and their individual pattern of health. A generally healthy, well-nourished child, fed on wholefoods and plenty of fresh fruit and vegetables, rather than on refined carbohydrates and an excess of sugary foods, who gets plenty of exercise and adequate rest, should produce a healthy response with moderate fever, followed by sweating and a good rash in eruptive infections. The infection should be resolved quickly and without complications. A body overloaded with toxins accumulated from a variety of sources including atmospheric pollution, chemicals in food and water, poor nutrition, sluggish elimination of waste products, insufficient sleep, too little fresh air and exercise, for example, is likely to suffer from lowered vitality and poor resistance to infection. What is of more significance therefore is the patient rather than the disease.

Herbal treatment is aimed at the individual child concerned. It is interesting that many of the herbs that are commonly used to treat infection not only encourage elimination of waste materials and toxins, but also provide a weakened system with vitamins, minerals and trace elements to boost general health. Children growing up today may well benefit from periodic times of cleansing the system of accumulated toxins, and a mild fever may well be an effective means of doing just this. It provides an opportunity to give the child's system a rest from eating solid food and the accumulation of more waste matter for a day or so, and allows the eliminative pathways a chance to throw off toxins through the increase in metabolism experienced with a fever. Sweating, a vital pathway of elimination, can be encouraged by giving the child warm infusions of diaphoretic herbs. Drinking plenty of liquid can not only encourage sweating, but also elimination via the kidneys and it is interesting that many of the herbs with diaphoretic properties, such as meadowsweet and elderflowers, also have a diuretic action. Herbs with mild laxative properties like dandelion root, liquorice, yellow dock root (*Rumex crispus*) and burdock, may also be helpful in some instances to speed the cleansing process and the resolution of infection. As long as the child is basically healthy and strong, most minor infections accompanied by a fever will be resolved without difficulty, and the child will be more robust as a result of this cleansing process.

Feed or starve a fever?

A child with a fever needs primarily to rest and secondarily to drink plenty of fluid and only eat lightly. Liquid is essential to encourage sweating, to cool the body and prevent dehydration. Warm or tepid water with a squeeze of fresh lemon juice can be given to the child to drink frequently. It is cooling and refreshing as well as antiseptic. Often the appetite will diminish significantly and the amount of food given should be determined by this. Heavy and oily foods should be avoided and light, nourishing soups are best. Those containing grains such as barley or rice, beans such as mung beans and vegetables such as spinach, cabbage, watercress and celery have an additionally cooling and cleansing effect. Over-concern by the parents to keep the child's strength up during illness may lead them to overburden the child's system with food at a time when he or she has little spare energy for digestion during the recovery process. It may well diminish the force of the natural healing process and slow recovery down or even predispose to complications.

If the temperature is no higher than 101–102°F (38.3–38.8°C) and the child is both comfortable enough and not prone to convulsions, it can be left to its own devices. If higher the temperature can cause the child to feel uncomfortable and quite unwell, and could if left lead to dehydration. Traditionally herbalists have recommended that the child is sponged down with tepid water, rose water or herbal infusions to exert their cooling effects until the fever subsides to at least 102°F (38.8°C).

TREATING FEVERS USING HERBS

Herbal infusions can be employed in a number of different ways. They can be given as warm drinks frequently through the day, they can be used for tepid sponging, poured into bath water or used as hand and foot baths. The following diaphoretic herbs can be used to encourage sweating and thereby to reduce fever, while at the same time encouraging the body's fight against the infection through their own antimicrobial actions. They can be used either singly or in combinations of several herbs together according to the child's taste and availability of the herbs:

- Basil (*Ocimum basilicum*)
- Boneset (*Eupatorium perfoliatum*)
- Chamomile (*Matricaria chamomilla*)
- Catnip (*Nepeta cataria*)
- Cinnamon (*Cinnamomum cassia/zeylanicum*)
- Coriander (*Coriandrum sativum*)
- Echinacea (*Echinacea angustifolia/purpurea*)
- Elderflower (*Sambucus nigra*)
- Ginger (*Zingiber officinale*)
- Hyssop (*Hyssopus officinalis*)
- Lavender (*Lavandula angustifolia*)
- Lemon balm (*Melissa officinalis*)
- Lemon grass (*Cymbopogon citratus*)
- Limeflowers (*Tilia cordata/europaea*)
- Meadowsweet (*Filipendula ulmaria*)
- Peppermint (*Mentha piperita*)
- Rosemary (*Rosmarinus officinalis*)
- Self heal (*Prunella vulgaris*)
- Thyme (*Thymus vulgaris*)
- Vervain (*Verbena officinalis*)
- Violet flowers (*Viola odorata*)
- Yarrow (*Achillea millefolium*).

Chamomile tea is a herb of choice for many herbalists when it comes to treating fevers in children. Not only does it enhance the immune response and reduce fever through its antimicrobial and diaphoretic properties, but it also relaxes the child sufficiently to ensure a good sleep. Rest is probably the single most beneficial factor in speeding recovery. It allows the healing energy of the body to concentrate on resolving the infection not being dissipated by other physical or mental activity. Lavender, lemon balm and limeflowers (*Tilia cordata/europaea*) work similarly. They are all pleasant tasting, which is a great bonus when treating children and can be drunk quite freely. Teas can be sweetened with honey if preferred.

Two paediatricians at Chicago University, Traismann and Hardy, ran some interesting trials using limeflowers (Weiss 1988). A total of 55 children with influenza symptoms were treated with limeflowers and bed rest and at most one or two aspirin tablets. Another 37 children were given the above as well as sulphonamides and a further 67 children were given only antibiotics. Those given only limeflowers and bed rest recovered most quickly and developed the least complications (e.g. middle ear infections). The children given antibiotics took longer to recover and developed more complications. The researchers came out ten to one in favour of limeflower tea. They recommended that trivial childhood illnesses are best not treated with such drugs except when complications developed, in which case they may be more applicable.

Garlic is renowned for helping the fight against infection and also for encouraging sweating. An older child may enjoy some chopped raw garlic in a teaspoon of honey or even on toast, if not, and for younger children, three garlic perles can be given per day with a drink. Garlic is one of the most effective antimicrobial herbs, acting on bacteria and viruses as well as parasites in the gut. It can be used for a wide variety of infections whether affecting the respiratory, digestive or urinary tracts (see also p. 30).

Warming spices like fresh ginger and coriander are excellent medicines for fevers and infections. By stimulating blood flow to the periphery, encouraging sweating and aiding the elimination of toxins via the skin as well as the digestive tract, they help the body resist infection and relieve fever. The volatile oils that lend these spices their characteristic taste and smell are highly antiseptic, activating immunity against bacterial and viral infection. Ginger root and coriander seeds can be decocted in water for 10–15 minutes and sweetened with honey if desired. They make delicious teas for children as long as they are not too pungent and can be drunk freely throughout the day. They are particularly useful during the early stages of fever.

Echinacea deserves a special mention as one of the most popular remedies to enhance resistance in all kinds of infections, particularly colds and flu. The chemical constituents found to be responsible for the positive effect of echinacea on the immune system include phenolic acids, flavonoids, essential oils, polyacetylenes, alkylamides, polysaccharides and steroids. Together these clearly have an interferon-like antiviral action and antiallergic properties. So echinacea can be taken at the first signs of any acute infection whether it is a sore throat, cold, chest infection, tonsillitis, cystitis or gastroenteritis. For best results $\frac{1}{4}$–$\frac{1}{2}$ tsp of the tincture needs to be taken in a little water every 2 hours. A cup of hot tea made from decocting half a teaspoon of the root in a cupful of water for 10 minutes, will stimulate blood flow to the skin, enhance sweating, and thereby reduce fever.

Meadowsweet (*Filipendula ulmaria*) is popularly known as the herbal aspirin. When crushed the flowers give off the characteristic smell of salicylic aldehyde, which when oxidized yields salicylic acid, from which acetylsalicylic acid or aspirin can be derived. Interestingly the name aspirin comes from the old Latin name for meadowsweet, *Spiraea ulmaria*. It is a cooling diaphoretic, bringing blood to the surface of the body to cause sweating. It is also mildly antiseptic and its anti-inflammatory and analgesic actions should help the child to feel more comfortable.

A popular infusion for enhancing sweating among children is the old-fashioned traditional English combination of yarrow, elderflowers and peppermint. The tea is light and refreshing and does not taste unpleasant, which is quite a consideration when it comes to treating children. They obviously have to be willing to take enough of the herbs for them to be adequately effective. Yarrow reduces fevers and clears toxins, heat and congestion by aiding elimination via the skin and the kidneys through its diaphoretic and diuretic actions. The volatile oils and resins have an antimicrobial and anti-inflammatory effect. Elderflowers are an ideal herb to take at the onset of any respiratory infection. They stimulate the circulation, enhance sweating and aid elimination of toxins via the skin and kidneys. They are well worth using to bring out the rash in eruptive infections and thereby speed the resolution of the infection. They have a decongestant action, excellent in colds, catarrh, sinusitis and bronchial congestion. Their relaxant effect on smooth muscle is helpful particularly where there is wheezing or asthma, to relieve bronchospasm and clear congestion. Peppermint has relaxing and analgesic properties, relieving headaches and malaise that accompany fevers. Like elderflowers, it increases the circulation, brings blood to the surface and enhances sweating. It too makes a good decongestant. The volatile oils are antibacterial, antiviral and antifungal and regarded as effective against the TB bacillus, herpes simplex and ringworm. A cupful of the hot infusion can be given every 2 hours.

Other herbs that increase resistance and help fight off infection include astragalus (*Astragalus membranaceus*) cat's claw (*Uncaria formentosum*), turmeric, Chinese angelica (*Angelica sinensis*), cleavers (*Galium aparine*), cloves, eucalyptus, hyssop (*Hyssopus off.*), liquorice, red clover (*Trifolium pratense*), thyme, oregano, rosemary, rose petals, wild indigo (*Baptisia tinctoria*). (For the treatment of infections underlying fever see also Immune System, p. 150.)

Propolis can be given in honey or a few drops of tincture in a drink. This is an antiseptic material which bees collect from tree sap to plaster over the hive to keep it clean and protected from infection. Certain substances from propolis such as flavonoids, help the body to make antibodies and enhance the work of white blood cells in killing harmful bacteria.

Should orthodox antibiotics be necessary for, for example otitis media/streptococcal throat infection, there are several things that can be recommended to help prevent side effects of, for example, diarrhoea, constipation, abdominal pain, candida proliferation. These include garlic, live yoghurt with *Lactobacillus* tablets, plenty of liquid to aid elimination, vitamin C, vitamin B and vitamin E.

AYURVEDIC APPROACH TO FEVERS/*JWARA*

Jwara is defined as a disease when obstruction to perspiration, increase in body temperature and pain all over the body occur together. It is classified according to stage of the disease: the first stage is known as *ama*; the second as *sama*; and the third as *nirama*. It is important to be aware of each stage as each one requires slightly different treatment.

- *Ama* stage: *Ama* accumulates in the stomach because of disturbed *Pachaka Pitta*.
- *Sama* stage: *Ama* locates into a specific site.
- *Nirama*: *Ama* in a particular site is eliminated from the body, through cleansing methods, (vomiting, sweating, purgation, etc.) and the temperature returns to normal.

The causes of fever (*Nidana*)

Disturbance of the *doshas*

- low digestive fire
- formation of *ama* which can result from incorrect eating, i.e. eating at the wrong time, eating too little or overeating, eating the wrong foods for one's constitution or devitalized, *ama*-producing foods
- over-exertion
- getting over-tired
- improper lifestyle.

The main *dosha* responsible for the development of fever (*Jwara*) is excess *Pitta* in body and mind. This may be caused through too much *Pitta*-increasing food (spicy, fatty, and sour foods, and red meat), lifestyle, weather, excess heat, frequent irritation, anger or other *Pitta* related emotions.

Pathogenesis/*Samprapti*

In the first stage (*ama* stage) incorrect eating or poor digestion causes a build up of *ama* in the stomach and the *doshas* (*Samana Vayu*, *Pachaka Pitta* and *Bodhaka Kapha*) to become disturbed. Excess *Pachaka Pitta*, the dominant *dosha* in the stomach, is carried with *Ama* to the liver and then to the first *dhatu*, *rasa dhatu*. *Vata* then circulates the *sama Pitta* (*Pitta* with *ama*) around the body causing fever and heat to be eliminated via the skin as this is the *rasa* site. The *sama Pitta* goes to the sweat glands and blocks them, causing a rise in body temperature, redness of the skin, fatigue, irritation and frequently constipation.

In the second stage (*sama stage*) known as relocation, the fever now varies according to the type of fever and can diversify according to whether it is *Vata*, *Pitta* or *Kapha* type of fever. *Sannipatik* fever involves all three *doshas*.

Prodromal symptoms (*Purva rupa*)

This is the first/*ama* stage when the accumulation of *ama* leads to the following symptoms: loss of appetite, unpleasant taste in mouth, belching, full feeling, lethargy, coated tongue, heaviness in the body. Ama increases *tamas* causing sleepiness, darkness and heaviness.

Symptoms/*Rupa*

This is the second/*sama* stage, when there is fever as well as specific symptoms including thirst, hot or burning sensation in body/stomach, vomiting, abdominal distension, constipation or obstructed urination. The fever goes up if food is eaten as it creates more *ama*, so fasting or very light eating is appropriate.

Vata type

Fever tends to start with feeling chilled, goosepimples and shivering, in the evening, around dusk or at dawn, times that are governed by *Vata*. The fever is generally not very high with little sweating and can be intermittent. There may be generalized aches and pains, backache, stiff joints, rigors, desire for warmth, constipation, with hard and dry stools, constant yawning, weakness, dry mouth with bad taste, dizziness, ringing in ears, loss of taste and hunger.

Pitta type

There tends to be a constantly high fever, and a feeling of heat inside and out. Stools, urine, eyes and skin feel hot. Symptoms are characterized by redness, heat, inflammation and as a result there is a thirst, sweating and desire for cold. There may be dizziness or faintness, acid stomach, diarrhoea, rashes, acrid or bad taste in the mouth, bad breath, restlessness, impatience and irritability. In children with a high fever there may be a tendency to delirium and febrile convulsions.

Kapha type

Fever tends to start with feeling chilled, goosepimples, cold symptoms, congestion, post nasal drip and cough. There is often shivering, a desire for heat, a feeling of heaviness, lethargy, sleepiness and slow-mindedness. There may be pallor, a dull headache, a bad taste in the mouth, loss of appetite,

excess saliva, constipation, nausea and vomiting. The fever can rise after eating and sleeping.

In the third/*nirama* stage, as toxins are returned to the digestive tract for elimination, there is sweating, low fever, the appetite returns and the body returns to normal.

Ayurvedic treatment of fevers

This involves:

- Lightening therapy (*langhana*) which means fasting, or eating a light diet
- Clearing of toxins from the digestive tract (*ama pachana*) (see p. 168)
- Prescribing herbal medicines (*bhesaja*)
- Use of laxatives for purgation (*virechana*).

Treatment in the first/*ama* stage:

1. Food (*ahara*): The patient should be given water, rice water or soup.
2. Activity (*vihara*): The patient should rest but not sleep as this creates more *tamas* and increases *Ama* and may push the fever up or prolong it further.
3. Medicines (*bhesaja*):
   - Dhasamula arishta is a well-known formula used at this stage, 15–30 ml twice daily
   - Coriander decoction. To make a (*sheeta*) decoction use eight parts coriander seeds (i.e. 90–100 g) to 8 cups water and simmer until 1 cup remains and sip through the day.

Treatment in the second/*sama* stage:

- All toxins need to be directed to *koshta*, the site for elimination, i.e. the gut and then *ama* is cleared, and the following medicines are appropriate.
- Chiretta
- Turmeric
- Ginger
- Long pepper
- Liquorice
- Neem
- Talisa (*Abies webbiana*)
- Sandalwood (*Santalum album*)
- Guduchi
- Amalaki
- Sitopaladi
- For *Pitta* and *Kapha* and fevers use Dhatree powder (Triphala, liquorice and senna).
- For *Vata* use castor oil.

In the third/*nirama* stage suitable cleansing medicines include,

- Dhatree churna
- In India doctors use castor oil enemas (2 cc castor oil 8 cc warm water (2:8 ml) are inserted into anal canal with syringe)
- *Ama pachana* (see p. 81)
- *Agni deepana*: Trikatu, Trikulu, Talisadi
- Triphala as a bowel cleanser and tonic for convalescence (*rasayana*) ($\frac{1}{4}$–$\frac{1}{2}$ tsp powder in a little warm water and honey at night).

General treatment for all dosha types

- *Andrographis paniculata* is a popular herb for treating fevers and an effective remedy for viral infections (Tillotson et al 2001). It is also known as kirata or Indian gentian. Thousands of years ago the Kiratas, a small tribe living in the Himalayan forests, used a bitter herb to treat fevers. The early Ayurvedic healers named it Kirata tikta, which means "the bitter herb of the Kirata people". It was used to treat a wide range of infections and to clear heat from the liver. When the British were in India, they used it to treat malaria and called it Indian gentian. It has been the subject of much scientific research, which has focused on its immune-enhancing properties, particularly since the publication of a Swedish study which reported its benefits in reducing symptoms of the common cold (Chopra and Simon 2000, p. 71). Other studies demonstrate this herb's ability to stimulate antibody production and cellular responsivity. By enhancing immunity, it can protect against a wide range of infections including tonsillitis, urinary tract infections, parasites, malaria and retroviruses.
- Tulsi (holy basil) is one of the favourite home remedies for relieving fevers and in fact it is considered to be "*jwaraagna*", destroyer of fevers. It is used for reducing pain and clearing congestion. Its anti-inflammatory and analgesic properties are well-documented $\frac{1}{2}$ tsp dried leaf powder can be given in a cup of hot water 3–4 times daily. Dr P.S. Phadke recommends a decoction with 100 g from leaves (a handful) with $\frac{1}{2}$ litre water. Decoct until $\frac{3}{4}$ cup remains:
  - For a child 6–12 years take 1 tsp 3–4 times daily
  - For a child 2–6 years $\frac{1}{2}$–$\frac{3}{4}$ tsp 3–4 times daily

  - For a baby 4–12 months $\frac{1}{4}$–$\frac{1}{3}$ tsp 2 times daily
  - For a newborn baby express milk into a tablespoon, and add $\frac{1}{4}$–$\frac{1}{3}$ tsp of the mixture feed in drops to baby (Phadke 2001).

- For fevers caused by gastrointestinal and respiratory infections a teaspoon of powdered turmeric added to a glass of hot milk can be given and raw sugar can be added to taste. If there is constipation add a teaspoon of warm ghee.
- For fevers with diarrhoea, especially in summer, bael sherbet alternated with the above tea is a popular Ayurvedic remedy (Phadke 2001). Powder of the dried pulp of bael fruit (bilva) is also used.

  To make bael sherbet: mix the pulp of three ripe bael fruit in 2 glasses of water. Add raw sugar to taste. Give to children 1–2 tbsp 3–4 times daily.

  Other fever recipes include:

1. 1 handful crushed mint leaves
   2–3 black peppercorns
   2–3 long peppers
   $\frac{1}{4}$ inch piece of ginger.
   Boil all the ingredients together in 2 cups water and simmer for 12–15 minutes. Cool, strain and divide into three doses to be taken at intervals through the day.

2. Tea made with the leaves of *Swertia chiretta* and stems can be given with honey to mask the bitter taste, three times daily.

3. 12 g dried Tulsi leaves
   3 g black pepper powder
   Combine ingredients to make a tea and use honey/palm sugar can be added to taste.

4. Tamarind – 1 tbsp tamarind extract in 1 glass boiling water. Cool, strain and add raw sugar and honey.

5. Lemon grass tea or a decoction of lemon grass leaves with ginger, sugar and cinnamon. 4 oz of the leaves to 1 pint boiling water.

6. In high fevers sandalwood paste is used on the forehead and is said to bring down a fever like a cool compress.

7. Guduchi *sattva* is a water-soluble powder-extract of the plant that is given 1 g twice daily in ghee or water for fevers and headaches.

8. The Bonduc nut (*Caesalpinia bonducella*) is useful for most types of fever. The juice of the fresh leaves is given, 1 oz with a pinch of black pepper three times a day.

9. An infusion of patol (*Trichosanthes doica*) taken with coriander seeds is another popular remedy for fevers (Dastur 1983, p. 84).

10. Decoction of black raisins and haritaki is considered very effective (Dastur 1983).

11. Strong decoction of bala root given with ginger is also popular.

For Vata type fevers:

1. Amritarishta. Contains guduchi (*Tinospora cordifolia*), dashmool (ten roots), jaggery, jeera (*Cuminum cyminum*) 15–30 ml twice daily in warm water.

   Vasant Lad (1999) recommends an infusion of equal parts ginger powder, cumin powder and myrrh (*Commiphora molmol*) powder steeped in boiling water for 10 minutes, taken to induce perspiration. $\frac{1}{2}$ teaspoon of the powder per cup of boiling water taken three times a day.

For Pitta type fevers:

1. Guduchi *satva* (water soluble extract) is cooling remedy for the treatment of all *Pitta* conditions.

2. Chandanadi is a formula given in India for fevers and burning sensation in hands, feet and eyes. It contains: chandan (sandalwood), tagar (*Valeriana walichi*), lauh bhasma (iron), pippali (*Piper longum*), haritaki (*Terminalia chebula*), shunthi (ginger), amalaki (*Emblica officinalis*).

3. Sitopaladi, (contains bamboo manna, pippali, cinnamon, cardamom) has a cooling effect, and is good for *Pitta* fevers (1.25–2.5 g three times daily in warm milk).

4. Vasant Lad recommends grating a raw onion and placing the pulp in a cool wet handkerchief and applying it to the forehead and the umbilicus. He states that this irritates the eyes which then produce tears and as they fall the fever comes down (Lad 1999).

5. Chiretta (*Swertia chiretta*) is excellent for fevers and infections.

For Kapha type fevers:

1. Tulsi, ginger, neem, and black pepper.
2. Pippali.
3. Sitopaladi. For flu and upper respiratory complaints.
4. Talisadi *churna* contains: black pepper; ginger; Talisa (*Abies webbiana*); pippali; manna of bamboo; cardamom; cinnamon; and cumin. This is given with honey for fevers and *ama pachana* as well as for coughs, colds, and phlegm.
5. Vasant Lad recommends an infusion made from 1 tsp of equal parts of ginger, cinnamon and fennel powder per cup of boiling water and drinking this three times daily (Lad 1999).

TREATMENT OF INFECTIOUS CHILDHOOD DISEASES

CHICKENPOX

A contagious viral infection, particularly prevalent in children under ten, chickenpox spreads by contact and droplet infection from talking, coughing, sneezing and laughing. The most infectious time is 1–2 days before the spots emerge and remains so until all blisters have dried up. This generally takes about a week. The incubation period is around 17–21 days. The most unpleasant symptom of chickenpox is the extreme itchiness, otherwise most children only feel mildly unwell. Infected adults tend to feel ill.

Treatment of chickenpox

- Children need to be given plenty of fluids even if they do not feel like eating much. Water with a squeeze of lemon or lime juice or herbal teas are recommended. An easily digested diet, high in vitamins and minerals to provide raw materials for the immune system, consisting of soups, casseroles and steamed vegetables, can be given when the child is hungry.

- Vitamin A and beta carotene, in red, green and yellow fruits and vegetables, helps healing of the skin. Vitamin C and bioflavonoids help to stimulate the immune system and to resolve fever in the initial phase of the illness. Hot lemon/lime drinks will help boost intake of vitamin C.

- Zinc, either in lozenge form or liquid doses of 15 ml, can be given once or twice a day to promote healing of the skin and to enhance the efforts of the immune system.

- Garlic and echinacea given regularly throughout the day will boost the immune response and both act as antiviral agents.

- Turmeric is equally useful ($\frac{1}{4}$–$\frac{1}{2}$ tsp of powder can be taken in hot water three times daily or the equivalent added to soups and drinks).

- For fever management if necessary, chamomile, boneset (*Eupatorium perfoliatum*), yarrow or lime-flower (*Tilia europaea*) can be given as warm infusions, sweetened if desired, $\frac{1}{2}$ cupful every 2 hours (see Fevers, p. 175). Chamomile, catnip (*Nepeta cataria*) or skullcap (*Scutellaria laterifolia*) are useful if the child feels particularly unwell or restless.

- To help clear the skin quickly and relieve itching: burdock, red clover (*Trifolium pratense*), rose petals, chamomile, elderflowers, and/or hearts-ease (*Viola tricolor*) can be given in infusions every 2 hours. Burdock root is rich in minerals and trace elements including iron, magnesium, silica, and zinc, as well as vitamin A. It has a detoxifying effect through its action on the liver, as well as its diaphoretic and diuretic properties, helping the body to eliminate toxins through sweat and via the kidneys. It helps to clear the skin and enhance immunity. In China burdock is valued for its ability to cool hot, inflammatory conditions and resolve fevers. By bringing out rashes to the surface of the skin, burdock can help to speed eruptive infections on their way. Red clover is also rich in minerals and trace elements including calcium, magnesium and potassium as well as vitamin C. It helps to detoxify the body and speed healing of the skin and is indicated in inflammatory skin conditions. The bitters stimulate the liver while the flavonoids have a diuretic action aiding elimination of toxins via the kidneys. Note: Red clover flowers contain salicylates.

Externally

- To soothe itching and speed healing of the skin, infusions of chamomile, chickweed, (*Stellaria media*) neem, lavender, marigold, raspberry leaves (*Rubus idaeus*) or St John's Wort (*Hypericum perforatum*) can be used to bathe the skin. Cool infusions are best, applied on cotton wool or a clean flannel or added to bath water.

- Tepid baths can be very soothing to the skin and help relieve itching. Oatmeal added to the water can also bring relief. A handful of raw oatmeal can be tied in a cloth or flannel and swirled around in the bath water. It can also be used to gently wash the skin, but care needs to be taken not to break the blisters.

- Aloe vera gel with a little turmeric powder mixed with it can be very effective.

- Dilute essential oils (chamomile, lavender and tea tree are all applicable) added to bath water may also relieve itching and help stop the development of secondary infection of the skin.

- Applications of distilled witch hazel or rose water can be particularly soothing.

- Decoctions of burdock, marigold, neem, turmeric, golden seal (*Hydrastis canadensis*) or yellow dock (*Rumex crispus*) can be sponged on to spots to relieve severe itching. If spots become infected, the skin can be bathed frequently with golden seal, marigold or neem (decoctions/infusions/ dilute tinctures).

- Once the blisters have dried and scabs have fallen off, comfrey (*Symphytum off.*) leaf ointment alternated with lavender oil will speed healing of the skin and help prevent scar formation. *Calendula* cream or oil and *Hypericum* oil, rubbing castor oil or vitamin E oil into the scars will also help.

- Children should be kept from exposing the skin to hot sun until the skin has completely healed as new skin can burn and scar easily.

- For blisters in the mouth diluted tinctures of myrrh (*Commiphora molmol*), *Calendula* or golden seal can be used to swab the mouth or as mouthwashes.

- Keeping the child as cool as possible is advisable for getting hot will involve increasing blood flow to the skin and aggravate itching. For this reason and to speed recovery it is best to keep the child quiet and discourage vigorous exercising and rushing about.

Ayurvedic approach

For prevention during an epidemic of chickenpox it is considered important to ensure that children keep the bowels open and give laxatives, such as liquorice root powder or decoction if necessary. A mixture of turmeric and tamarind (*Tamarindus indica*) seeds can be given twice daily to enhance immunity.

Amalaki (dried fruit powder and the juice of fresh fruit) is used as a prophylactic.

Treatment of acute infection

- Trikatu with juice of the leaves of Bonduc nut (*Caesalpinia bonducella*) is given at first signs of infection.
- A mixture of juice of leaves of Bonduc nut and amalaki juice with honey and sugar is another traditional prescripton ($\frac{1}{4}-\frac{1}{2}$ tsp of powder twice daily in warm milk or ghee).
- To reduce the severity of an attack, a decoction of shatavari is given with milk.
- Juice of tamarind leaves with turmeric and water and juice of gotu kola leaves with honey help cool heat and clear the skin.
- Holy basil leaf juice or an infusion of the dried leaves also clears heat and helps resolve infection.

Externally

- A paste of neem leaves mixed with water can be used externally.
- Turmeric paste, or paste of roots of khus khus (*Vetiveria zizanoides*) grass relieves itching.
- A paste of sandalwood can also be applied to the body to cool heat and itching.
- Rice flour has a cooling and soothing effect. It can be thickly dusted all over the affected area.
- Triphala decoction serves as a good wash for skin and eyes; as does a decoction of coriander seeds (Dastur 1983, p. 220).
- Water boiled with neem leaves, Kasondi (*Cassia occidentalis*), khus khus grass, sandalwood and dhamasa (*Fagonia cretica*) is used for bathing to relieve heat and irritation and speed healing of blisters.

MUMPS

A viral infection affecting the salivary glands and parotid glands, mumps is spread by contact with infected saliva and so is less contagious than measles or chickenpox. It rarely occurs under the age of 2 and is most common between 5–15 years of age. It takes 2–3 weeks to incubate and is infectious for about 6 days before the glands swell up, until 3 days after they go down. Swelling of the face can cause pain on swallowing, dry mouth, and discomfort while eating and talking. Sharp or acid foods such as lemon juice may aggravate the inflammation of the salivary glands. Swelling takes 3–7 days to recede, during which time the child may feel slightly unwell or fairly normal.

Treatment of mumps

- Because mumps causes pain when chewing and swallowing, food may need to be liquidized, and given as soups, juices and smoothies.
- Giving citrus fruits/drinks is best avoided as they can be painful to swallow.
- Drinks given throughout the day can include spring water, hot water or dilute teas of red clover (*Trifolium pratense*) marigold, thyme or cleavers (*Galium aparine*).
- Foods rich in beta carotene and vitamin C, which help to resolve viral infection and enhance the efforts of the immune system, are recommended.
- Zinc lozenges or 15 ml of liquid zinc can be given for 7–10 days to enhance immunity.
- Turmeric, garlic, black pepper and ginger can be added to soups and hot drinks to boost immunity.
- Garlic and echinacea will help stimulate the immune system to resolve infection, and can be combined with boneset (*Eupatorium perfoliatum*), basil, limeflowers (*Tilia europaea*), yarrow, chamomile, peppermint, lemon balm or elderflowers to reduce fever and inflammation.
- Chamomile or catnip (*Nepeta cataria*) tea is recommended if a child is restless and uncomfortable.
- Red clover, cleavers and marigold help reduce swelling of the parotid glands and can be given as teas or dilute tinctures every 2 hours during acute infection.

Externally

- Discomfort of the affected area around the neck and ears can be eased by gentle massage with dilute essential oils of chamomile, eucalyptus, lavender or thyme. A base of warm castor oil or sesame oil for the essential oils can be soothing to swollen glands.

- A few drops of these oils could also be added to hot water for steam inhalations and for compresses to be applied to the area. Dilute oils can also be added to bath water.

- Compresses using hot infusions can also be applied to relieve swelling and discomfort. Red clover, poke root (*Phytolacca decandra*), marigold, cleavers, mullein and lobelia (*Lobelia inflata*) are all suitable. The compresses should be replaced every 20–30 minutes and can be left on overnight.

- A hot water bottle against the painful side can alleviate pain. Compresses soaked in the above herbal infusions can be wrapped around the hot water bottle.

Ayurvedic approach

- In India, the milky juice from the stem or the root of gullara (*Ficus racemosa*) is applied to swollen glands (Dastur 1983, p. 102).

- Holy basil leaf juice or tea helps to relieve pain and swelling and reduce any accompanying fever, as it has analgesic as well as febrifuge properties.

- A paste made from holy basil leaves and sandalwood powder can be applied to the affected areas to relieve pain and inflammation.

- Fruit pulp (or leaves) of tamarind as a poultice will soothe inflammation and swelling and help to relieve pain. It has been shown in research (Williamson 2002) to have antiviral properties.

- Long pepper or black pepper can be given ($\frac{1}{4}$ tsp of the powder in hot water with honey). Pippeline, a constituent of pepper, has analgesic and anti-inflammatory properties and enhances antiviral immune mechanisms and specifically antigen-specific protective response (Phadke 2001, p. 90).

- Liquorice is also used, and has soothing and anti-inflammatory properties.

- Half a teaspoon of turmeric powder in hot water is useful for its antimicrobial and anti-inflammatory properties.

- Other useful antiviral herbs include: garlic, ginger, rose petal, amalaki, coriander, neem, centella, haritaki and ashwagandha.

MEASLES

Measles is a highly contagious viral infection spread by droplet infection, which tends to occur in epidemics. The incubation period is between 8–14 days from exposure, but a child may be infectious 7 days after being infected until 10 days after the rash begins. The seriousness of measles is related largely to the high risk of complications following the initial infection. It is often characterised by a high fever, which resolves gradually once the rash has developed fully. If the temperature rises again and the child seems unwell there could be a secondary infection. Complications of measles include eye damage, pneumonia, middle ear infection, bronchitis and more rarely encephalitis.

Treatment of measles

As in all infectious diseases with fever, the body's efforts to throw off the infection need to be supported, helping to resolve the disease quickly with a minimum of complications.

- The child needs to rest and drink plenty of fluids.

- Bright sunlight is best avoided as measles often causes heightened sensitivity to light.

- Vitamin A, beta carotene and vitamin C support the immune system and help speed resolution of viral infections. Research has demonstrated that vitamin A supplementation, particularly during acute measles or in children under two, may improve the outcome and recovery rate. When children are low in vitamin A the mucous membranes throughout the body become more susceptible to infection. The measles virus is more able to infect and damage these susceptible tissues. During a measles infection our stores of vitamin A can decrease significantly; if it decreases to the point of deficiency this can predispose to eye damage, secondary respiratory disease and diarrhoea (What Doctors Don't Tell You 1994).

- Zinc lozenges/15 ml liquid zinc will also support the immune system.

- To enhance immunity garlic and echinacea can be given at the first signs of infection every 2 hours.

- These can be combined with other herbs to encourage perspiration and help resolve the fever. Boneset (*Eupatorium perfoliatum*), lemon balm, chamomile, catnip (*Nepeta cataria*), elderflowers, limeflowers (*Tilia europaea*), peppermint and yarrow are all cooling and can be given through the day.

- These can also be used as hand and foot baths especially if the child is loathe to drink very much due to discomfort in the mouth or throat. Infusions of these or dilute essential oils of either lavender, chamomile, basil or eucalyptus can be added to bath water. Oils can also be used in room sprays or vaporizers.

- Olive leaf extract and elderberry are other useful antivirals.

- At the first signs of illness compresses of ginger, burdock or thyme can be applied to the skin to help bring out the rash and so alleviate the child's discomfort.

- Burdock and peppermint tea help to bring the rash out and can be given to the child every 2 hours until the rash subsides.

- For inflamed eyes, infusions of chamomile, rose, eyebright (*Euphrasia off.*) elderflowers or yarrow made with spring or distilled water, can be used to bathe the eyes 2–3 times a day. The tea needs to be tepid to avoid further irritation of the eye.

- If the child is irritable or restless and has trouble getting comfortable, chamomile or catnip tea may provide some relief.

- Solid food is best avoided until the fever has subsided.

Ayurvedic approach to treatment of measles

When there is an epidemic of measles certain prophylactic measures are recommended:

- The bowels should be kept open and the child not allowed to become constipated and a little powdered liquorice can be given daily as a preventative.
- The child should be protected from exposure to hot sun.
- Sugar, mustard and asafoetida (*Ferula asafoetida*) and other substances with heating properties are contraindicated.
- Coconut water is recommended for cooling.

Useful prescriptions include:

- Infusion of neem leaves, cumin seeds and raw sugar, $\frac{1}{4}$ tsp of each to a cup of boiling water.
- Infusion of black raisins, coriander seeds and chiretta (*Swertia chiretta*) leaves to be given in the morning.
- Powder of equal parts tamarind seeds (*Tamarindus indica*) and turmeric $\frac{1}{4}-\frac{1}{2}$ tsp in warm water three times daily.
- A traditional recipe is composed of: Catechu (*Acacia catechu*), triphala, neem bark, leaves of kadve padval (*Trichosanthes doica*), guduchi and vasa (*Adhatoda vasica*).
- Infusion can also be given of safflower flowers (*Carthamnus tinctorius*). Infuse $\frac{1}{2}$ oz of flowers in 1 pint of boiling water given in 3 doses.
- Rice flour on the skin is very soothing.

GERMAN MEASLES (RUBELLA)

German measles is a viral infection that can be so mild as to pass unnoticed by child and parents and may not require treatment. It is an important eruptive infection however, due to the risk it poses to the unborn child when contracted by a pregnant woman. For this reason blood tests to ascertain immunity to Rubella are taken in teenage girls.

- If a fever develops, teas of chamomile, elderflowers, limeflowers, peppermint or yarrow can be given.
- Add *Calendula* or cleavers, which aid the efforts of the lymphatic system and echinacea to enhance immunity.

- Externally dilute oils of lavender, thyme or rosemary can be massaged into swollen lymph nodes.
- If the skin is itchy and the child seems irritable, the skin can be bathed with infusions of burdock, chamomile, chickweed (*Stellaria media*) lavender or yarrow.
- Distilled witch hazel and rosewater make good alternatives.

CANDIDIASIS (*CANDIDA ALBICANS*)

- *Candida albicans* is a fungus which naturally lives in the intestines with billions of bacteria, mostly lactobacillus, which fulfil a variety of functions including synthesis of vitamins. Candidiasis or overgrowth of *Candida albicans* tends to occur in children depleted from tiredness, stress, poor diet or other illness. It is particularly prevalent in children frequently prescribed antibiotics which disturb the gut flora.

- There is increasing awareness that candida overgrowth may account for a variety of chronic symptoms including food allergies, fatigue, behavioural problems, bloating, bowel disturbances and itching. In the gut the fungus can produce root-like extensions (rhizoids) which penetrate the gut lining and enable whole proteins and allergens as well as intestinal toxins to pass through the gut into the bloodstream (leaky gut syndrome). This contributes to the development of food allergies including eczema, asthma, migraine, recurrent infections, catarrh and bowel problems. Yeast cells attach themselves to the mucous membranes in the body from mouth to anus and in the genitourinary tract. They can affect the whole system causing e.g., fungal infection of toenails, genital pruritis and athlete's foot. Intestinal candida can also produce toxins that once absorbed affect immune and endocrine systems and inhibit T-cell function, producing an allergy to intestinal yeasts, such as yeasts and moulds on foods, bread, etc.

Causes of candida overgrowth include:

- Antibiotics, which destroy lactobacillus but not candida.
- Sugar, which feeds yeast and suppresses the immune response.

- A high carbohydrate diet, as incomplete digestion of carbohydrates provides yeast in the gut with a plentiful food supply. It is important to replace simple with complex carbohydrates.
- Drugs such as cortisone encourage yeast infection.

CHRONIC FATIGUE SYNDROME

Apart from feeling tired, lethargic and out of sorts following a viral infection, a child may experience symptoms such as bowel disturbances and pain, wind, nausea, headaches and depression which suggest post viral or chronic fatigue syndrome. Chronic fatigue syndrome is often associated with lowered immunity related to poor function of the thymus gland, and to nutritional deficiencies, particularly of vitamin A, vitamin B, zinc and magnesium. It can also be linked with food allergies and candidiasis.

Treatment of candidiasis and post viral syndrome

Treatment is aimed at enhancing general immunity, combating yeast infection in the gut and its effects elsewhere in the body, and raising nutritional status.

- Lactoacidophyllus as a supplement or in live yoghurt, as well as garlic and olive oil will aid re-establishment of the normal bacterial population of the gut.

- Avoiding mould-containing foods, yeast in marmite and bread, mushrooms, fermented foods such as vinegar, cheese, and malt extract, sugar and junk food is advised as these will encourage proliferation of yeast infections.

- To help combat infection, antifungal herbs (see Immune System, p. 150) can be taken as well as grapefruit seed extract: 4 drops stirred into a glass of water three times a day. This should be followed with food to avoid queasiness (Landis and Khalsa 1998, p. 392).

- Berberine-containing herbs kill yeast and activate macrophages (Landis and Khalsa 1998), they inhibit leaky gut syndrome and combat bacterial infection. These include barberry root (*Berberis vulgaris*), Oregon grape root (*Berberis aquifolium*), and golden seal root (*Hydrastis canadensis*).

- Other antifungal herbs include: thyme (*Thymus vulgaris*), cloves (*Eugenia caryophyllus*) and cinnamon (*Cinnamomum cassia*). Perilla leaf (*Perilla frutescens*), onion (*Allium cepa*) and garlic (*Allium sativum*) inhibit germination rate of spores from *Aspergillus flavus* and *Cladosporium cladospoiroides*. Burdock root (*Arctium lappa*) and chameleon plant (*Houttuynia cordata*) also help inhibit candida proliferation in the gut. They can be combined with general immune enhancing herbs (see Immune System, p. 150).

- Rose, fennel, (*Foeniculum vulgare*), hyssop (*Hyssopus off.*), marjoram (*Oreganum marjorana*), marigold, turmeric, rosemary, tulsi and myrrh (*Commiphora molmol*) can also inhibit fungal infection and help re-establish normal bacterial population of the gut.

- For fungal infection of the toenails soak the feet in warm water to soften the nails. Then cut them short, straight across and apply tea tree oil mixed with equal parts of neem oil.

- For oral thrush I have found that an infusion of marigold, sage (*Salvia off.*) or thyme as mouthwash three times daily, works very well.

- Alternatively one can use a drop of essential oil thyme/turmeric/marjoram in 20 ml thyme tincture. Use $\frac{1}{4}$–$\frac{1}{2}$ tsp diluted with a little water to swill around the mouth or 1–2 ml marigold, thyme, myrrh or sage tincture diluted in water as a mouthwash.

ALLERGIES

An allergic reaction is an exaggerated immune response to an allergen, which produces symptoms related to the release of chemicals such as histamine. Plasma cells in the body produce antibodies, immunoglobulins, which have a memory. When an allergic reaction occurs, immunoglobulins are formed that bind to mast cells lining the mucous membranes, such as those in the respiratory and gastrointestinal tracts, ready to form a complex with the allergen when the person is exposed to the same substance again and attach to the surface of various cells in blood vessels and tissues. When this occurs, histamine, leukotrienes and other irritant cytokine chemicals and prostaglandins are released, and these give rise to allergic symptoms.

The term atopy implies a susceptibility to develop immediate allergies on exposure to certain substances such as atopic eczema, asthma and hayfever. Classic allergic symptoms include:

- inflammation of the nasal passages
- over-production of mucus and irritation of the eyes that characterize hayfever
- inflammation of the digestive tract producing diarrhoea
- asthma
- urticaria
- eczema.

Allergens come into contact with the body's tissues in several different ways.

By mouth

Babies and children can react to foods or drugs. Milk, eggs, shellfish, nuts, wheat, and strawberries are common allergens and penicillin can often cause a drug reaction. Symptoms can vary widely, ranging from:

- swelling of the face
- stomach aches
- nausea
- intestinal problems
- bloating
- gas
- constipation
- vomiting
- diarrhoea
- urticaria
- wheezing
- failure to thrive.

Some children have specific allergies only to one food such as tomatoes or shellfish. Some react only to large amounts of the incriminated food while others require just a few molecules to set off the allergic response.

Airborne allergens

Some children react to inhaled substances including: household chemicals, environmental pollutants,

Table 7.1 Symptoms of allergy

In a baby	In a toddler	As children get older
Frequent crying	Frequent respiratory	Similar reactions to adults
Feeding difficulties	or ear infections (The incidence	which may follow the pattern of
Colic	of these can diminish significantly	allergic relatives including:
Constipation or diarrhoea	if milk produce is reduced in or omitted	
Eczema, urticaria, or other rashes	from the diet)	• Chronic eczema
Dry skin or persistent nappy rash	Stomach aches	• Hayfever
Insomnia and irritability	Mood swings	• Asthma
Restlessness	Temper tautrums	• Bowel problems
Constant apparent hunger	Constipation (diarrhoea)	• Headaches or migraines
Frequent possetting	Flatulence	• Urticaria
Mucous congestion, leading to	Eczema	• Tonsilitis
problems such as bronchiolitis,	Tonsilitis	
croup and frequent respiratory	Croup	
infections		

pollens, dust, animal dander and moulds. Symptoms can develop such as

- fatigue
- itching or inflamed eyes
- sneezing
- chronic mucus
- headaches
- rhinitis
- congestion of the throat or chest
- coughing, wheezing and eczema occurring during hayfever season.
- Hayfever/allergic rhinitis can be triggered by different kinds of pollens in trees, grass and flowers.
- Animal dander, moulds, mildew, fungus, dust and smoke are common allergens. Long-term irritation and inflammation are a drain on the immune system's resources and make the allergic child generally more susceptible to infections and a vicious circle of allergic response and respiratory infection can develop with little relief in between.

Through the skin

External sources of allergens such as environmental substances, household chemicals, and biological washing powders can cause rashes on contact. Wool, various plants, creams, bases and ointments such as lanolin, strong sunlight and extreme cold can all act as triggers.

Allergic responses tend to vary with age. Broadly speaking babies react to skin contact and food. The delicate skins of babies can react to wool, baby lotions and ointments, nylon, rubber pants, disposable nappies and washing powder. Their immature digestive tracts can react to foods such as formula feeds, substances that come through the breast milk including milk produce, wheat, eggs and nuts. Toddlers react to these as well as to infections and older children react to all of these as well as what they inhale, such as grass pollen and house dust mite (Table 7.1).

Children who exhibit allergic symptoms as a baby may "outgrow" their allergies but unless their underlying tendency is addressed there is a strong likelihood that other symptoms related to allergy appear at a later date.

Factors contributing to allergies

Pollution

The cause of an allergic reaction does not lie simply in the specific allergen itself, be it grass pollen, the house-dust mite or any other, but rather in the factors that compromise the efficient functioning of a child's immune system. Breast milk contains immunoglobulins which protect the baby's immature immune system and provides vital substances for the development of immunity including gamma linoleic acid, zinc, selenium, interferon, iron and antioxidants. However, probably as a result of nutritional deficiencies and pollution, breast milk does not appear to protect in the same way as it used to and many breast-fed babies are becoming allergic to substances coming through the milk, although they are far less prone to allergies than those fed on formula milk. Drugs and toxins such as pesticides, herbicides, drug residues in foods, and many other chemicals and heavy metals in the environment from food, water and air, pass through the breast milk to the baby, where they can interfere with normal immune function. Caffeine, alcohol and nicotine can all play a part. Many toxic substances, insecticides and dioxin for instance collect in fish, eggs and meat. Vegetarian and vegan mothers have lower levels of hazardous chemical in their milk compared with meat and fish eaters. However, the benefits of breast-feeding still far outnumber those of bottle-feeding, so breast is still best, especially for the first 4–6 months of life, until the baby's immune system is more mature. Research has shown that breast-feeding at this time boosts immunity and minimizes allergic tendencies and sets the pattern for the future, reducing the likelihood of allergy and autoimmune disease such as Crohn's disease and ulcerative colitis in older children and adults.

Poor diet and nutritional deficiencies

Dietary deficiencies of protein, essential fatty acids, vitamins and minerals, notably zinc, can disrupt the formation of prostaglandins and antibodies by a child's developing immune system. It appears that children suffering from allergies require more essential fatty acids than normal children. This may be due to faults with the metabolism of EFAs, meaning that dietary linoleic acid (LA) is not converted to its usable form, gamma linoleic acid (GLA) and so is not available for the immune system. This inherited tendency is most apparent in children with eczema, asthma and hayfever and is often overcome by adding GLA to the diet, as well as plenty of foods rich in EFAs. Should allergic symptoms persist, a deficiency of either vitamins or minerals necessary for production of enzymes involved with EFA metabolism may be present. This may be caused by eating nutrient-depleted foods or foods that rob the body of nutrients or block their availability to the body.

Digestive problems

Proper function of the digestive tract and liver are vital to prevention and treatment of immune problems and susceptibility to allergies. Digestive problems such as poor elimination, *Candida* overgrowth and enzyme deficiency can lead to an accumulation of toxins in the gut and poor absorption of nutrients and predispose to allergies. Poor absorption means that nutrients consumed providing raw materials for the immune system are not being adequately absorbed. Irritation and inflammation created in the gut wall, from *Candida* for example, can render it more permeable to toxins from the intestines as well as to whole proteins from foods, predisposing the child to food allergies.

Stress

Emotional difficulties, stresses at home or at school should be taken into consideration and as much support provided as possible. Stress has a well-documented effect on the function of the digestive tract and could account for enzyme deficiency in many instances. Acute stress appears to enhance the immune response, but chronic stress can lead to immunosuppression. Mechanisms for this process may involve reduced lymphocyte mitogenic response and a decrease in the number of lymphocytes by means of increased apoptosis (Shi et al 2003).

Drugs

This includes overuse of antibiotics that can suppress immune function and cause disruption of the gut flora. This can lead to abnormal bowel overgrowth and candidiasis and digestive disturbances such as chronic constipation and diarrhoea and result in absorption of toxins into the system, which further compromises immunity.

Genetic problems

These include damage to chromosome 6 which governs immunity and can cause recurring infections and inherited susceptibility.

Treatment of allergies

When treating allergies it is obviously important to address the underlying issues contributing to allergies and treat accordingly. It is important to ascertain which allergens are responsible for the reaction and to remove them as far as possible to allow the child some respite while treatment is instigated. It is not enough to identify the allergen and remove it, for the malfunctioning immune system remains unchanged, relieved of a burden temporarily, only to turn its attention at a later date to another substance to which the child is frequently exposed. This is confirmed by the fact that many infants that are found to be cow's milk allergic and are fed on soya products instead, can sooner or later begin to react adversely to soya as well. It is the child that needs treatment, not the allergen.

Having said this, an external or atmospheric allergen may be difficult to identify and remove from contact with the child, e.g. pollen in the atmosphere during the hayfever season. However, if a child reacts to environmental allergens, there are usually food substances to which the child also reacts and these are far easier to manipulate once identified. Generally speaking if the offending food items are removed, the child is better able to cope with the environmental allergens. Removing wheat (a member of the grass family) from the diet during the hayfever season often means that grass pollen can be better tolerated by the respiratory mucus, and hayfever symptoms can be reduced if not eliminated. Similarly, removal of milk products from the diet may mean that a child who reacts to the dander of a pet with rhinitis or asthma, may be able to hug their pet without suffering the normal consequences of sneezing or wheezing.

Identifying food allergies can present challenges as symptoms can develop up to 3 days after ingestion. Cravings are a classic sign. When children crave milk it is usually a sign of allergy/addiction. Food substances most likely to cause reactions include:

- wheat
- milk produce
- pork
- beef
- eggs
- sometimes chicken
- oranges and other citrus fruits
- peanuts
- potatoes

- tomatoes (also often peppers and aubergines which are in the same family)
- maize
- gluten (a protein found in oats, wheat, barley and rye)
- food additives
- agricultural chemicals, such as pesticides and herbicides in foods
- aspartame
- fungi and yeasts on foods
- chocolate
- tea and coffee
- cane and beet sugar
- salicylates (Table 7.2).

The offending foods are best omitted from the diet for 2 months, allowing time for symptoms to abate, and then gradually reintroduced in small amounts once every 5 days. If there is no recurrence of symptoms, the food can be then given at more frequent intervals, every 4 days, then 3 and so on, and then in increasing amounts. Should symptoms develop, the food needs to be removed again completely until they clear, and then reintroduced more gradually. It is best to maintain treatment of the child using herbs until the food can be tolerated in reasonable amounts on a regular basis. This can take months and sometimes even years. The longer the offending food is removed from the diet the better the child is able to tolerate it later. Care needs to be taken by parents to ensure that the removal of foods does not nutritionally compromise their children's diet. Some food allergies are called fixed, as they tend to last for life, such as egg, strawberries, shellfish and penicillin.

It is generally possible to treat a child with allergies successfully even if the allergens cannot be identified and removed, but it may take longer. Every child needs to be treated as a whole; attention should be paid to the underlying causes of allergy and these may differ from one child to another. Diet, stress levels, temperament, constitution, environment, exposure to harmful chemicals, sleep, exercise and fresh air are all important considerations in a child's life. Added to this, specific weaknesses or imbalances such as a weak digestion or an inherited tendency to allergy, can all play their part. By improving the function of the immune system using herbs and proper nutrition,

Table 7.2   Salicylates

Allergic reactions to salicylates	Salicylates are found in the following fruits	Salicylates are found in the following herbs
Asthma	Raspberries	*Filipendula ulmaria*
Eczema	Pineapple	*Silybum marianum*
Hyperactivity	Sultana grapes	*Hydrastis canadensis*
Urticaria	Strawberries	*Eleutherococcus senticosus*
Gastro-intestinal problems	Sultanas	*Withania somnifera*
Headaches	Raisins	*Hypericum perforatum*
Recurrent mouth ulcers	Currants	*Echinacea angustifolia/purpurea*
Irritability	California dates	vitex *Agnus castus*
		Glycyrrhiza glabra
		Panax ginseng
		Ginkgo biloba
		Taraxacum radix
		Trigonella foenum-graecum
		Foeniculum vulgare

the general health and vitality of the child should improve, reducing susceptibility.

Herbs can be prescribed to nourish the body, particularly the immune system, and to balance the digestive tract and combined with gentle methods to minimize symptoms associated with inflammation and swelling.

- A combination of echinacea and liquorice is often used for the prevention and relief of hayfever. Both inhibit IgE-mediated allergic responses that give rise to the irritation and inflammation of the airways, while they provide symptomatic relief through their anti-inflammatory and decongestant properties respectively.

- Recommendations for boosting the immune system (see p. 160) can be followed using immune and digestive tonics such as liquorice, turmeric, pippali and ginger.

- Immune tonics such as echinacea, astragalus (*Astragalus membranaceus*), liquorice, ginseng (*Panax ginseng*) ginger, pippali, garlic and guduchi can be given; also chamomile, lemon balm, eyebright (*Euphrasia off.*), ginkgo (*Gingko biloba*), feverfew (*Tanacetum parthenium*), red clover (*Trifolium pratense*), wild yam (*Dioscorea villosa*), and yarrow, which will help quieten allergic reactions. These can be given as teas or dilute tinctures and may need to be taken over several months for good effect.

- Digestive herbs can be taken an hour or so prior to food to enhance flow of digestive enzymes. Ginger tea, hot lemon and honey, or a handful of seeds to chew (not for younger children who may choke) either cumin, coriander, fennel or caraway, prepare the digestive tract for food and help break down of foods efficiently to reduce risk of large undigested molecules, especially whole proteins passing through the gut wall to be misinterpreted as foreign invaders by the immune system, giving rise to an allergic response.

- Chamomile and yarrow can be given daily as a tea. They help soothe the allergic response and inhibit the production of histamine.

- Essential oils of chamomile, lemon balm and yarrow can be used in a variety of ways, in the bath, as inhalations and for massage, diluted in a base using 1–2 drops of oil per 5 ml of base oil.

- Nettles (fresh is best) provide relief for hayfever and are said to act much like an antihistamine. They can be added to soups, stews or teas to help to calm the allergic response.

- The severity of the inflammatory response can be diminished by vitamin C with bioflavonoids and magnesium, which have antihistamine action and can be given through diet or as supplements to older children.

- Quercetin is a bioflavonoid found in citrus fruits that helps to inhibit secretion of histamine, leukotrienes and prostaglandins. Other flavonoid-containing foods and herbs could also prove helpful as they have anti-inflammatory, antioxidant, immuno-regulating properties and capillary strengthening effect (Landis and Khalsa 1997).

- Triphala is one of the best Ayurvedic remedies for allergies and helps to clear out accumulated *Kapha* ($\frac{1}{2}$ tsp in hot water last thing at night for general immune support and in the morning to clear congested airways).

The following Ayurvedic herbs are used to enhance immunity in the general treatment of allergies (Box 7.1).

Box 7.1   Herbs used in the general treatment of allergies

Ashwagandha
Shatavari
Neem leaves
Turmeric
Eclipta
Boswellia (*Boswellia serrata*)
Vasa (*Adhatoda vasica*)
Anthrapachaka leaf (*Tylophora indica*)
Guduchi
Ginseng (*Panax ginseng*)
Tulsi

References

Chopra D, Simon D 2000 The Chopra Centre Herbal Handbook. Rider, London, p. 71

Dastur JF 1983 Everybody's Guide to Ayurvedic Medicine. DB Taraporevala Sons & Co. Private Ltd, Bombay

Lad V 1999 The Complete Book of Ayurvedic Home Remedies. Judy Piatkus Ltd, London

Landis R, Khalsa KPS 1998 Herbal Defence against Illness and Ageing. Thorsons, London

Phadke PS 2001 Home Doctor. Silverdale Books, Leicester, England. p. 90

Shi et al 2003 What Doctors Don't Tell You. Satellite House, London SW19 4E2

Tillotson AK, Tillotson NH, Robert A Jr 2001 The One Earth Herbal Sourcebook. Kensington Publishing Corps, New York

Weiss RF 1988 Herbal Medicine. Beaconsfield Publishers Ltd, England, p. 231

What Doctors Don't Tell You. Sept 1994 vol. 5, no 6 Satellite House, London

Williamson E 2002 Major Herbs of Ayurveda. Churchill Livingstone, London

Chapter **8**

The digestive system

CHAPTER CONTENTS

The main function of the digestive system is to convert the natural resources from around us into energy for every cellular action that keeps us alive. Our health largely depends on how well we are able to digest, absorb and utilize the nutrients from our food. While food conversion provides energy, it also requires energy to perform all the essential biochemical reactions involved in the process of digestion. If the digestive energy is weak or disturbed, problems arise, which can cause symptoms involving the digestive tract itself such as stomach aches, diarrhoea or constipation, as well as those affecting general health and energy, such as lethargy, headaches, irritability, inability to concentrate, disturbed sleep and lowered immunity.

Optimum functioning of the digestive tract depends on several factors. First, regular peristaltic movements require sufficient dietary fibre to push food through the gut so that we can evacuate food residues as well as the waste products of metabolism. Poor elimination leads to a toxic state of the bowel, which then becomes prone to infection and the spread of toxins to the rest of the body. The condition of the bowels can fundamentally affect general health and give rise to a wide variety of problems. Antigens and toxins from bowel bacteria have been related to development of a number of diseases (Murray and Pizzorno 1990).

Secondly the digestive tract is influenced by the nervous system. There is constant interaction between the brain and the digestive tract, making the process of digestion very susceptible to the effect of mind and emotion, personality and constitution. The autonomic nervous system regulates blood flow to and from the digestive tract, as well as the secretion of digestive juices. Stress can, for example, reduce the flow of digestive enzymes and thereby reduce digestion and absorption or it may cause excess hydrochloric acid in the stomach, which can irritate and inflame the lining of the stomach or intestine. An upset at home or school or too much excitement can disrupt digestion and cause symptoms such as tummy aches and colic.

The right diet is vital to the health and normal function of the digestive tract. Over-refined foods, excess sugar, fizzy drinks, ice creams and fried foods, as well as indigestible foods such as bread, cheese, red meats, can all irritate and create disturbances.

AYURVEDIC APPROACH

Just as our bodies are made up of the five elements, earth, water, fire, air and ether, so too is the food we eat. Our digestive power enables our bodies to utilize the five elements in food, to extract the nutrients and transform them into bodily elements through the process of digestion. According to Ayurveda, most diseases arise from poor functioning of the digestive system. Our appetite and our ability to digest and absorb nutrients with the help of digestive enzymes is known as *agni* or "digestive fire" and this is central to health. Maintaining the balance of the digestive fire is the key to preventative health, as well as to the treatment of all digestive problems.

The various mechanisms of the human body produce energy to enable perception, action and expression. This energy is represented by the element of fire. *Agni* is a Vedic term meaning burning, transforming, or perceiving, from the root *"ang"* to burst forth. *Agni* has all the qualities of fire: hot, dry, light, fragrant, subtle, mobile and penetrating. It is increased by hot, fragrant spices like ginger, black pepper and cayenne as these have a similar nature. There are many different types of fire in the body (*Jatharagni*), the main form of which is digestive fire.

Five elemental fires: Bhutagnis – Each of the five elements has its own digestive fire. These reside in the liver, responsible for turning digestive fire into *Agni* that corresponds to each of the five elements necessary for building up the respective tissues in the body. If their functioning is impaired the respective element in the body will not be formed correctly. Substances such as ghee or aloe vera gel help regulate elemental digestive fires.

Seven tissue fires: Dhatuagnis – Each of the seven *dhatus* has its own digestive fire, responsible for proper formation of that tissue. When *agni* is too low, too much tissue of an inferior nature will be formed. When it is too high insufficient tissue will be formed.

According to Ayurveda, when *agni* is sufficient it prevents the build up of toxins in the body, the mind and senses are clear and acute and we have the energy to direct our lives in a positive direction. When deficient it causes a build up of toxins in the body which gives rise to dullness, heaviness, stagnation and cloudiness of mind and perception.

Digestive fire (*agni*) works on the food mass that has been swallowed and liquefied. It separates the pure or nutritive part of the food (*sara*) from the waste material (*kitta*). This it breaks down into the forms of the five elements. These in turn are absorbed and transferred to the liver where the elemental *agnis* turn them into the respective elemental tissues for the body. The earth elements digested and transformed from the food serve to build up the basic bulk or protein of the body, like the muscles. The water element builds up the vital fluids, plasma, blood and fat. The fire elements build up the enzymes and haemoglobin. The air elements build up the bone and nerve plexuses. The ether elements build up the mind and senses. *Prana Vayu* helps in digestion of food. *Samana Vayu* controls peristaltic movements and absorption of food. *Apana Vayu* controls defecation and expulsion of gases.

Thirteen forms of *Agni*

Jatharagni

This is the digestive fire which imparts energy to all the secretions and enzymes in the process of digestion and resides in the stomach and small intestine. It is not simply responsible for digesting and absorbing nutrients from food but also for destroying pathogenic micro-organisms in the gut. If the digestive fire is low and digestion incomplete as a result, partially digested or undigested food ferments and breeds toxins in the gut, thereby compromising the immune system.

There are four different conditions of *agni*:

1. Variable (*Vishama*)
2. High (*Tikshna*)
3. Low (*Manda*)
4. Balanced (*Sama*).

Vishamagni

Digestive fire tends to be variable in *Vata* types with their fluctuating nature and nervous digestion. It is caused by over heavy/light diet and activities which increase *Vata* and in turn it causes vataja disorders. As a result, high *Vata* types can be alternately very hungry and not hungry at all and sometimes they digest well and at other times may suffer distension, gas, constipation, diarrhoea,

heaviness of abdomen, borborygmi, colicky pain and tenemus. After a while *vishamagni* becomes low digestive fire (*mandagni*) and the ability to digest well diminishes.

Tikshnagni

Digestive fire is usually high in *Pitta* types, evidenced by a strong appetite, good powers of digestion without gaining excessive weight. *Agni* can be overly increased by eating hot spicy food in hot weather, and by activities which increase *Pitta*, and in turn it disrupts digestive enzymes and causes *Pittaja* disorders. If *agni* is too high a child will eat more, digest quickly, the metabolic rate is fast, and the child may be prone to febrile disorders, hypoglycaemia, irritability, headaches, nausea, stomach aches and diarrhoea.

Mandagni

Agni is usually low in *Kapha* types who have dull but constant appetites, slow metabolism, tending to hold weight even without eating excessively. *Mandagni* is caused by diet and activities which increase *Kapha* including eating too much, heavy, oily and sweet foods (not ghee), sedentary lifestyle and excessive sleep. In turn low digestive fire leads to *Kapha* disorders such as mucus congestion and a tendency to frequent colds and coughs. Weak digestive power means that it takes a long time to digest even a small quantity of food, causing a feeling of dullness, heaviness in the stomach, a tendency to coughs, breathlessness, a feeling of heaviness in body, excess saliva, nausea, lethargy, and sleepiness after eating. Symptoms are worse with *ama* causing, for example joint pain, headache, sinusitis and lassitude.

Samagni

Digestive fire is balanced when the *doshas* and emotions are balanced and is indicated by regular and moderate appetite with good powers of digestion promoting good health. Children with *Samagni* can tolerate hunger, heavy food, irregular or excessive food intake and still preserve good digestive fire.

When *agni* is normal mild, *Sattvic* spices such as cardamom, turmeric, coriander and fennel can be given to children through their diet to maintain the health of the digestive tract. *Agni* can also be maintained by regular exercise, yoga, deep breathing (*pranyama*), meditation, and proper eating.

Ill health develops as a result of either excess, deficient or abnormal *agni*, which all eventually become low digestive fire. Weak *agni* lowers immunity as *ama* is formed from poor digestion and obstructs the channels (*srotas*) throughout the body.

The undigested food mass: *Ama*

If digestive fire is low it leaves a residue of undigested or partly digested food that can accumulate, stagnate and ferment. This is known as *ama*, from the root "*am*", to harm or weaken. Its formation and accumulation is said to be the beginning of the disease process for all diseases. It weakens the defence system and lowers resistance to diseases starting from the common cold. Hence *agni* is the key to health.

Agni is increased by pungent, sour and salty tastes and a small amount of bitter taste. Early trials demonstrated that the bitter taste stimulated gastric secretion though only when the herb was tasted. Later trials on a patient with an occluded oesophagus and a gastric fissure found that both salivation and gastric secretion increased in line with each other (Mills and Bone 2000). As an example of the gastric-stimulating effect of pungent tastes, a double blind trial on human volunteers found that black and red pepper significantly increased parietal and pepsin secretion (Myers et al 1987).

To raise digestive fire: *Agni deepana*

Spices are the best thing for increasing *agni*. They generally have the same qualities as *agni*, being hot, dry, light and fragrant.

Popular remedies for raising digestive fire include:

- Trikatu (ginger, long pepper and black pepper)
- Trikulu (clove, cinnamon, cardamom)
- Pippali
- Ginger
- Hingwastaka (lavan (salt), hing (asafoetida), trikatu, ajmoda, kalijeera, jeera).

To clear toxins: *Ama pachana*

Bitter and pungent herbs generally have the ability to clear *Ama* from the gastrointestinal tract. Remedies for cleaning toxins include:

- General use for all three doshic types: Triphala which is a mixture of amalaki, haritaki, bibhitaki
- For *Vata*: haritaki; hingwastaka; lavan bhaskar; five salts
- For *Pitta*: guduchi and ginger; coriander; amalaki
- For *Kapha*: Triphala guggulu; Trikatu.

Stages of digestion

According to Ayurveda there are three stages of digestion. The first stage is governed by *Kapha* and takes place in the mouth and stomach. It involves saliva and the alkaline secretions of the stomach and is responsible for the extraction of the water and earth elements from the food eaten. *Kapha* predominant children may tend to have an excess of these secretions and may be prone to symptoms such as nausea, bringing up mucus, profuse salivation and poor appetite, especially if they eat too many sweet and salty foods.

The second stage is ruled by *Pitta* and involves the acid secretions from the stomach and small intestine. Here the fire element is extracted. Eating too much sour, salty and pungent foods can increase these secretions and give rise to burning stomach pains, nausea and diarrhoea.

The third stage is ruled by *Vata* and takes place in the large intestine and involves the formation of stools. Here the air and ether elements are extracted from foods. Eating too much light, dry, astringent, bitter or pungent foods will increase *Vata* and give rise to symptoms such as wind, bloating, abdominal pain and constipation.

PROBLEMS AFFECTING THE DIGESTIVE TRACT

The digestive tract in Ayurvedic medicine is known as the *annavahasrota* and the problems arising in this *srota* include:

- *Agni manda*: low digestive fire
- *Ajeerna*: indigestion

- *Arochak*: nausea
- *Grahani*: colitis
- *Chardi*: vomiting
- *Krumi*: pathogens, bacteria, worms, etc.

LOW DIGESTIVE FIRE: *AGNI MANDA*

Doshas involved: *Kledaka Kapha, Samana Vayu, Vyana Vayu, Pachaka Pitta*.

Agni manda is considered the main cause of all other diseases in the body. It causes the formation of *ama* and affects all other kinds of *agni* as they are nourished by the *agni* of the digestive tract.

Causes of low digestive fire

1. Dietary: irregular food intake in terms of time and quantity, fasting, excessive amounts of food, heavy food, fatty foods, e.g. cheese, hot, spicy foods, dry, raw and unripe fruits, very cold food/drinks, too much liquid which dilutes digestive juices, strong tea and coffee, incompatible food, stale or contaminated food.
2. Iatrogenic: misuse of purgatives or enemas.
3. Debility due to illness, disease of the digestive tract such as gastroenteritis or chronic diarrhoea.
4. Environmental factors: the seasons, time, abnormal seasons, hot moist climate, etc.
5. Suppression of natural urges, emotional problems.
6. Disturbance of the *doshas*.
7. Constitution.

Pathogenesis: (Samprapti)

When *Samana Vayu* is deficient it cannot ignite the digestive fire, when excessive it blows it out. *Pachaka Pitta* is responsible for *agni*. Low *Pitta* means not enough *agni*. Too much *Pitta* means it burns itself out leading to low digestive fire. When *Kledaka Kapha* accumulates in the digestive tract it causes low digestive fire. One or more of the above dietary causes aggravates the *doshas*. The aggravated *doshas* disturb normal *agni*. The disturbed *agni* aggravates the *doshas* and the vicious circle continues.

Symptoms include indigestion, anorexia, heaviness in abdomen, lethargy, restlessness, flatulence, belching, bad breath, foul-smelling faeces, disturbed sleep and irritability.

Treatment for disturbances of *agni*

For vishamagni: Vata shamana

Oily (e.g. ghee), mild spicy, sour and salty foods and medicines help to balance digestive fire when combined with a light diet. In India they use an oil enema intermittently, using sesame oil or Dashamula oil. Formulae used include: Hingwastaka churna (asafoetida, ginger, cumin, rock salt, etc.) LavanaBhaskar churna, $\frac{1}{8}-\frac{1}{4}$ tsp with warm ghee before meals (see Formulae, p. 302) Lashunadi vati (garlic compound tablets). Vehicle/*anupana*: warm water/ghee.

For tikshnagni: Pitta shamana

Hot spices should be avoided and digestive bitters such as chamomile, guduchi, dandelion root, rosemary and amalaki with their cooling properties can be taken. Heavy, cold, unctuous and sweet foods are useful (see *Pitta* reducing diet). Purgatives are used intermittently, once every 2–4 weeks, for example Triphala and Darthree.

Sandalwood, amalaki and shatavari cool *Pitta*. Chiretta lowers digestive fire without increasing toxins. Vehicle/*anupana*: cool water/ghee.

For mandagni: Kapha shamana

A light diet (see Detoxification diet, p. 166) is recommended. Incompatible or excess foods, irregular eating, heavy food should be avoided. Warm water or honey is best as an *anupana* (vehicle). In India they prescribe emetics to clear *Kapha* quickly and effectively from the stomach. Here we use expectorants and warming spices as a gentler approach.

To stimulate *agni* and the secretion of the digestive juices, appetizing, digestant, bitter, pungent and astringent foods and medicines are given. Spices are particularly good and the following formulae and herbs are indicated: Trikatu, cayenne, ginger, pippali, chitrak (*Plumbago zeylanica*), musta (*Cyperus rotundus*), guduchi (*Tinospora cordifolia*), bilva fruit (*Aegle marmelos*), and asafoetida (*Ferula asafoetida*).

Spices also digest *ama*, astringent, bitter and pungent herbs also dry excess liquid mucus which can dampen digestive fire. Hingwastaka churna,

Trikatu and ginger are effective *ama* reducing remedies.

A light diet is recommended.

INDIGESTION: *AJEERNA*

Causes include:

1. Drinking too much cold water which lowers *agni*.
2. Overeating, incorrect food and eating between meals (which confuses digestive fire), improper time for meals, eating when stressed, angry or too late at night.
3. Suppression of natural urges, for example not eating when hungry, are seen to damage digestive power.
4. Incorrect sleep pattern such as sleeping in day, not sleeping well at night, working at night can all affect digestion.

The above all lower *agni*, and as a result *ama* develops and combines with whichever *dosha* is predominant in the stomach, *Vata*, *Pitta* or *Kapha* and gives rise to indigestion.

Pathogenesis: (Samprapti)

Low digestive fire causes *Ama* accumulation in the stomach. The breakdown of food is not complete, due to poor functioning of *Samana Vayu* which inhibits digestion and absorption. This leads to nutritional deficiencies and absorption of toxins into the system. There is indigestion, lethargy, feeling heavy and sluggish, excess salivation, a bad taste in the mouth and a coated tongue.

Signs and symptoms: (Rupa)

Kapha type

The first stage of indigestion involves *ama* and *Kapha*, and is known as *Ama Ajeerna*.

The symptoms of *Kapha* and *ama* include: heaviness, lethargy, coated, greasy tongue, sluggish bowels. There may be stomach pain, loss of appetite, fullness of the stomach, a bad taste in the mouth, increase of saliva/mucus, and fluid retention.

Pitta type

The second stage of indigestion involves *ama*, *Kapha* and *Pitta* and is known as *Vidagda*.

Kapha and *ama* accumulated in the stomach affects *Pachaka Pitta*, causing wind, belching, acid regurgitation, bad breath, heat, burning sensation, nausea, vomiting, thirst, irritability, anger, heartburn and sweating.

Vata type

The third stage of indigestion involves *ama* and all three *doshas* and is known as *Vishtabda*.

This involves *ama*, *Samana Vata* and *Pachaka Pitta*. Accumulated *ama* blocks movement in the stomach, and disturbs *Samana Vayu* which moves either up or down affecting *Apana Vayu* or *Udana Vayu*. This can lead to pain, and symptoms such as belching, wind, bloating, diarrhoea, vomiting, headache, IBS symptoms, piles, and spastic colon.

Treatment of indigestion

Kapha type: *Ama Ajeerna*

Give a little warm water with warming herbs to raise digestive fire and increase *Vata*, decrease *ama* and *Kapha*. Useful formulae of warming herbs include:

- Trikatu consisting of: ginger, long pepper and black pepper
- Trikulu consisting of: cinnamon, cardamom, cloves (take 1 tsp of powder in hot water)
- Talisadi (see Formulae, p. 302)
- Ajwan, or ajwan powder (*Trachyspermum ammi*)
- Ajmoda (*Carum roxburghianum*)
- Ginger juice.

Pitta type: *Vidagda*

Gentle purgation with Triphala, is recommended. Useful herbs include amalaki, guduchi, coriander, cumin, turmeric, fennel. Remedies are best taken in ghee or water. Chamomile, rose, peppermint and lemon grass tea will cool heat and soothe irritation.

Vata type: *Vishtabda*

Gentle laxatives: haritaki, and Triphala are recommended. For *agni deepana* (raising digestive fire): cumin, pippali, ginger, Trikulu or ajwan are helpful. Enemas are recommended in India: 2 cc castor oil and 8 cc warm water, or Triphala decoction (*kasaya*).

General treatment of indigestion

- *Agni deepana*: Raise digestive fire using: hing-wastaka, trikulu: cinnamon, cardamom, cloves, pippali churna with honey or ginger (see also p. 196).
- *Ama pachana*: Clear toxins using: Triphala, haritaki with raw sugar; amalaki and raw sugar (medicines are given with sugar to speed absorption) and ginger tea (see also p. 168).

WEAK DIGESTION

If a child has a weak stomach (which corresponds to the Ayurvedic concept of low *agni*), foods will not be digested easily and the stomach will be upset by a number of foods or combinations of foods. Food intolerances and allergies may develop.

A weak stomach can be constitutional, inherited from a member of the family or related to a difficult birth or other illness that has lowered the child's vitality because the vital energy of the body has been directed to healing elsewhere. The child may seem lethargic, look pale and thin, have a pale tongue and a poor appetite. There may be a tendency to constipation or diarrhoea, with particles of undigested food observable in the stools.

It is important to enhance digestion by using herbs and to respect the child's weakness by giving easily digested foods in moderate rather than over-large meals that might impose too much work on the digestion. Red meats, cheese and raw foods are best avoided as they are hard to digest, especially in the evenings. Excess milk products and foods containing sugar are also best avoided. Warm foods are more easily digested than cold, raw hard foods, so soups, stews and casseroles are better than salads.

Herbs can be given to strengthen the stomach for children with weak digestion who are prone to stomach upsets and vomiting episodes. Cardamom, ginger, angelica, cloves, coriander, dill, fennel or spearmint taken in warm tea will enliven the digestion and stimulate the flow of digestive juices, thereby enhancing digestion. These can be used singly or in combination and sweetened with honey if desired.

A combination of fennel and chamomile is particularly useful to calm the stomach and to soothe a distressed child.

ANOREXIA/NAUSEA: *AROCHAKA*

According to Ayurveda there are five causes (*nidana*) for loss of appetite:

1. Excess *Vata*
2. Excess *Pitta*
3. Excess *Kapha*
4. Imbalance of all three *doshas* (*Tridosha*)
5. Mental, (caused by grief, fear, anger, etc).

According to The Ayurvedic Encyclopedia (Swami Sada Shiva Tirtha 1998), an excess of the *doshas*, individually or combined or mental stress blocks the *srotas* that carry food, such as the oesophagus and stomach, causing reduced interest in food. Imbalance of the *doshas* in the digestive tract causes low digestive fire and *ama*. The tongue is coated with a layer of *ama* which covers the taste buds. This results in loss of taste or a bad taste in the mouth. There is little appetite due to low digestive fire, there may be nausea, and food eaten gives no satisfaction.

Signs and symptoms: (Rupa)

With loss of appetite and nausea there may be a variety of symptoms depending on which of the above causes is involved:

- *Vata*: Vomiting, an astringent taste in the mouth, weight loss, fear, anxiety, insomnia, abdominal pains, constriction in the throat, difficulty swallowing and a choking feeling.
- *Pitta*: A bitter or sour taste, bad breath and heartburn.
- *Kapha*: A sweet or salty taste, a coated feeling in the mouth, vomiting, excess saliva or mucus, itching, heaviness of the body, water-brash, lethargy and fatigue.
- *Tridosha*: Abnormal taste or absence of taste and any of the above symptoms.
- Mental: Worry, anger, dullness, or other emotion associated with a particular *dosha*.

Treatment of anorexia/nausea

Digestive herbs, such as cardamom, ginger, or ginger and lemon in equal parts can ease nausea, clear toxins and enhance digestion. Tea can be sipped through the day.

- For *Vata*: Herbal tea made with pippali and cardamom powders can be sipped through the day. A prescription combining pippali, raisins, rock salt, ginger and medicated wine is taken in India as an appetizer to stimulate appetite.

- For *Pitta*: Herbs such as guduchi, amalaki, chiretta and fresh ginger can be given in ghee.
- For *Kapha*: Fennel or pippali mixed with honey can be helpful.

Tonics can be given once nausea/vomiting has stopped and the tongue has cleared, such as Chyawan prash and ashwagandha.

Nervines such as gotu kola, sandalwood (*Santalum album*), jatamansi (*Nardostachys jatamansi*) and ashwagandha help to address underlying tension that disturbs the digestion. Sandalwood oil can be applied to the forehead to relieve tension and anxiety.

A light diet is recommended as well as massage, using sesame oil applied to the feet and head for *Vata* and *Kapha*, and gotu kola oil for *Pitta* conditions.

VOMITING: *CHARDI*

The ease with which children vomit depends to a certain extent on their age. Babies vomit easily due to overfeeding, wind, weak digestion, indigestible foods or infection. Toddlers vomit due to overeating, indigestible food, stomach upset, allergic reaction, infection, weak digestion, over excitement, emotional upset or cold/cough with copious phlegm which has been swallowed and accumulated in the stomach. By establishing the cause treatment implemented will obviously be more effective.

Treatment of vomiting

If a child has overeaten or reacted badly to food eaten there is vomiting of largely undigested food. In a baby this happens immediately after a feed. In an older child it could be several hours later and typically at night. There is usually a stomach ache and nausea, which builds up gradually to vomiting. Herbal teas can be given, taken slowly in sips so that they do not come straight back up again. Chamomile, fennel, lemon balm, ginger, cinnamon, cumin are all suitable herbs. Spearmint, patchouli and basil will all help to quell nausea and settle the stomach. These can be given as teas or dilute tinctures (5–10 drops of tincture in a glass of water).

For infections, herbal teas and tinctures can be given to help resolve infection swiftly and to settle the stomach. Chamomile, ginger, lavender, lemon balm, spearmint and thyme all have antimicrobial and carminative properties. Honey water spiced with ginger or cinnamon is excellent. Garlic with its strong antimicrobial properties is also an effective remedy in this instance.

Herb teas, spring water or hot water with a squeeze of lime can be sipped frequently through the day to prevent dehydration. A pinch of salt and 5 ml of glucose in a glass of water will help to replace electrolytes lost through vomiting.

Gastroenteritis is normally a result of viral infection in the digestive tract causing inflammation. In a natural response the digestive tract tries to rid itself of the irritant through diarrhoea, vomiting or both, which generally lasts 24 hours and resolves itself. When defences in the gut are low it can last longer and be associated with fever or malaise. Spanish tummy or travellers' diarrhoea often occurs as the digestive tract struggles with new foods and micro-organisms. Garlic taken daily will help to combat over-proliferation of harmful microbes and prevent gastroenteritis. Three to five drops of grapefruit seed extract in a glass of water can be given three times daily, as a preventative measure.

To treat gastroenteritis, herbal teas can be sipped through the day to settle the stomach and help to resolve infection quickly. Chamomile, lemon balm, yarrow, spearmint, fennel (*Foeniculum vulgare*), thyme, basil, cinnamon, ginger and oregano (*Oreganum vulgare*) are all rich in volatile oils with antimicrobial properties and have the added advantage of carminative actions relieving spasm and discomfort. Neem, garlic and atricidal are also excellent remedies with powerful antimicrobial properties.

COLITIS/IBS: *GRAHANI*

The classic IBS symptoms of abdominal pain and bloating, wind, irregular bowels, constipation and diarrhoea or alternating attacks of both, a sense of incomplete evacuation and mucus in the stools are frequently relieved by changes in diet and gentle herbal therapy. Interestingly, a recent Cochrane Review of treatment of recurrent abdominal pain in children concluded that there is little evidence to suggest any current drugs are effective in managing this condition (Huertas-Ceballos et al 2002).

There is often a relationship to be found between IBS symptoms and food intolerance. A recent review concludes that dieticians may have a very positive role to play in IBS (Dapoigny et al 2003). If offending substances such as wheat and dairy products, citrus fruits and junk foods are removed from the diet the symptoms can often improve dramatically. A recent trial found that lactose maldigestion may well be a contributory factor in children with IBS, and lactose avoidance in these children may reduce medication use to relieve symptoms (Gremse et al 1999).

However it may be difficult to return the child to the diet without repercussions, so it is important to understand the causes of the disruption of the digestion and seek to remedy those as far as possible. Amongst these emotional upset, pressure at school, family problems, for example, can all play a part, combined with poor diet and irregular eating habits. The link between IBS, mood disorders, anxiety and depression is well established (Solmaz et al 2003), and experience shows that treating the nervous system can have a very beneficial effect on IBS (see Nervous System, p. 246). Removing junk foods, orange juice and chocolate from the diet certainly can reduce stress symptoms and relaxing herbs such as chamomile, lemon balm, hops and lavender not only calm the nerves but are excellent for stress-related digestive problems.

Aromatic herbs and spices such as fennel, ginger, cardamom and angelica (*Angelica archangelica*) are very helpful, acting to enliven the digestion, enhance secretion of digestive juices, relieve tension and spasm in the gut and clear toxins. Where there is more of a tendency to constipation, antispasmodics like wild yam (*Dioscorea villosa*) and mild laxatives such as liquorice are helpful, while astringents like tormentil (*Potentilla erecta*), rose and agrimony (*Agrimonia eupatoria*) will tone the bowel where there is a tendency to diarrhoea. Although yet to be tested in a controlled trial, a small post-marketing surveillance study concluded that the effectiveness of artichoke leaf for IBS was rated highly and tolerability was good (Walker et al 2001).

Ayurvedic approach

According to Ayurveda IBS falls into the category of *grahani*, disturbed function of the intestine. The functions of *Pachaka Pitta* and *Samana Vayu* are altered due to disturbance of *agni*. According to Vasant Lad (Lad 1999) *Vata* pushes *Pitta* into the colon.

The underlying causes of *grahani* are as follows:

- Irregular eating habits
- *Asatmya* (intolerable food)
- Incompatible foods such as bread and bananas, milk with fish, milk with sour fruits, fruits with potatoes
- Heavy, cold, dry foods
- Debility due to other illness
- Excessive food intake
- Suppression of natural urges
- Over-exertion
- Misuse of medicine, antibiotics, etc.
- Disturbances in season and time
- Food poisoning
- Giardia, amoeba and other pathogenic microorganisms
- Low digestive fire
- Mental stress and strain, grief, sorrow, etc.

It is also said to be caused by a history of diarrhoea which causes the digestive fire, *Pachaka Pitta*, to be taken out of the intestine by *Vata*, leading to low digestive fire.

Exciting causes: (Viharja)

Low digestive fire (*mandagni*) disturbs the function of the intestine and affects digestion and absorption of food. This leads to an accumulation of toxins (*ama*). *Sama Vayu* (*Vata and ama*) does not convert and digest food properly, the separation of food and toxins is incomplete, causing sticky *ama*. *Ama* combines with food causing acidity, foul-smelling stools, often with undigested food, pain, debility and malaise. Bowels are sometimes solid, other times liquid, depending on the disturbance of *agni* and the intestine. There is usually wind, bloating, cramping pain, and there can be food allergies, and loss of weight due to poor absorption.

With diarrhoea (*atisara*) caused by food poisoning, infection, etc., *Pachaka Pitta* leaves the duodenum with the *Vata*. Digestive fire goes, causing low *agni* until it recovers. The stomach becomes full of undigested food, when this reaches the duodenum it causes *grahani*/malabsorption. A reduction of bile can cause pale fatty stools that smell offensive and float. There may be low energy, lethargy and hunger as the *dhatus* need nutrition and stimulate the appetite. Weight loss occurs as the tissues (*dhatus*) are not being properly nourished due to poor absorption.

Prodromal signs (*purvarupa*) include: thirst, laziness, debility, slow digestion, a feeling of heaviness in the body, excess salivation, loss of taste, abdominal distension, undigested food in the stool, wind, pale floating stools and spasm/tenesmus.

Symptoms (*rupa*) include: undigested food/large stools, constipation/tenesmus, diarrhoea, wind, cramp-like pain, offensive-smelling stool with *ama*, irritation, debility and stomatitis.

According to Ayurveda there are different types of *grahani*: *Vata* type, *Pitta* type, *Kapha* type and a type where all three *doshas* are involved:

- When *Vata* is disturbed (*Vataja*), symptoms will tend to be variable. There may be dry skin, dry mouth and pharynx, thirst, bloating, noises in the ear, pain in the abdomen, back, groin and neck, loss of weight, debility, anal fissures, depression or anxiety.

- When *Pitta* is disturbed (*Pittaja*), there may be foul-smelling belching and flatus, heartburn, thirst, heat, irritability, fever, yellow, liquid or foul-smelling stools.

- When *Kapha* is disturbed (*Kaphaja*), there may be slow digestion, a feeling of fullness, loss of taste, nausea, vomiting, mucus or stickiness in the mouth, bronchial catarrh, heaviness in chest and abdomen, foul-smelling eructations.

Treatment of IBS/colitis: *Grahani*

When treating *grahani* the diet needs to be light and easy to digest. Heavy, indigestible foods such as bread, cheese, red meat, cold, raw foods should be avoided. Generally herbs to improve digestive fire, i.e. digestives and appetizers such as ginger and bilva are used to treat *grahani*. Vasant Lad (Lad 1999) recommends 1 tsp of psyllium husk and $\frac{1}{2}$ cup of yoghurt 1 hour after the evening meal, or 1 tsp of flax seed boiled in 1 cup of water

and drunk at bedtime. To clear *ama* from the digestive tract use *ama pachana* (see also above).

For *Vata* type:

- Ginger, long pepper, chitrak (*Plumbago zeylanica*), and dashmula can be used. Lavanabhaskar (contains five salts as well as fennel, long pepper, black cumin, cinnamon leaf, talisha, rhubarb root, pomegranate seeds, cinnamon and cardamom) decreases high *Vata*, and increases *agni*. Hingwastaka (a compound medicine containing asafoetida, ginger, black pepper, and rock salt) is recommended $\frac{1}{2}$ tsp in warm water 1 to 2 hours before lunch and supper. Shatavari and ashwagandha both calm *Vata*. Fennel, cumin, cardamom, Trikulu (clove, cinnamon, cardamom), sesame oil, ghee, sour and salty foods are all recommended.

- Haritaki or Triphala $\frac{1}{2}$ tsp at night in hot water before bed can be given as laxatives and bowel tonics.

For *Pitta* type:

- Amalaki (*Emblica officinalis*) and coriander water are very good for cooling *Pitta*, as is sandalwood powder prepared in ghee. It is often mixed with fennel, long pepper, black pepper, and cloves. Turmeric (*Curcuma longa*), guduchi (*Tinosporia cordifolia*) is a bitter tonic worth using for a whole range of digestive problems. Manjista (*Rubia cordifolia*), gokshura (*Tribulis terrestris*), shatavari (*Asparagus racemosus*), neem (*Azadirachta indica*), rice water, bitter and sweet foods, and chirayata (*Swertia chiretta*) are applicable.

For *Kapha* type:

- Ginger, honey, Trikatu, (a compound that contains black pepper, long pepper, and ginger) specific for low *agni* and high *ama*, turmeric, Hingwastaka, ginger and lime juice can be used. Also cardamom, cinnamon, cloves, sandalwood, cumin, nutmeg, rock salt, ajwan and pippali. Fasting and eating bitter, pungent and astringent foods is advised with gentle purgation using Triphala.

There are two herbs that deserve special mention in the treatment of *grahani*:

- Shatavari: *Asparagus racemosus*, the roots and succulent tubers of the wild asparagus, is one of the prime rejuvenating medicines in Ayurveda. A member of the same family as the common asparagus, shatavari has nutritive properties and has cooling, soothing and lubricating properties recommended for overheated and depleted conditions of body and mind. Its taste is sweet and bitter and it is balancing to *Pitta* and *Vata*. Traditionally respected as a digestive aid, its cooling properties are effective in relieving inflammatory conditions, soothing irritated tissues and curbing diarrhoea and IBS. Modern research has borne this out and demonstrated its ability to soothe heartburn and indigestion (Dalvi et al 1990). Shatavari also enhances immunity and has been shown to improve macrophage activity in response to *Candida albicans* (Rege and Dahanukar 1993). The nourishing effect of shatavari is useful for people who are depleted by chronic bowel problems and who have lost weight. It is available in powder and capsule form. When used for treating digestive problems take $\frac{1}{2}$ tsp of the powder in half a cup of warm milk after each meal. It mixes well with equal parts of amalaki and liquorice.

- Amalaki: *Emblica officinalis*. Also known as Indian gooseberry, amalaki is considered the best herbal medicine for rejuvenation in Ayurveda, and forms the basis of the most famous Ayurvedic tonic, Chayawanprash. This is one of the best sources of antioxidant vitamins, and apparently the juice of the amalaki fruit possesses almost 20 times as much vitamin C as orange juice. Although the taste of amalaki is predominantly sweet, it contains five out of the six tastes, missing only salty and so it is appropriate for balancing all three *doshas*. It is famous as a remedy for all *Pitta* problems and is frequently used with equal amounts of haritaki and bibhitaki in the traditional formula Triphala, a gentle bowel tonic. Triphala is particularly helpful for chronic constipation as well as IBS; $\frac{1}{2}$ tsp of the powder can be taken last thing at night in warm water.

Herbs can be given to strengthen the stomach for children with weak digestion who are prone to stomach upsets and vomiting episodes. Cardamom, ginger, angelica, cloves, coriander, dill, fennel or spearmint taken in warm tea will enliven the digestion and stimulate the flow of digestive juices, thereby enhancing digestion. These can be used single or in combination and sweetened with honey if desired.

A combination of fennel and chamomile is particularly useful to calm the stomach and to soothe a distressed child.

When a child is upset or overexcited, the sympathetic nervous system causes a rush of adrenaline (epinephrine) and all the resultant physical changes that accompany stress or excitement, including the flow of energy away from the digestive system. Digestion obviously works better when the child is relaxed and the parasympathetic nervous system comes into play. As a result of the stress, food is not digested well and sits in the stomach, which if it is very tense, can forcibly throw it out. Children are often prone to vomiting before tests or exams, if they are anxious or unhappy, if there is something they "just cannot stomach" or are "sick and tired of". In this instance the child requires love, patience and understanding and perhaps some help from a school counsellor or a family therapist depending on the origin of the distress. Relaxing herbs that support the nervous system can be very beneficial. Chamomile, catnip, hops, rosemary, lavender and lemon balm are all particularly applicable to stress-related digestive problems. Wild oats, skullcap (*Scutellaria lateriflora*) and vervain (*Verbena officinalis*) are all nourishing to the nervous system.

The lining of the stomach naturally secretes mucus to protect the stomach walls, so that the acid and enzymes digest only the food and do not corrode the sensitive lining. This mucus can become excessive, either through irritation of the stomach from not eating properly or through swallowing mucus from the respiratory system during an infection, such as a cold/cough. This results in the accumulation of gastric catarrh, which inhibits normal function of the stomach and interferes with efficient digestion of food (this would equate with a *Kapha* disturbance of the digestion). It can give rise to periodic vomiting as the body tries to clear the phlegm. In this case the vomit is watery and resembles mucus, either white, yellow or green. The child will have an accompanying stomach ache and nausea for a few days, and look pale. Interestingly the main Ayurvedic approach to treatment of such a problem would be the use of herbal emetics. Here the body is using this cleansing method on its own accord.

To treat gastric catarrh, the catarrhal condition of the respiratory tract will need to be resolved using expectorants (see Respiratory System, p. 218). All mucus-forming foods need to be avoided until the child is properly better (see p. 219). Herbal teas can be given to clear the catarrh, such as angelica, cardamom, cinnamon, elderflowers, fennel (*Foeniculum vulgare*), ginger, meadowsweet (*Filipendula ulmaria*), spearmint. Golden seal (*Hydrastis canadensis*) (from sustainable sources only) is one of the best remedies in this instance but because it is very bitter it can only be given in very small amounts to children. Three to five drops of tincture added to a pleasant-tasting infusion of one of the above aromatic herbs can be tried. The above herbs can also be given in sips frequently through the day during bouts of vomiting.

Once the vomiting has stopped and the stomach is working again, cinnamon and ginger will help to re-establish the normal bacterial population of the gut.

Ayurvedic approach to vomiting: *Chardi*

Vomiting is caused by aggravation of either *Vata*, *Pitta*, *Kapha*, or all three *doshas*. It can also be related to stress or upset, ingested toxins, unwanted food, and pathogens (*krumi*), i.e. infection. As a result *Pachaka Pitta* with its liquid and acidic properties and *Kledaka Kapha* are both disturbed by *ama* causing *Sama Pitta* and *Sama Kapha*. According to the Ayurvedic Encyclopedia (Swami Sada Shiva Tirtha 1998), upward moving *Udana Vayu* becomes aggravated and affects all the *doshas* causing them to move upwards.

Prodromal signs: (Purvarupa rupa)

These include nausea, salty taste in the mouth, excess salivation, loss of taste and appetite.

Signs and symptoms: (Rupa)

These will vary according to the predominant *dosha* involved:

- *Vata*: Vomiting of food causes pain in the umbilical region, back and ribs, regurgitating occurs a little at a time, with an astringent taste and frothy substance, emitted only with difficulty and force. Vomiting is associated with belching, coughing, dry mouth, head pain, hoarseness and exhaustion. Vomiting caused by parasites, *ama* and pregnancy can also be caused by *Vata*.

- *Pitta*: Vomit is brown, green, or yellow. It may be blood flecked, sour or bitter tasting and hot. Thirst, fainting, heat or burning sensation may be experienced.

- *Kapha*: Vomit is oily, thick, cold and mucousy, sweet or salty tasting and comes out in a large or continuous quantity. The face can swell and there may be an accompanying cough and sleepiness.

- *Tridosha*: Symptoms of all three *doshas* appear.

Treatment: (Chikitsa)

When treating vomiting follow general guidelines for balancing the predominant *dosha* involved (see p. 83). Haritaki with raw honey or castor oil with boiled milk reduces the upward motion of the *doshas* and can be given in all cases. Fennel, patchouli (*Pogostemon patchouli*) and coriander are also good remedies for all types.

- *Vata*: Bilva, barley, cardamom, cloves, coriander, ginger, raspberry, bamboo manna (vamsha lochana), pippali, black pepper and garlic will clear toxins and help balance *Samana Vata*.

- *Pitta*: For excess *Pitta* in the stomach Ayurvedic doctors use emetics with sweet herbs like liquorice to cleanse the stomach. Afterwards a mixture of cooked barley with raw honey and cane sugar or basmati rice with green lentil soup is given. Neem, chirayata (*Swertia chireta*), bilva, coriander, raspberry leaves, spearmint, vamsha lochana (*Bambusa bambos*) are all indicated. Grapes and coconut are useful foods. Powders of amalaki, bala and sandalwood may be mixed with food. Peppermint, rose, coriander, chamomile and lemon grass are excellent taken as teas.

- *Kapha*: Useful herbs include cardamom, bilva, cloves, ginger, Triphala, musta (*Cyperus rotundus*), and raspberry leaves (*Rubus idaeus*) mixed with raw honey. In India an emetic made with a decoction of pippali (*Piper longum*), neem (*Azadirachta indica*) and rock salt is recommended to cleanse the undigested food toxins (*ama*), from the stomach. Afterwards at meal time, barley is given with neem and yoghurt/water (1:3).

- *Tridosha*: Herbs, foods and other therapies advised for each *dosha* are used. The season, time of the day, strength of the person and their digestion are all taken into consideration when deciding which is the dominant *dosha* that requires treatment first.

Long-term vomiting greatly aggravates *Vata* so a *Vata* reducing diet is generally used to restore balance and strength (see Enhancing Immunity, p. 166).

TRAVEL SICKNESS

Ginger is an effective remedy for travel sickness in which *Samana Vata* is disturbed by the movement and rebels! It can be taken as crystallized ginger and chewed as a preventative either before the journey or as nausea arises. It can also be added to food, such as ginger biscuits, taken as ginger tea, ginger beer or dilute ginger tincture. Ginger is well established for treating many forms of nausea. A recent review looked at six studies including postoperative nausea, seasickness, morning sickness and chemotherapy-induced nausea, which overall favoured ginger over placebo for treating nausea (Ernst and Pittler 2000).

Other antinausea herbs including chamomile, fennel, lemon balm, meadowsweet and spearmint will all help settle the stomach and can be chewed or sipped as teas when required.

Essential oils of aniseed (*Pimpinella anisum*) cinnamon, fennel, ginger, melissa or spearmint can be used for inhalation; a few drops on a handkerchief or on clothes can be very effective.

The Neiguan point (two fingers width from the wrist crease) can be massaged or sea bands which exert pressure on the point can be worn, to help to prevent nausea.

DIARRHOEA: *ATISARA*

Diarrhoea occurs when the intestines are irritated and the bowel muscles contract more frequently and intensely than usual, causing griping and pain as the body attempts to rid itself of the irritant. The food residues do not stay long enough in the bowel for water and electrolytes to be reabsorbed, so the bowel

movement is watery. In the short term there is risk of dehydration and temporary electrolyte imbalance. In the long term there is risk of additional nutritional disturbance because of poor absorption of vital nutrients. Acute diarrhoea tends to last 24 hours and arises from a number of different causes:

- Diarrhoea with nausea, vomiting, malaise and fever is most commonly caused by infection by *E. coli*, *Salmonella* and *Campylobacter*. Mild gastroenteritis often develops on trips abroad when it takes the gut a while to adjust to the change of food and micro-organisms. Precooked meals and eggs harbouring *Listeria*/*Salmonella* can cause food poisoning.

- Overeating the wrong foods, i.e. those that are hard to digest including greasy foods, rich creamy sauces, spices, or even over-indulgence of otherwise healthy foods, such as too much roughage in grains, fruit or vegetables can irritate the gut and produce loose stools.

- Eating too much cold food and drink such as ice cream, fruit juices and milk from the fridge, salads, especially cucumber, can be a strain on the stomach, which prefers to be warm. The child is usually quite well apart from the loose stools.

- Diarrhoea often accompanies infections elsewhere in the body in which case there will be fever, and malaise as well as other symptoms, a cold/cough/rash for example. Where there is infection elsewhere, a chest infection for example, for which the child has been prescribed broad-spectrum antibiotics, this could upset the normal bacterial population of the gut and allow pathogenic bacteria to proliferate resulting in bowel infection and diarrhoea.

- Stress or over-excitement can cause diarrhoea with tummy aches on a short-term basis.

Chronic diarrhoea

This can have several causes including:

- Food intolerance or allergy, commonly to milk or wheat products. If diarrhoea is pale in colour and foul smelling it could indicate coeliac disease involving gluten intolerance. Thread worms (see p. 210) and candidiasis (see p. 185) can also cause chronic diarrhoea. If a child is run down from other illness, frequent antibiotics or stress, it can weaken the digestion and cause the bowel to be over-sensitive to foods and easily irritated, giving rise to diarrhoea. A recent acute bowel infection can lead to chronic irritation/inflammation.

- Chronic non-specific diarrhoea tends to be seen mostly in children between the ages of 3 months and 6 years. Despite frequent passage of stools containing undigested food particles the children can appear quite well and to thrive normally. It is considered primarily a motility problem but may be the early signs of IBS. Involuntary diarrhoea resulting in a child frequently soiling underwear can be related to chronic constipation. Hard stools can block the bowel but some liquid stool can get past it.

Treatment of diarrhoea

Herbal remedies with antimicrobial actions can be given every hour or two in acute diarrhoea and three times daily in chronic problems. If there is infection with accompanying fever see fever management (see Treatment of Fevers, p. 175).

Antimicrobial herbs

Berberis vulgaris, Berberis aristata (daruharidra) and *Hydrastis canadensis* contain the alkaloid berberine which is known to be an effective antimicrobial against a number of diarrhoea causing organisms (Cernakova and Kostalova 2002, Taylor and Greenough 1989).

Garlic appears to act as a broad-spectrum antibiotic both on Gram-positive and Gram-negative bacteria. It is effective against a number of pathogenic intestinal bacteria and furthermore appears to be active against antibiotic-resistant bacteria whilst not resulting in resistance to itself (Sivam 2001). It can be given as a juice (made by chopping raw garlic and leaving it covered with honey for an hour or two) or in capsules.

Echinacea tincture $\frac{1}{4}-\frac{1}{2}$ tsp can be given in a little water, every 2 hours in acute diarrhoea and three times daily in chronic cases. Chamomile, thyme, ginger, cinnamon, fennel are all mildly antiseptic and help to relax the bowel muscles and relieve griping, and can be taken similarly. If the child feels cold and looks pale, ginger tea is especially helpful with its warming, antispasmodic and antimicrobial properties. It is good for chronic diarrhoea where it is related to low vitality and digestive weakness. (From an Ayurvedic perspective this would correlate with low digestive fire.)

For general treatment of diarrhoea astringent herbs taken as teas/tinctures can be combined with carminatives to relax the gut and soothe griping and pain. Tannins in the astringent herbs tone the mucosa of the gut, protecting it from irritation and inflammation. Astringent herbs include agrimony, rose, blackberry leaves, American cranesbill (*Geranium americanum*), oak bark, meadowsweet, shepherd's purse (*Capsella bursa-pastoris*), tormentil (*Potentilla erecta*) and thyme. Carminative herbs include cardamom, cumin, cinnamon, fennel, ginger and spearmint. Unsweetened blackcurrant/bilberry juice contains astringent tannins and a high vitamin C content. Lemon juice will also exert an antimicrobial effect on the gut and can be pleasant as well as effective when combined with ginger. Simmer $\frac{1}{4}-\frac{1}{2}$ tsp of grated fresh ginger in a cup of water for 5–10 minutes. Add juice of $\frac{1}{2}$ lemon and sweeten with honey if desired.

Demulcent herbs soothe and calm the irritated gut lining, they are easily digested and nutritious. Such herbs can be combined with astringent, carminative and antimicrobial herbs and include: comfrey leaf (*Symphytum off.*), marshmallow (*Althea off.*), Iceland moss (*Cetraria islandica*), linseed (*Linum usitarissimum*), psyllium seed (*Plantago psyllium*) and slippery elm (*Ulmus fulva*). Slippery elm can be sucked as tablets or given as powder made into gruel by mixing with warm water or rice milk and honey if preferred. Adding a pinch of cinnamon/ginger powder can make it more palatable.

Two drops of essential oil of either chamomile, geranium or sandalwood in 1 tsp sesame oil can be massaged lightly over the abdomen (always in a clockwise direction in the direction of the natural movement of the bowel) to relax and soothe the digestive tract. Thyme oil is highly antiseptic and can be added to water and sprayed into the room as a disinfectant or used in a vaporizer.

Dietary advice

In acute diarrhoea, particularly with fever, it is best not to give food or milk, just fluids and to fast the child for a few hours. Once the appetite has returned and the child feels a little better, fruit with astringent properties such as bilberries, blackcurrants, apples or pears, can be given, preferably cooked and warm as cold food is harder to digest and better avoided.

Brown rice cooked until very soft can be given mixed with honey and natural live yoghurt with a pinch of cinnamon or ginger powder can be mashed with banana to help re-establish the normal bacterial population of the gut and prevent further infection. Sprigs of spearmint can be added to rice/yoghurt to calm the stomach and quell griping. A spicy "lassi" can be made using $\frac{1}{2}$ cup natural live yoghurt and $\frac{1}{2}$ cup spring water and a pinch each of ginger, cardamom and cinnamon.

Once the bowel has completely settled down, normal eating can be resumed. Meals are best taken regularly and snacking between meals discouraged. Cold foods are best avoided to aid recovery of the digestive tract. Light, easily digested foods are recommended. Garlic capsules/juice can be given to re-establish the normal gut flora. Garlic contains the prebiotic fructo-oligosaccharide, fermentation of which in the intestine has been shown to increase numbers of bifidobacteria (Chow 2002).

Ayurvedic approach to diarrhoea: *Atisara*

Loose motions, diarrhoea are known in Sanskrit as *Atisara* and involves all three *doshas* which are deranged due to low digestive fire and *ama*.

Causes: (Nidana) of diarrhoea

Causes include drinking excessive amounts of water, excess consumption of pungent, dry, fatty, hard, cold or unaccustomed foods, eating before the last meal is digested and eating at unusual times.

Other causes include food poisoning, suppression of natural urges, intestinal parasites, changes of lifestyle and seasonal changes.

Pathogenesis: (Samprapti)

When accumulated *Vata* in the gastrointestinal tract becomes aggravated it causes *Kapha* (water) to move downward, from the stomach dampening the digestive fire. This causes the faeces to become watery and produces diarrhoea. If *Pachaka Pitta* is aggravated it liquefies the food, which is not digested properly and in its unabsorbed state it is passed out.

Prodromal symptoms: (Purvarupa rupa)

These may include prickling pain in the chest, rectum and alimentary tract, weak body, constipation, gas and indigestion.

Signs and symptoms: (Rupa)

- *Vata*: Small quantity of watery faeces are expelled with noise, severe pain and difficulty. Stools may be frothy, thin, rough, slightly brown and frequently expelled. There may be a dry mouth and straining.
- *Pitta*: Stools may be yellow, green, mixed with blood and foul smelling. Thirst, faintness, perspiration, burning sensation, painful elimination and burning may present as accompanying symptoms.
- *Kapha*: Stools can be solid, slimy, pale, mucusy, fatty, frequent, heavy, foul smelling and difficult to pass followed by pain, sleepiness and poor appetite.

Diarrhoea can be present with or without *ama*. With *ama* stools sink, and have a foul smell and can be associated with intestinal gurgling, undigested food particles and excess salivation. When food is not properly digested and *ama* accumulates, the *doshas* combine with *ama* and become deranged. They then travel in the channels, weakening *dhatus*, *malas*, and causing frequent multicoloured faeces and abdominal pain.

Treatment: (Chikitsa)

Diarrhoea caused by excess *doshas* with undigested food and *ama* needs to be eliminated. Initially astringent herbs and foods are not used to stop diarrhoea with *ama* until the toxins are expelled with the stool. If diarrhoea is stopped while *ama* is still in the body it may cause further problems such as haemorrhoids, oedema, fever, etc. It is best to allow the *ama* diarrhoea to be eliminated, even to induce it through the use of haritaki. Children should avoid drinking too much fluid as this will aggravate the problem.

The primary concern is to rekindle the digestive fire. Ginger, coriander, bilva, musta (*Cyperus rotundus*), haritaki, calamus, pippali, chitrak, and sour pomegranate are used to enhance digestion. Later bala, gokshura (*Tribulus terrestris*), bilva and rock salt are combined with foods and drinks to strengthen the constitution. One part yoghurt mixed with three parts water (lassi) also promotes digestion. Alternatively, either a mixture of pippali with honey or a mixture of chitrak (*Plumbago zeylanica*) with lassi is recommended.

For general treatments useful herbs include pippali, ginger, coriander, haritaki, calamus, gokshura, bilva and fennel.

For *Vata* and *Kapha*:   bala, gokshura, bilva, ginger, coriander, calamus, pippali, chitrak, sour pomegranate, Dashmul, amalaki, ghee and rock salt taken with foods and drinks are given to strengthen the digestion and the constitution. Where there is pain, gas retention, a desire to pass urine or stool but inability to do so, bilva, pippali, ginger, cane sugar and sesame oil can be given.

Pitta: chiretta (*Swertia chireta*), katuka (*Picrorrhiza kurroa*), bilva (*Aegle marmelos*), sandalwood, lotus seeds, mango taken with raw honey, ghee and rice water are all used. Goat's milk is also given in *Pitta* diarrhoea.

After the bowels are cleared a *Pitta* reducing diet is recommended (see Immune System, p. 149) as *Pitta* increasing foods at this time may lead to further bowel inflammation. Should this occur boiled goats' milk with raw honey and cane sugar can be given.

For clearing *ama*: gentle laxatives can be given if the child is strong. After this light meals are recommended including barley gruel with bala, shatavari and gokshura. Green lentils are said to improve digestion. If diarrhoea continues use digestives like Trikatu and astringents like lotus seeds, red raspberry and haritaki.

For thirst, boiled water with musta and sandalwood (endangered plant, only obtain from sustainable sources) is used.

For pathogenic micro-organisms treatment with immune-boosting herbs like guduchi is indicated. Treat as for *Pitta* diarrhoea.

In chronic diarrhoea, should the anus become inflamed through frequent movements, ghee can be applied followed by neem oil or sandalwood oil.

CONSTIPATION

Children are particularly prone to constipation at certain times, including times of transition, the change over from breast-feeding to other sources of milk, the introduction of solid food, potty training and beginning playgroup or school. As well as the recognized factors such as poor diet and lack of dietary fibre, constipation can be due to a number of other factors which require attention if it is to be treated successfully.

Poor bowel habits

If the urge to pass a stool is ignored by a child who is in a hurry to eat breakfast and rush off to school or is engrossed in something more interesting, it may be another 24 hours before another urge arises. Even if the call to stool is heeded, the child may still be too preoccupied to take the time to evacuate properly and a residue remains which gradually builds up, and as it stays in the large bowel so it loses moisture and becomes harder to pass. Once a child has experienced the painful passing of a hard stool, he/she will be reluctant to do so again and so the constipation may get worse.

Eating habits

Junk foods, sugar and excess animal protein cause putrefaction in the bowel, while irregular eating or eating while doing something else, such as sitting in the car, can disturb digestion and predispose to constipation.

Lack of exercise

Exercise is required to promote healthy circulation of blood to the bowel muscles for them to work efficiently. Too little exercise, and too much sitting around either at school, at computers or watching TV can contribute to constipation.

Food intolerance

Specific intolerances to, for example, wheat, gluten, milk, can irritate the gut, causing tension and spasm of the bowel muscles, and inhibiting peristalsis.

Illness

If a child is ill or feverish, or there has been vomiting causing loss of water from the body, the bowel will compensate by absorbing water from the stools. This is not true constipation, only a temporary state, as the bowels should return to normal once the child recovers.

Emotional factors

Worry, anxiety and stresses of all kinds can lead to tension in the bowel muscles. This may occur during transition from one stage to another. The child may feel insecure and "hold on" in this case to the stool. The overflow and soiling that can result from constipation can further add to family stresses, social and psychological problems thereby aggravating emotional problems.

Vitamin and mineral deficiencies

These can play a part in erratic bowel movements, particularly vitamin C and magnesium deficiency and aluminium excess.

Fluid intake

Insufficient fluid intake can cause hard dry stools which are difficult to pass, and can disturb the bacterial population in the gut, predisposing to further bowel problems.

The autointoxication that results from constipation can result in lethargy, poor concentration, irritability, poor sleeping habits, headaches and muscle aches.

Treatment of constipation

A child's diet should contain sufficient fibre to bulk out the stool and encourage evacuation as well as discourage the growth of putrefactive bacteria in the gut. Figs, prunes, raisins, apricots, desiccated coconut, rhubarb, watercress, parsley and honey are all high in fibre and help to keep the bowels moving.

There are many children who suffer from constipation and other bowel problems related to wheat intolerance. Gluten allergies can also occur in children, not necessarily manifesting as frank coeliac disease but causing a variety of bowel problems. Gluten is found in wheat, oats, barley and rye. Milk allergies can also be implicated. Avoidance of

suspected foods can be instigated on a temporary basis and any improvement observed.

It is important to balance the intestinal bacteria by giving the child plenty of live yoghurt, olive oil and garlic (raw or in juice or capsules). Anything other than ripe bananas, which actively encourage beneficial bacteria, added to yoghurt will destroy many of the benign bacteria. Alternatively, grapefruit seed extract or acidophyllus tablets can be given to improve transit time of food through the bowel by balancing the intestinal flora in the same way.

Children need to be encouraged to play outside or take regular and active exercise such as swimming, bicycling, riding, walking and dancing.

Herbal treatment

It is inadvisable to give laxatives as the sole means of treatment, because children's bowels, like those of adults, may become habituated to their use. However, to soften the stools and help evacuate hard, impacted faeces and clear out the system, they can be used in the short term as long as attention is paid to background causes such as diet, bowel habits as well as any emotional problems that are brought to light, to deal effectively with the problem.

Bulk laxative herbs moisten and bulk out the stool contents and help to push them along the gut for evacuation. Psyllium seeds and linseeds are both good bulk laxatives. 1 tsp/5 ml of seeds in a cup of warm water left for a few minutes for the seeds to swell into a gel, can be given before bed. Psyllium seeds have been compared with other laxatives in an open, multicentre trial of 381 patients. This concluded that they were an effective treatment and "associated with better stool consistency and reduced incidence of adverse events compared with lactulose or with other laxatives" (Dettmar and Sykes 1998). Such laxative herbs contain mucilage, a substance that attracts water to it and so helps to moisten the bowel and acts as a lubricant, helping to clear the gut of hard, impacted stools. Mucilaginous herbs also soothe an irritated gut and lessen the impact of food intolerances. They include slippery elm which can be given as tablets or powder, made into a gruel by mixing with equal parts of warm water or rice, oat, almond milk and a pinch of cardamom/cinnamon/ginger powder. Other mucilaginous herbs include marsh-mallow and comfrey leaf, which can be given as teas or dilute tinctures.

Other herbs can be given which are stimulating to the bowels and are useful for children who tend to be sluggish or sedentary and their bowel muscles rather inactive. These include butternut, dandelion root, liquorice root and yellow dock root, 5–10 drops of tincture can be given in water either at night before bed or three times daily after meals depending on the extent of the problem.

Relaxing herbs are indicated for tense/anxious/overactive children with tight, contracted bowels. These include chamomile, fennel, dill, cardamom, catnip, ginger, spearmint and thyme. Once the bowel muscles are more relaxed, normal peristaltic movements should resume (see also Nervous System, p. 245).

A teaspoon of honey/molasses in a cup of ginger tea first thing in the morning makes a pleasant-tasting and nutritious remedy for mild constipation. Honey and lemon can also be given. Alternatively, apricots mashed with a little honey are effective for moving the bowels.

Abdominal massage can be helpful and the element of therapeutic touch between parent and child is particularly healing to an anxious or insecure child. Dilute oils of either chamomile, ginger, black pepper, fennel, lemon balm, basil, lavender or rosemary can be used in a base of sesame oil and the abdomen massaged gently clockwise in the direction of the bowel movements last thing at night before bed.

If laxative herbs need to be given to a child on a regular basis, it means the cause of the problem is not being addressed. There may be food intolerance, in which case the suspected foods need to be omitted from the diet for 3–4 weeks at least to give time for the bowels to respond positively.

Ayurvedic approach

Defecation is a downward action for which *Apana Vata* is responsible. If the movement of *Apana Vata* is disturbed or blocked, the downward direction is reversed and constipation will occur. As the main site of *Vata* is the lower abdomen, including the bowel, constipation tends to occur when there is an increase of *Vata dosha* and often afflicts *Vata* predominant children. Stools are dry, the rectum is constricted and there is wind and bloating. The best time for elimination, according to Ayurveda, is first thing in the morning, and *Vata* predominant children need to be encouraged to pass a bowel movement on a regular basis in the morning.

Causes: (Nidana) of constipation

Changes in routine and diet, excess dry or cold weather, tension, fear and anxiety, suppression of natural urges, especially ignoring the call to stool, overexertion, tiredness, staying away from home, travelling abroad, dryness of the bowel caused by excess *Vata* and aggravated by insufficient fluid and oil intake and excessive hard, dry, cold and indigestible food which lower digestive fire are all cited. A daily massage with sesame oil, followed by a warm bath or shower, works well, paying particular attention to massaging the lower abdomen in a clockwise direction. Ayurvedic doctors recommend sesame oil enema under medical supervision.

A quarter of a teaspoon of Triphala powder (*churna*) given in hot water at night, has a mild laxative and bowel cleansing action and does not create dependency.

WORMS

Three types of worms can occur in children: threadworms, roundworms and tapeworms. The latter is more unusual and is generally not treated with herbs. Some children are more prone to worms than others. If the digestive system is functioning well and the enzymes secreted sufficiently, and peristaltic movements are regular, making for efficient bowel habits, there is less likelihood of worms being able to survive in the bowel.

Treatment of worms

It is important to treat the digestion as a whole, paying attention to symptoms indicative of imbalance such as wind, pain, constipation or diarrhoea and to treat accordingly. Raising the digestive fire with warming digestives such as ginger, cinnamon, cardamom and pepper makes a good start to treatment.

Foods and herbs can be given that are toxic to worms. These include garlic: give 1–2 cloves chopped finely in a spoonful of honey or in a little warm milk 30 minutes before breakfast. Also raw onions, pumpkin seeds, raw carrots and carrot juice, a pinch of cayenne pepper added to cooking/in yoghurt, apples, desiccated coconut and raw turnip. Ground pumpkin seeds in grated carrot for breakfast makes an effective recipe.

Sweets and sugary foods and refined carbohydrates should be avoided as worms thrive on these and such foods are more likely to predispose to constipation, which will further encourage proliferation of worms. Live yoghurt can be given every day to enhance general health of the bowel and discourage putrefaction. Lacto acidophyllus and grapefruit seed extract are useful supplements.

Useful anthelmintic (to expel worms) herbs include:

> wormwood (*Artemisia absinthium*)
> southernwood (*Artemisia abrotanum*)
> balmony (*Chelone glabra*)
> gentian (*Gentiana lutea*)
> vervain (*Verbena off.*)
> pennyroyal (*Mentha pulegium*) and
> sage (*Salvia off.*)
> (all of the above should be avoided by pregnant women)
> spearmint
> thyme
> aniseed (*Pimpinella anisum*)
> blue flag (*Iris versicolor*)
> fennel (*Foeniculum vulgare*)
> self-heal (*Prunella vulgaris*)
> echinacea.

When treating older children add a tiny pinch of cayenne to teas/tinctures. Research from Egypt found that *Inula helenium* and *Artemisia santonica* have both been shown to be promising anthelmintics against the common intestinal roundworm *Ascaris lumbricoides* (El Garhy and Mahmoud 2002). A useful recipe is 1 part balmony, 1 part spearmint, 1 part aniseed and $\frac{1}{2}$ part wormwood.

Many of the anthelmintic herbs are strong and bitter tasting. They can be taken in small doses with more aromatic herbs to disguise their taste, such as fennel and spearmint and sweetened with a little apple concentrate or honey. They are best taken first thing in the morning $\frac{1}{4}-\frac{1}{2}$ a cupful of tea at a time on an empty stomach, so that they have more impact on the intestines than they would if they were diluted by food. Another dose can be taken before each meal through the day as well. Repeat this for 1 week. If a child cannot be persuaded to take $\frac{1}{4}-\frac{1}{2}$ a cupful, they can be given sips as frequently as possible through the day or diluted in fruit juice. Alternatively the herbs can be ground and given in a teaspoon of honey or molasses. Other laxative foods and herbs such as liquorice or dandelion root can be given to speed the expulsion of worms from the gut. Stools need to be checked daily for expelled worms to see if the treatment is effective. Repeat treatment after 2 weeks to ensure expulsion of worms that were eggs or just hatched at the time of the initial treatment.

Calendula or neem cream, or a couple of drops of either eucalyptus, lavender, tea tree (*Melaleuca alternifolia*) or thyme oil in cream base can be applied to the anus at night to prevent the worms from laying eggs and to relieve itching. Children need to be made aware of proper hygiene, washing hands frequently in hot soapy water especially before eating and after touching pets. They need to be persuaded not to scratch an itching anus. Closely fitted underwear or pyjamas will help. Fingernails need to be cleaned daily.

Ayurvedic approach

Causes of worms include:

- drinking infested water
- low digestive fire
- eating excess sugar
- improper food combining
- insufficiently cooked foods
- poor hygiene.

When worms are associated with increased *Vata*, garlic, basil, psyllium husks, oregano, thyme, black pepper, bay leaves, cardamom, asafoetida, cinnamon, mustard, cloves and haritaki are all indicated.

When associated with *Pitta*: amalaki, bibhitaki, neem, psyllium husks, kutki, and daruharidra (*Berberis aristata*) and pomegranate can be given.

When associated with *Kapha*: bibhitaki, neem, garlic, basil, oregano, thyme, cinnamon, cardamom, clove, black pepper, bay leaves, mustard, rosemary, pomegranate, asafoetida are all indicated.

It is important to raise digestive fire and clear *ama* (see Immune System, p. 149) so that the bowel becomes an inhospitable environment for further worm infestation. Spices can be added to cooking to increase digestive fire.

Neem/sesame oil can be applied to the rectum. A neem/sesame oil enema is generally recommended by Ayurvedic physicians.

References

Cernakova M, Kostalova D 2002 Antimicrobial activity of berberine – a constituent of *Mahonia aquifolium*. Folia Microbiol (Praha) 47(4): 375–378

Chow J 2002 Probiotics and prebiotics: A brief overview. J Ren Nutr 12(2): 76–86

Dalvi SS, Nadkarni PM, Gupta KC 1990 Effect of *Asparagus racemosus* (Shatavari) on gastric emptying time in normal healthy volunteers. J Postgrad Med 36: 91–94

Dapoigny M, Stockbrugger RW, Azpiroz F, et al 2003 Role of alimentation in irritable bowel syndrome. Digestion 67(4): 225–233

Dettmar PW, Sykes J 1998 A multi-centre, general practice comparison of ispaghula husk with lactulose and other laxatives in the treatment of simple constipation. Curr Med Res Opin 14(4): 227–233

Ernst E, Pittler MH 2000 Efficacy of ginger for nausea and vomiting: a systematic review of randomized clinical trials. Br J Anaesth 84(3): 367–371

El Garhy MF, Mahmoud LH 2002 Anthelminthic efficacy of traditional herbs on *Ascaris lumbricoides*. J Egypt Soc Parasitol 32(3): 893–900

Gremse DA, Nguyenduc GH, Sacks AI 1999 Irritable bowel syndrome and lactose maldigestion in recurrent abdominal pain in childhood. South Med J 92(8): 778–781

Huertas-Ceballos A, Macarthur C, Logan S 2002 Pharmacological interventions for recurrent abdominal pain (RAP) in childhood. Cochrane Database Syst Rev (1): CD003017

Lad V 1999 The Complete Book of Ayurvedic Home Remedies. Judy Piatkus Limited, London

Mills S, Bone K 2000 Principles and Practice of Phytotherapy. Churchill Livingstone, London

Murray MT, Pizzorno J 1990 Encyclopaedia of Natural Medicine. Little, Brown and Company, London

Myers BM, Smith JL, Graham DY 1987 Effect of red pepper and black pepper on the stomach. Am J Gastroenterol 82(3): 211–214

Rege NN, Dahanukar SA 1993 Quantitation of microbicidal activity of mononuclear phagocytes: in vitro technique. J Postgrad Med 39: 22–25

Sivam GP 2001 Protection against *Helicobacter pylori* and other bacterial infections by garlic. J Nutr 131(3s): 1106S–1108S

Solmaz M, Sayar K, Kavuk I 2003 Psychological factors in the irritable bowel syndrome. Eur J Med Res 8(12): 549–556

Swami Sada Shiva Tirtha 1998 The Ayurveda Encyclopedia. Ayurveda Holistic Centre Press, New York

Taylor CE, Greenough WB 1989 Control of diarrheal diseases. Annu Rev Public Health 10: 221–244

Walker AF, Middleton RW, Petrowicz O 2001 Artichoke leaf extract reduces symptoms of irritable bowel syndrome in a post-marketing surveillance study. Phytother Res 15(1): 58–61

Chapter **9**

The respiratory system

THE FUNCTION OF THE RESPIRATORY SYSTEM

To ensure sufficient intake of oxygen it is vital for children to have a fully functioning respiratory system, to have plenty of fresh air and exercise every day and that they breathe properly. The quality of the air breathed in is also of vital importance. Children's lungs are delicate organs susceptible to external factors including heat, dust, moulds, pathogenic micro-organisms and chemical irritants. The pollution in the air, cigarette smoke, carbon monoxide, lead from car fumes, etc., becomes pollution in their lungs, which is then carried in the blood all round the body.

According to Western medicine the main function of the lungs is the exchange of oxygen and carbon dioxide and the maintenance of acid–base in the body. We also know that the air we breathe is not only vital to our physiological functioning, but also to our more subtle processes. In India air is called "prana", the breath of life. Not only are we breathing in gases vital for normal functioning of our cells and tissues, but we are also taking in the energy of the atmosphere around us which radiates from the trees and other green plants and ultimately from the sun. Correct breathing is vital for our nerves and muscles to permit relaxation and ensure rest, as well as encouraging a clear alert mind. In many cultures and religions the use of the breath is central to spiritual practices such as yoga and meditation and traditional movements like Qi Gong and Tai Chi.

Most adults inhale and exhale between 10 and 15 times each minute, while children respire faster in response to their greater need to provide energy to every cell as it functions and multiplies. This allows for the rapid growth and development and the high levels of vitality that characterize childhood. While a healthy respiratory system is vital for the normal development of every child, the immaturity of children's lungs and the fact that they possess fewer alveoli than mature adult lungs, means that children are particularly prone to respiratory problems, which of course can compromise the adequate exchange of oxygen and carbon dioxide in the lungs necessary for optimum health.

PREVENTING RESPIRATORY PROBLEMS

The origin of respiratory illness may arise from the respiratory system itself, as it is open to the external environment via the nose and mouth and so it is vulnerable to airborne irritants and infection. It also functions, in conjunction with other pathways of elimination of waste products, the skin, the bowels and the urinary tract, as an organ of elimination. If the body is overloaded with toxins, it can impose a greater burden on the respiratory system and this can lead to problems. If waste products are not eliminated efficiently via one pathway, the others are over-worked. If digestion is poor and diet is over-heavy and devitalized, it can lead to accumulations of toxins in the gastrointestinal tract. Constipation means these toxins are not being eliminated efficiently from the bowels and creates an overload of toxic matter to be excreted elsewhere. This may cause an accumulation of catarrh in the respiratory tract and predispose to further respiratory problems (Donovan 1988). It is also possible that stress, anxiety and other emotions can be expressed through the lungs. They have been associated with tension in the bronchial system and lowered immunity, which can predispose to chest infections and asthma. It is therefore important that the overall health of each child is ascertained through careful case history-taking when treating respiratory problems.

When considering preventative health, pollution in and out of the home requires careful consideration. It is quite possible that pollution in the home poses even more of a threat than those outside. Household moulds, bacteria, dust, damp, tobacco and household chemicals all impose their influence in the lungs. Washing bedclothes in hot water will kill dust mites, a dehumidifier will help to resolve problems from damp such as household moulds and fungi, and an efficient vacuum cleaner with a good filter will help to minimize dust, animal dander, moulds and bacteria. Certain houseplants, notably devil's ivy (*Epipremum aureum*) and the Boston fern (*Nephrolepis exalta*) are recommended by a Dr Wolverton of NASA (Tillotson et al 2001, p. 410) to reduce air pollution and toxins including fungal toxins in the home. Non-toxic cleaning materials, available mostly from health food shops, are clearly preferable to those containing potentially toxic chemicals, while clothes made of natural fibres tend to cause fewer problems than man-made materials such as polyester, although wool can be a problem for children suffering from allergies.

HERBS FOR THE RESPIRATORY SYSTEM

The herbal approach to the treatment of respiratory problems is first and foremost prevention through diet, lifestyle and herbs to maximize immunity and resistance to respiratory infections. A diet high in fresh, organic fruit and vegetables to maximize vitamin, mineral and antioxidant intake will benefit lung function. Carotenoid-rich foods like carrots, tomatoes, apricots, winter squash and red peppers are particularly good (see also Enhancing Immunity, p. 166).

Herbs such as echinacea, garlic, thyme, liquorice, ginger and turmeric all have effective immunostimulatory as well as antimicrobial actions and would all be applicable here. Research concerning children with recurrent respiratory tract infections indicates a tendency to show reduced immune function with particular depression in numbers of T lymphocytes. Treatment aimed at stimulating antibody and T-cell function in 117 children with recurrent respiratory infections produced beneficial results (Prusek et al 1987). Pulmonary macrophages play a key role in defence against respiratory infection (Gordon and Read 2002), and stimulation of macrophage response appears to be a mode of action of echinacea (Bauer 2002) and garlic. Both garlic and echinacea have been shown to be effective in respiratory tract infections, and have been recommended in the treatment of children (Bauer 2002, Andrianova et al 2003).

Propolis is another excellent anti-infective agent and is particularly effective in the prevention and treatment of upper respiratory infections of children such as tonsillitis and sinusitis (Mantle 2004, p. 51). A group of preschool children and schoolchildren were treated during the cold season of 1994–1995 with an aqueous propolis extract which had a rich content of flavonoids. In relation to acute and chronic inflammatory diseases of the upper airways, the analysis of the data obtained pointed out the favourable effects of this local treatment, expressed by lowering of the number of cases with acute or chronic symptoms, and decrease and sometimes suppression of the viral–microbial flora carriage of the upper airways (Crisan et al 1995).

AYURVEDIC APPROACH

The lungs are the primary site of *Kapha*. According to Ayurveda phlegm is produced in the stomach and then accumulates in the lungs (Frawley 2000, p. 195). Most respiratory disorders are therefore *Kapha* problems. *Kapha* predominates in childhood which accounts for why these problems abound in children. *Kapha* predominant children will be particularly prone. By reducing *Kapha* foods (see p. 68) particularly in *Kapha* seasons (winter and early spring) and using *Kapha* reducing herbs (those that are warming, light and dry, see p. 14), many respiratory problems can be prevented.

The lungs are also pervaded by air (*Vata*) when *prana* enters the body. *Vata* disturbance can lead to spasm of the airways as well as lowered immunity, predisposing to colds and coughs. Immunity will generally be lowered by insomnia, stress, anxiety and grief and low digestive fire (see Immune System, p. 150).

Pitta disorders of the lungs can also occur and tend to be accompanied by fever and infection. Most severe infections such as bronchitis and pneumonia involve *Pitta*. This may reflect a system overloaded with toxins and heat, and infection represents the body's effort to throw these out.

Low digestive fire causing accumulation of *ama* tends also to predispose to mucus, regardless of the *dosha* involved. So raising digestive fire is always a consideration when treating respiratory disorders (see Digestive System, p. 196).

Useful Ayurvedic herbs for the respiratory system include:

- Liquorice – throat and larynx tonic
- Sitopaladi (see Appendix, p. 302)
- Chiretta.

Children are more prone to upper respiratory infections by one of 200 odd rhinoviruses or other micro-organisms that can infect the lungs, than anything else. If they are treated speedily with simple dietary measures and herbal remedies combined with rest and nurture, there is less risk of complications requiring antibiotic treatment (which can be reserved for more serious conditions for which there is no better alternative). This is particularly important if the child has a history of catarrh or chest problems or asthma. It has to be borne in mind that many other infectious diseases begin with cold symptoms before other characteristic symptoms emerge, the rash with measles, the whoop with whooping cough for example, and early treatment may lead to a speedier resolution.

TREATING THE COMMON COLD

When using herbs to treat the common cold, the aim is to support the body's fight against the infection and speed recovery, while at the same time relieving the often annoying symptoms.

Echinacea is one of the prime cold remedies that has received much press coverage over the last few years. Research shows preparations made from the pressed juice of the flowering aerial parts of *Echinacea purpurea* are an effective supportive treatment of common viral infections of the upper respiratory tract and can diminish the severity and the length of common colds significantly (Bauer 2002). Taking 2.5 ml of the tincture at the onset of infection and taken every 2 hours until all symptoms have cleared, can certainly stop a cold from progressing.

At the *first signs* of infection, hot herbal infusions (sweetened with honey or flavoured with unsweetened blackcurrant/apple juice or liquorice if required) can be given to ease the symptoms and if taken every 2 hours can speed infection on its way. Equal parts of the four following herbs or any of them given singly as hot infusions can be taken in the same manner:

1. Yarrow stimulates the circulation and induces sweating, helping to reduce fevers, clear toxins, decongest the airways and soothe aches and pains.

2. Peppermint is a stimulating aromatic decongestant. It helps to clear the airways and reduce fever.

3. Elderflower is an effective decongestant and expectorant. Taken in hot infusion it helps to relieve catarrh and fever, flu and sinusitis. Research indicates that elderberry extract is active against both influenza types A and B (Zakay-Rones et al 1995).

4. Boneset (*Eupatorium perfoliatum*) is one of the best remedies to relieve aches and pains, reduce fever and clear catarrh.

- Turmeric is another effective antimicrobial; $\frac{1}{4}$ tsp can be mixed with honey and taken off the spoon or stirred into hot water every 2 hours.

- Garlic is an excellent remedy for all respiratory infections if children can be persuaded to take it. Research has demonstrated that garlic is effective for non-specific prevention of acute respiratory infections in children (Andrianova et al 2003). It can be given as capsules, juice, chopped into a teaspoon of honey or made into a dip and given every 2–3 hours.

- Agrimony (*Agrimonia eupatoria*) and eyebright (*Euphrasia off.*) are rich in tannins with astringent properties. They help to protect the mucous membranes from irritation caused by cold viruses and to dry catarrh and reduce swelling of congested mucous membranes.

- Eucalyptus, basil, lemon balm, hyssop (*Hyssopus off.*), pine (*Pinus sylvestris*), rosemary and thyme all contain volatile oils with antimicrobial properties. They also stimulate mucous membranes and with their expectorant properties help loosen and clear phlegm.

- Coltsfoot (*Tusilago farfara*), hyssop, mullein or thyme in hot infusion will also help clear phlegm in the throat or chest.

- Chamomile is useful in all children's infections, helping to soothe a fractious child and promote rest and sleep, which in turn aids speedy recovery. Research has demonstrated chamomile's ability to provide sedative as well as spasmolytic effects (Avallone et al 2000). Chamomile contains antimicrobial volatile oils which help to resolve infection, reduce fever and clear catarrhal congestion (Carle and Isaac 1987).

- If there is a sore throat or an irritating cough, demulcent herbs can be added to prescriptions to soothe irritated mucous membranes and help loosen phlegm, making it easier to clear. These include marshmallow (*Althea off.*), liquorice, comfrey leaf (*Symphytum off.*) or mullein. Research has demonstrated that marshmallow root and leaf have antimicrobial actions against a number of infections including *Pseudomonas aeruginosa*, *Proteus vulgaris* and *Staphylococcus aureus* (Mantle 2004).

- If the throat is painful and there are swollen or tender lymph glands, marigold, cleavers (*Galium aparine*) or blue flag (*Iris versicolor*) can be combined with other chosen herbs.

- A decoction of warming spices makes a very palatable drink and is also effective especially when there is copious catarrh and/or a blocked nose (Box 9.1).

Local applications

Gargles or throat sprays made from undiluted lemon juice, raspberry leaf (*Rubus idaeus*) tea, sage (*Salvia off.*), tea with a teaspoon of cider vinegar or $\frac{1}{2}$ tsp tincture of myrrh (*Commiphora molmol*) in a little water, can be used several times a day.

Herbal infusions can be added to bath water and used for hand and foot baths, especially if a child is reluctant to drink. A mustard foot bath may be an old-fashioned remedy but it is helpful when it comes to throwing off a cold. A dessertspoonful of dry mustard powder is added to

---

Box 9.1   Common cold recipe

$\frac{1}{2}$ oz fresh ginger root, sliced
1 stick of cinnamon
3 cloves
3 black peppercorns
3 cardamom pods.

Place in a pan and cover with 1 pt/600 ml of cold water. Bring to boil, cover and simmer for about 20 minutes. Strain, sweeten with honey if desired and give hot every 2 hours.

---

2 pints/1200 ml hot water and the feet soaked for 5–10 minutes twice daily. Cover the head with a hat/towel to increase body heat. Powdered cinnamon, cloves, cardamom and ginger can be used in the same way.

Inhalations

The combined mucus-clearing and antiseptic effects of steam and volatile oils make inhalations an excellent treatment for respiratory infections. Inhalations two or three times a day using a few drops of essential oil in a bowl of hot water are suitable for children over the age of 4 as long as a parent is present. Putting a towel over the head stops the volatile oils from escaping into the atmosphere and makes the inhalation more effective. For younger children the same oils can be used in a vaporizer and placed in a bedroom at night to ease congestion of the airways and to disinfect the atmosphere. Chamomile, clove, eucalyptus, rosemary, rose, lavender, pine, basil, lemon and thyme oil are all excellent antiseptics and help to clear the airways. They can be used singly or in combination. Essential oils of eucalyptus, basil, rose, lavender or pine can be diluted in a base of sesame oil (2 drops per 5 ml) and massaged into the chest, neck, throat or feet or added to bath water.

Dietary treatment

A child with a cold is best fed on light, easy to digest food, so that most of the body's energy can be directed to resolving infection as opposed to the process of digestion. Soups, vegetables, stews and casseroles, fruit and vegetable juices are all suitable and dairy produce, sugar, red meat and grains (including bread) are best avoided. Leeks, garlic and onions all enhance the immune system's fight against infection with their pungent and antimicrobial properties and can be added liberally to the diet. Foods containing vitamins A and C will help the body to throw off a virus. Hot lemon and honey drinks can be given freely to help clear catarrh and soothe a sore throat and chest. Blackcurrant tea is rich in vitamin C and bioflavonoids. Supplements of vitamin C with bioflavonoids, 100 mg 3–5 times a day, 1 teaspoon of cod liver oil and 5 mg zinc lozenges three times daily can be given until the child recovers (McElroy and Miller 2003).

Ayurvedic treatment of colds

Ginger tea (sweetened with honey if required) sipped throughout the day can be very effective for reducing general cold symptoms and stopping a cold in its tracks.

A randomized, double-blind study using an extract of a well-known antiviral herb *Andrographis paniculata* on 158 patients demonstrated that this herb was highly effective in "reducing the prevalence and intensity of the symptoms in uncomplicated common cold beginning at day two of treatment. No adverse effects were observed or reported." (Tillotson et al 2001, p. 413).

It is possible to be more specific in treatment of a common cold using Ayurveda:

Vata type colds are characterized by sneezing, scanty mucus, a dry cough, hoarseness, restlessness and insomnia. There may also be generalized aches and pains, headache, and pain in the joints.

- Diaphoretic herbs (as for *Kapha*) can be given combined with demulcent herbs like bala, shatavari, ashwagandha and liquorice.
- Sitopaladi is an excellent remedy and $\frac{1}{4}$–$\frac{1}{2}$ tsp can be mixed into a teaspoon of honey and a little warm water or milk and given three times daily.
- Other suitable herbs include slippery elm and astragalus (*Astragalus membranaceus*).

Pitta type colds can be associated with fever, sore throat, yellow mucus, diarrhoea, flushing and irritability.

- *Pitta* reducing herbs such as gokshura, punanarva (*Boerhavia diffusa*), coriander, fennel (*Foeniculum vulgare*), spearmint and other cooling diaphoretics can be used.
- Echinacea, burdock and yarrow are also useful.
- Sitopaladi in honey and chiretta are particularly indicated. I have often used them in my practice at the onset of respiratory infections with success.

Kapha type colds involve more tiredness, lethargy, congestion and copious mucus, which is thick, white or clear. *Kapha* and *ama* reducing herbs and foods are indicated here.

- Ginger, cinnamon (*Cinnamomum* spp.), pippali, tulsi, liquorice, echinacea, mint, cloves (*Eugenia caryophyllata*), yarrow, elderberry, ajwan (*Trachyspermum ammi*), burdock, lemongrass (*Cymbopogon citratus*) are all suitable as they are expectorant and diaphoretic and help induce sweating. They are best given as hot teas regularly through the day.
- Like the above a tea made with lemon juice, fresh ginger and raw honey will help to clear phlegm and resolve infection.
- Sitopaladi is excellent, $\frac{1}{2}$–1 tsp in honey 3–4 times daily.

Dairy products, sweets, fried foods, herbal tonics such as shatavari and ashwagandha, and yeasted breads are best avoided as they all increase *Kapha*.

CHRONIC CATARRH

While it is normal for a child to have catarrh for a few days after a cold until the irritated mucous membranes are fully recovered, in some children the catarrhal stage persists chronically for weeks, months or longer. There are several reasons why this could occur.

- Irritation of the airways by atmospheric pollution, cigarette smoke, dust, petrol fumes, dry air from central heating, carbon monoxide, etc. (de Jongste and Shields 2003).
- A poor diet, junk foods, excess milk products, sugar, refined carbohydrates, and wrong food combinations can cause constipation and putrefaction in the bowels allowing toxins to be circulated in the bloodstream. Mucus or catarrh is one way the body can discharge some of its toxic overload.
- Allergy to milk/wheat can cause chronic catarrh and predispose to frequent respiratory infections, colds, sore throats, chest and middle ear infections.
- Sinusitis can cause chronic catarrh as well as postnasal drip and an accompanying irritating cough.

Herbal treatment of chronic catarrh

- Echinacea is indicated where there is chronic infection in the sinuses.
- Astringent herbs such as marigold, elderflower, eyebright (*Euphrasia off.*), thyme and plantain can

be used, which tone the mucous membranes and protect them from irritation and reduce phlegm.

- Aromatic herbs with a high volatile oil content have stimulating and antimicrobial properties and help to loosen sticky mucus, making it easier to expectorate. Chamomile, peppermint, thyme, ginger, hyssop (*Hyssopus off.*) and basil are good examples of these.

- Warming spices including ginger, cloves (*Eugenia carophyllata*), cinnamon (*Cinnamomum* spp.), caraway (*Carum carvi*) and black pepper (*Piper nigrum*) in hot tea will enhance digestion and cleanse toxins from the gastrointestinal tract, as well as stimulate clearing of mucus from the respiratory tract.

- Essential oils can be used in inhalations or vaporizers, a few drops can be mixed in a base oil of sesame for massage of the face around the frontal and nasal sinuses. Chamomile, lavender, lemon, pine, basil, eucalyptus and peppermint are all suitable.

- For sluggish bowels it is well worth using bowel cleansing herbs for a week or two on commencing treatment, such as liquorice, dandelion root, linseed (*Linum usitatissimum*), psyllium seeds (*Plantago psyllium*), (see Constipation, p. 208). Garlic in the form of capsules/juice/raw can be given daily to clear putrefactive bacteria from the bowel as well as to clear catarrh and sinus infection.

Dietary suggestions

For the first few days of treatment the child is best fed only on a light diet consisting largely of fruit and vegetables, soups and herbal teas. Mild spices such as cumin, coriander, turmeric and ginger can be added to these to help clear congestion. For the next 2–3 weeks they should avoid sugary foods, red meat, milk products and excessive amount of grains, particularly wheat and bread, as far as possible. Dried fruit such as prunes and apricots can be given to keep the bowels moving. The child needs to drink plenty to encourage elimination of toxins through the kidneys. Hot lemon and honey and hot unsweetened elderberry or blackcurrant juice help to break down thick mucus.

The skin presents a huge area available for the excretion of waste products through the pores by sweating. If this major pathway of elimination is not employed through regular vigorous exercise, which warms the body and encourages sweating, then more pressure is put upon other pathways of elimination. For this reason children need to take plenty of vigorous outdoor exercise.

There also needs to be enough fresh air in the house, especially in winter when infections abound, windows are rarely opened and children may be reluctant to play out in the cold. Bowls of water placed near radiators in centrally heated houses may help to reduce drying of the atmosphere which can cause irritation of mucous membranes and render the child more susceptible to catarrh. An ionizer may help to reduce the harmful effects of the atmosphere on delicate mucous membranes. Sweat therapy is advised using diaphoretic and expectorant herbs prepared as a tea, including cinnamon, ginger, pippali, tulsi, liquorice and sitopaladi $\frac{1}{2}$–1 tsp in honey 3–4 times daily.

Ayurvedic approach

The nose is the gateway to the rest of our breathing apparatus through which we inhale fresh air and *prana*. It is therefore of utmost importance that a child is able to breathe freely. An excess of mucus which blocks the passageway is seen predominantly as an excess of *Kapha dosha* brought about generally by over consumption of *Kapha* foods and especially wheat products, dairy products, salt and sugar. This can be exacerbated by other *Kapha* increasing factors such as cold, damp weather, sedentary lifestyle, sleeping too much and, most importantly, by low digestive fire. (For general treatment of *Kapha* see p. 68.)

- Warming spices are the best way to raise digestive fire and clear excess *Kapha* from the system. Suitable spices to be given three times a day as hot teas include: ginger, pippali, cinnamon, cloves, caraway (*Carum carvi*), coriander, ajwan (*Trachyspermum ammi*) and black pepper. A teaspoon of ajwan seeds with a pinch of rock salt stirred into a little hot water will also help to raise digestive fire.

- Hingwastaka (see Appendix p. 302) makes a suitable formula and $\frac{1}{4}$–$\frac{1}{2}$ tsp can be given in a little hot water twice daily, before lunch and dinner.

- One of the best remedies for clearing mucus is $\frac{1}{4}-\frac{1}{2}$ tsp of turmeric powder stirred into hot water twice a day. Alternatively $\frac{1}{2}$ tsp of turmeric can be boiled with $\frac{1}{8}$ tsp of ajwan seeds for 10 minutes and a teaspoon taken in a teaspoon of honey 2–3 times a day.

- A tea made from a teaspoon of dried holy basil leaves with a pinch each of clove and cinnamon powder sweetened with a little honey, will help to clear mucus.

- Another useful prescription is a $\frac{1}{2}$ tsp each of liquorice and ginger powder simmered in a cup of water for 10 minutes.

- A steam inhalation of ajwan is also an effective way of relieving nasal congestion. A tablespoonful of ajwan seeds can be added to $\frac{1}{2}$ a small pan of boiling water, simmered for 5 minutes covered, removed from the heat and then the steam inhaled. This is suitable for older children under adult supervision but for younger children the pan can be left in a safe place nearby for the steam to fill the room the child is in. Eucalyptus leaves or a few drops of the essential oil can be used similarly.

SINUSITIS

If the sinuses become congested and inflamed following a cold, flu or chronic catarrh, this can predispose to a sinus infection, either viral or bacterial. The resultant pain and swelling around the nose and eyes, as well as headaches and even toothache, can be quite distressing for children. Nasal congestion, sinusitis, postnasal drip and the irritating cough that can accompany it respond well to herbal treatment and dietary changes.

Chronic sinusitis can also be related to overproduction of mucus in an attempt by the body to cleanse itself of toxins that are not being adequately eliminated elsewhere. Lack of fresh air and exercise, constipation and insufficient fluid intake and urination can all be contributory factors.

Sinusitis can also be caused by atmospheric pollution such as passive smoking. Alternatively blockage and infection in the sinuses can be related to over-production of mucus due to food intolerance, most often to cow's milk and milk products.

Atopic diseases such as rhinitis are a common feature of cow's milk allergy (Iacono et al 1998).

A diet that reduces mucus, avoiding milk, sugar, wheat and excess red meats, and includes plenty of fresh fruit and vegetables, seeds, and essential fatty acids is recommended. The Hay diet is often helpful in clearing chronic catarrh. It involves avoidance of combining proteins with carbohydrates and acid fruits with carbohydrates in the same meal. Once the sinusitis clears normal eating can gradually be resumed.

Treatment of sinusitis

- For sluggish bowels dandelion root, liquorice, psyllium (*Plantago psyllium*) or linseed (*Linum usitarissimum*) are all helpful. Syrup of figs, cooked prunes and apricots will also stimulate bowel function.

- Herbs such as yarrow, limeflowers (*Tilia europaea*), ginger, catnip (*Nepeta cataria*), peppermint, chamomile, lavender, hyssop (*Hyssopus off.*), thyme, lemon balm and basil taken as hot teas stimulate the circulation to the periphery and increase sweating and thereby elimination of toxins through the pores.

- Herbs rich in volatile oils not only stimulate the linings of the sinuses, helping to loosen and shift the mucus, but also have antimicrobial properties that help to resolve the accompanying infection in the sinuses. These include aniseed (*Pimpinella anisum*), chamomile, fennel (*Foeniculum vulgare*), rose, ginger, hyssop (*Hyssopus off.*), lavender, peppermint, rosemary and thyme. These are best taken as hot infusions (sweetened with honey/liquorice/apple concentrate if desired) three times a day. They can be taken singly or in mixtures, blended to suit the child's taste.

- Essential oils of the same herbs along with pine, lemon and eucalyptus can be used for steam inhalations and to make nose drops. As well as the antimicrobial properties of the oils, many constituents in the oils such as chamazulene in chamomile have potent anti-inflammatory actions (Safayhi et al 1994). For a steam inhalation a few drops of oil can be added to a bowl of hot boiled water, using a towel over the child's head to stop the volatile oils and steam from escaping. This can be done morning and night. To make nose drops add 1–2 drops of the chosen essential oils per 5 ml of base oil such as sesame oil, warm the oil and massage the facial area around the sinuses and insert 2 drops into each nostril morning and night.

- Once the mucus starts to loosen and drain, the sinusitis should clear fairly quickly. If not, astringent herbs like agrimony (*Agrimonia eupatoria*), elderflowers, marigold, rose petals, eyebright (*Euphrasia off.*) and golden rod (*Solidago virgaurea*), as well as demulcent herbs like marshmallow (*Althea off.*), comfrey leaf (*Symphytum off.*), mullein and Iceland moss (*Cetraria islandica*) can be given internally as infusions to soothe the irritated mucous membranes.

- For a particularly persistent sinus infection combined with general tiredness, irritability and malaise, immune-enhancing and antimicrobial remedies including echinacea, myrrh (*Commiphora molmol*), turmeric, chamomile, garlic or wild indigo (*Baptisia tintoria*) are indicated.

- Drinks of hot lemon and honey, elderberry and blackcurrant juice will also help to loosen the mucus congestion while supplements of vitamin C, zinc, garlic and cod liver oil will help to build resistance to infection.

Ayurvedic approach

Sinusitis is most likely to be a *Kapha* problem with involvement of *Pitta* and will be aggravated by *Kapha* foods (particularly cold drinks, dairy produce; see p. 147) and cold, damp *Kapha* weather. However the other *doshas* can also be involved.

- *Vata* type: there will be signs of *Vata* imbalance such as wind, constipation, restless sleep, low weight, scanty mucus, sinus pain and headaches.
- *Pitta* type: there will be signs of *Pitta* imbalance such as heat, yellow phlegm, tendency to fever, inflammatory problems and irritability.
- *Kapha* type: there will be signs of *Kapha* imbalance such as lethargy, feeling of heaviness, foggy-mindedness, laziness, excess saliva, loss of sense of smell and thick mucus.

Ayurvedic treatment

For general treatment use fresh ginger tea or freshly grated ginger pulp with a teaspoon of honey 2–3 times a day to help to raise digestive fire, clear toxins and reduce excess *Kapha*.

- For *Vata*: ginger, bala, astragalus (*Astragalus membranaceus*), garlic, pippali, basil, angelica (*Angelica archangelica*), are suitable. Trikulu, and Sitopaladi are useful formulae (see Appendix p. 302).
- For *Pitta*: mullein, bala, mint, guduchi, amalaki, chamomile, neem, and turmeric.
- For *Kapha*: calamus, neem, turmeric, ginger, pippali, basil, fenugreek (*Trigonella foenum-graecum*), garlic and onions. Sitopaladi and Trikatu are useful formulae.

Salt water made from adding $\frac{1}{2}$ tsp of sea salt to a cup of warm water can be drawn (or poured using a netty pot) up into one nostril and eliminated through the other and then repeated on the other side. This rather unpleasant form of treatment, suitable for older children, is excellent. Nasal drops using the same saline solution is preferable for younger children. Two or three drops in both nostrils am and pm.

SORE THROATS

The defences of the throat can be vulnerable to a number of different pathogenic micro-organisms, viral and bacterial, either in the nose, the sinuses, the mouth or the lungs as well as by general systemic health. Sore throats, like all other symptoms, need to be seen in the wider context of the child's general health and well-being, not simply the micro-organisms involved. An infection will develop only where the environment is hospitable for the microbes to settle and multiply.

One common cause of a mild sore throat on waking is central heating, as it causes low humidity. At night during sleep the mucous membranes of the nose dry out and swell, congesting the nose and causing mouth breathing. The low humidity irritates the mucous membranes in the throat causing discomfort. Placing a dehumidifier/vaporizer in the bedroom should easily remedy this.

When tonsils, adenoids and other lymph glands around the throat become swollen and painful, they are merely doing their work, along with other lymphatic tissue in the body, to defend the body from infection. Lymphocytes produced by the tonsils and adenoids are the first line of defence against airborne pathogens that are inhaled through the nose and mouth. Once the underlying causes of swollen lymph glands are resolved, the swelling will gradually subside.

Ayurvedic approach

According to Ayurveda there are three types of sore throats.

- *Vata* type: the throat is dry, irritated and associated with wind and constipation and hoarseness.
- *Pitta* type: the throat is red, swollen and inflamed, the pain can be severe as in a streptococcal infection.
- *Kapha* type: a sore throat occurs with congestion and phlegm.

Treatment of sore throats

Most infections affecting the throat are viral, though the more serious infections tend to be bacterial. Herbs can be used in both bacterial and viral infections but obviously care needs to be taken with children with acute sore throat, swollen glands and fever, because of the risk of complications of a streptococcal throat infection. If a child has a sore throat with runny nose or eyes, slight cough and nasal congestion, it is more likely to be a viral infection, but if the child has only a severe sore throat and swollen glands with or without fever and malaise, but no accompanying upper respiratory symptoms, it is more likely to be a bacterial infection (see also Treatment of Infections, p. 180).

- Antimicrobial herbs including chamomile, basil, cat's claw (*Uncaria tormentosa*), self-heal (*Prunella vulgaris*), thyme, garlic, turmeric, wild indigo (*Baptisia tinctoria*), myrrh (*Commiphora molmol*), cinnamon, ginger, garlic and onion can be used to enhance the efforts of the immune system to fight off infection. Propolis is also recommended.

- Many herbs traditionally used for sore throat such as those containing rosmarinic acid (e.g. sage and rosemary) have antiviral action (Petersen and Simmonds 2003).

- Honey itself has antiviral action, supporting the traditional lemon and honey cure.

- Echinacea and garlic can be given every 2 hours. These can be combined with remedies that specifically help the cleansing work of the tonsils such as cleavers (*Galium aparine*), marigold, blue flag (*Iris versicolor*), burdock, dandelion root and golden seal (*Hydrastis canadensis*).

- Tinctures/infusions of thyme, sage (*Salvia off.*), rosemary, myrrh, golden seal and propolis can be used as gargles or in throat sprays.

- Antiseptic essential oils can be used for inhalations/vaporizers, to disinfect the room, including rosemary, eucalyptus, pine, lemon or thyme.

- For fever management elderflowers, limeflowers (*Tilia europaea*), chamomile, yarrow, lemon balm, peppermint can be given as teas throughout the day.

- Demulcent herbs to relieve heat and discomfort in the throat, such as mullein, liquorice, marshmallow (*Althea off.*), coltsfoot (*Tussilago farfara*) and slippery elm (*Ulmus fulva*) can also be given.

Ayurvedic approach

- *Vata* type sore throats require warming and soothing herbs such as ginger, cinnamon, cardamom, haritaki, liquorice, slippery elm, amalaki, anise (*Pimpinella anisum*) and garlic. Tea of liquorice, ginger, cinnamon in equal parts ($\frac{1}{2}$ teaspoon of mixture powder) in hot water can be taken three times daily.

  - Gargle: salt and warm water is suitable or $\frac{1}{2}$ tsp turmeric powder in warm milk.

  - Massage of sesame oil or ghee medicated with liquorice or calamus can be applied to the throat.

- *Pitta* type sore throats require cooling, detoxifying antimicrobials including katuka (*Picrorrhiza kurroa*), guduchi, chamomile, liquorice, amalaki, bibhitaki, fennel (*Foeniculum vulgare*) and lemongrass.

– Gargle: sandalwood: 2.5 ml of tincture/2.5 g of powder or $\frac{1}{2}$ tsp turmeric powder or $\frac{1}{2}$ tsp of neem tincture in $\frac{1}{2}$ cup of warm water or $\frac{1}{2}$ cup of neem infusion are all suitable.

- *Kapha* type sore throats require warming diaphoretics, expectorants, decongestants and astringents. Useful herbs include ginger, bibhitaki, basil, lemongrass (*Cymbopogon citratus*), haritaki, garlic, cinnamon, coriander and turmeric. Drinks of hot lemon and honey will help to soothe the throat.

   – Gargle: sandalwood/turmeric in hot water (see above).

Sitopaladi and chiretta can be taken generally by all types, $\frac{1}{4}-\frac{1}{2}$ tsp in hot water or a teaspoon of honey three times daily, as well as Triphala powder, $\frac{1}{4}-\frac{1}{2}$ tsp in hot water with honey at night.

TONSILLITIS

Tonsils and adenoids provide a first defence against atmospheric pollution and infection entering the body through the mouth and nose. They also filter poisons in the bloodstream and those draining from the nose and sinuses. When they become swollen, inflamed and painful during an infection, they are responding to an increased demand for their cleansing work in an attempt to throw it off. The tonsils in so doing are fulfilling their protective role by inhibiting the spread of infection further into the body. For this reason the surgical removal of the tonsils should only be a last resort.

Tonsillitis can be both acute and chronic. Acute tonsillitis flares up in response to a viral or a bacterial infection, and tends to occur when there is low vital energy, excess toxins in the body and catarrhal congestion. It frequently heralds or accompanies a cold or flu virus, laryngitis or mumps. When bacterial, the onset is sudden with a severe sore throat and swollen neck glands, often with a fever, but with no or few other upper respiratory symptoms. The *streptococcal bacterium* involved can, in rare cases, affect the kidneys (causing nephritis) or the heart (in rheumatic fever). This means that the first signs of bacterial infections require prompt action.

Treatment of tonsillitis

At the first signs of infection, hot infusions can be given, and there are several different herbs that could be applicable:

- Antimicrobial herbs to support the work of the immune system: echinacea, garlic, self-heal (*Prunella vulgaris*), wild indigo (*Baptisia tinctoria*), cat's claw (*Uncaria tormentosa*), burdock, turmeric, golden seal (*Hydrastis canadensis*) and ginger.

- Depurative herbs to enhance the work of the lymphatic tissue in its cleansing work: cleavers (*Galium aparine*), self-heal, marigold and blue flag (*Iris versicolor*).

- Diaphoretic herbs to induce sweating and reduce fever if necessary: chamomile, catnip (*Nepeta cataria*), peppermint, elderflowers, limeflowers (*Tilia europaea*) and yarrow.

- Tannin rich herbs to astringe the mucosa and reduce accompanying catarrh and inflammation: agrimony (*Agrimonia eupatoria*), chamomile, elderflowers, ground ivy (*Nepeta hederacea*), plantain, thyme, marigold, blackberry (*Rubus fructicosus*) and raspberry (*Rubus idaeus*) leaves.

- Demulcent herbs to soothe and relieve painful tonsils: coltsfoot (*Tussilago farfara*), comfrey leaf (*Symphytum off.*), marshmallow (*Althea off.*), liquorice and mullein (Rau 2000).

A useful recipe and one that I use frequently for children with tonsillitis, is equal parts of cleavers (*Galium aparine*), echinacea, ground ivy (*Nepeta hederacea*), plantain and thyme as an infusion with a teaspoon of thyme honey. Give one cupful 3–6 times daily.

Propolis is also an effective remedy (active against 46 strains of *Streptococcus pyogenes*) and can be combined with these herbs (Bosio et al 2000).

Local applications

Gargles or throat sprays can be made using pure lemon juice, herbal infusions or a teaspoon of tincture diluted in warm water of chamomile, turmeric, myrrh (*Commiphora molmol*), golden seal (*Hydrastis canadensis*), sage (*Salvia off.*) or thyme (Hwang et al

2003). These can be used every 2 hours if the throat is very painful; otherwise three times a day.

Inhalations using essential oils of chamomile, lemon, pine, eucalyptus, lavender or thyme can be helpful. The same oils can be used in vaporizers, diluted in sesame oil for massages or added to water for compresses applied to the throat and neck.

Dietary treatment

Follow treatment for fevers (see p. 175). Children should avoid dairy produce, sugar, grains and animal produce for a week and have plenty to drink. Hot lemon and honey, honey and cider vinegar, herbal teas, ginger juice or carrot and apple juice, elderberry juice, blackcurrant tea or juice (unsweetened) are all helpful during infection to enhance immunity, and to relieve the sore throat and catarrh. They can be continued for a few days after the acute symptoms are gone as they increase resistance to further infection.

Supplements of a teaspoon of cod liver oil daily, 100 mg natural vitamin C tablets every 2–3 hours and one or two garlic capsules every 2 hours can be given until the child is well again.

Ayurvedic approach

In Ayurveda tonsillitis is known as *tundikeri* and is said to be precipitated often by constipation.

- Hot fomentations applied to the area are recommended and the tonsil area kept warm.
- Decoction of Babula bark (*Acacia arabica*) with rock salt can be used as a gargle.
- Fenugreek (*Trigonella foenum-graecum*) leaves or seeds, and tamarind leaves (*Tamarindus indica*) can also be used for making gargles. Fenugreek contains soothing mucilage and essential oils with analgesic properties. Tamarind leaves also have a demulcent action and antimicrobial properties (Phadke 2001).
- Liquorice, *Alpinia galanga* (kulanjana), and calamus root powder combined together with honey to form a paste are used as a "lick" for children to soothe infection and inflammation.
- *Acacia catechu* is given internally in pills (Khadiradi vati) to be sucked 2–3 a day.
- A handful of fresh rose petals boiled in a cupful of water, strained and sweetened with honey

can be sipped warm as tea to relieve the pain (Phadke 2001).

Chronic tonsillitis

It is important to establish the background causes of chronic tonsillitis before embarking on treatment, so that these are properly addressed. Chronically inflamed or pus-filled tonsils may not be able to continue efficiently with their cleansing work and as a result a child can be run down and prone to other illnesses. It is possible that the tonsils are being overworked by toxins draining from elsewhere, such as chronic catarrh in the sinuses or ears, or by allergic response, possibly to milk produce. The child may be depleted from, for example, poor diet, digestive problems, sluggish bowels and pollution in the atmosphere, particularly passive smoking. Chronic tonsillitis can also be related to frequent use of antibiotics for treatment of acute bouts. There may also be emotional factors involved – the throat area is related to the voice and its use in the expression of emotions and communication. If there are unexpressed or suppressed emotions, such as anger, grief, unhappiness or frustration, these could cause problems involving the throat.

Treatment of chronic tonsillitis

- As in the treatment of acute tonsillitis, herbs for the immune system, such as neem, elderberry juice, turmeric, thyme, echinacea and garlic, can be combined with remedies to support the lymphatic system, such as cleavers (*Galium aparine*), red clover (*Trifolium pratense*) or marigold and herbs to astringe the mucous membranes such as raspberry leaves (*Rubus idaeus*), ground ivy (*Nepeta hederacea*), thyme, self-heal (*Prunella vulgaris*) or plantain.
- In addition, extra herbs, such as blue flag (*Iris versicolor*), burdock, celery seed (*Apium graveolens*), marigold, and nettles need to be used to help the body eliminate toxins.
- Gargles or throat sprays using sage (*Salvia off.*) and thyme can be used morning and night, myrrh (*Commiphora molmol*), propolis and turmeric are also suitable.
- Regular massages or compresses, applied to the throat area, can be given, using strong infusions

of the herbs used for teas or from essential oils of rosewood or thyme in a base of sesame oil.

- The diet should be light and easy to digest with plenty of fresh fruit and vegetables, seeds and unrefined oils. Milk produce should be avoided altogether, preferably for a few months, as long as plenty of other calcium-containing foods are included in the diet. Sugar, refined carbohydrates and red meats should be kept to a minimum.
- Supplements of vitamin C, 500 mg daily, a teaspoon of cod liver oil, and garlic capsules, two twice daily, can be given until the problem is resolved.
- The child will need plenty of nurturing, rest and sleep, regular gentle exercise and fresh air.
- Grapefruit seed extract and probiotics are useful after antibiotics for acute bouts of tonsillitis.

In Ayurveda the herb of choice for chronic tonsillitis is agastya (*Sebenia grandiflora*) $\frac{1}{2}$ tsp of the powdered lead/bark is used with honey twice daily over a period of 6 months.

LARYNGITIS

Infection and inflammation of the larynx can develop from infection in the mouth, throat or nose, or postnasal drip during a cold. It may also occur with tonsillitis or bronchitis. Irritation from a dusty or smoke-laden atmosphere, excess use of the voice as in singing, talking or shouting can also contribute to inflammation.

Treatment of laryngitis

- Steam inhalations have a soothing effect on the larynx. Essential oils added to hot water, with their antiseptic and anti-inflammatory properties can help relieve pain and inflammation. Chamomile, eucalyptus, thyme, rose, lavender, pine, rosewood and sandalwood are all suitable.
- The same oils can be used for compresses applied regularly to the throat and chest, or in massage oils.
- Herbal infusions can be given using chamomile, catnip (*Nepeta cataria*), turmeric, burdock, self-heal (*Prunella vulgaris*), coltsfoot (*Tussilago farfara*), echinacea and marshmallow (*Althea off.*) flavoured with liquorice or honey. Give a half to one cupful every 2 hours.

- Garlic and echinacea can also be given every 2–3 hours.
- Propolis is also useful.
- Hot lemon and honey drinks, or blackcurrant tea can be alternated with the herbal tea.
- Keep the air in the room as moist as possible, and the child discouraged from talking to allow the larynx to recover quickly.

Ayurvedic approach

Laryngitis can be caused by exposure to cold wind, or over-use of the voice which aggravates *Vata*, or through congestion caused by excess *Kapha* descending from the nose or from inflammation and congestion in the bronchial tubes related to excess *Pitta*.

With excess *Vata* there will be a dry throat, loss of voice and hoarseness. With excess *Pitta* there will be yellow mucus, inflammation, fever and with excess *Kapha*, a swelling of the throat with much mucus.

- *Vata*: anti-*Vata* diet is recommended and demulcent herbs including shatavari, liquorice, bala, marshmallow (*Althea off.*) as well as warming herbs such as ginger, cardamom and cinnamon; $\frac{1}{2}$ tsp of calamus ghee three times daily is recommended by David Frawley (Frawley 2000).
- *Pitta*: anti-*Pitta* diet and bitter herbs such as turmeric, katuka (*Picrorrhiza kurroa*), burdock and barberry (*Berberis aristata*) are recommended. Sudarshan taken with ghee is also effective.
- *Kapha*: anti-*Kapha* diet with expectorant and decongestant herbs such as thyme, elecampane (*Inula helenium*), ginger, yarrow, and calamus is recommended.
- Triphala can be taken at night as a general treatment.

CROUP

When the larynx is swollen and inflamed, it can go into spasm and in small children can obstruct the passage of air and cause croup – with its characteristic barking or whistling sound made as the child tries to breathe through a tense wind-pipe and past inflamed vocal cords. Babies and small children are more likely to develop croup as their air passages are so narrow and more easily become blocked with mucus when they are inflamed.

Croup can be caused by various viral or bacterial infections, including the common cold and bronchitis. The typical symptoms begin after a child goes to bed with slight cold symptoms. During sleep, mucus runs down the throat, irritating the larynx, causing it to swell and go into spasm. The child wakes coughing and often struggling to breathe freely. Tension caused by ensuing fear only makes the situation worse.

Treatment of croup

- For acute bouts a bowl or kettle of steaming water nearby, or a hot tap turned on in the bathroom creates a steamy atmosphere, which can soothe the air passages and relax spasm in the throat. Herbs and oils can be added to the boiling water to soothe the inflamed larynx, clear the mucus and relax the spasm.

- The combined antispasmodic (Achterrath Iuckermann et al 1980), anti-inflammatory (Safayhi et al 1994) and antimicrobial (Carle and Isaac 1987) properties of chamomile make inhalations of tea or essential oil an excellent treatment. Sips of chamomile tea to relax the child may also be helpful.

- Birch (*Betula alba*) leaves, eucalyptus leaves, lavender flowers or pine needles (*Pinus sylvestris*) and oils of eucalyptus, lavender or pine are also effective. A few drops of essential oil can be added to water and sprayed into the room, or dropped on a damp towel on the radiator or in a bowl of water, or used in a vaporizer, diluted in a base oil and in the bath or for hand and foot baths. Essential oils can be mixed with sesame oil (1 drop per 5 ml oil) and rubbed into the chest, throat or back, or used in compresses to apply frequently to the head or chest.

- Infusions made from chamomile, catnip (*Nepeta cataria*), thyme, coltsfoot (*Tussilago farfara*), horehound (*Marrubium vulgare*), or marshmallow (*Althea off.*) with wild cherry (*Prunus serotina*), can be given to the child to drink in sips (or in a bottle for a baby).

- A useful recipe for croup, to clear the phlegm and reduce spasm, is an infusion of equal parts of catnip, coltsfoot, liquorice, horehound and wild cherry. A tablespoonful can be given every 30 minutes until the breathing is better.

- During the following day or two, herbal teas of chamomile, thyme and marshmallow, hot lemon and honey, or a little cider vinegar in a glass of warm water can be given.

For ongoing treatment

It is important that the bowels are kept open to help clear the toxins contributing to infection and phlegm. Sesame oil, with a few drops of lavender or chamomile oil, can be rubbed into the chest and a cup of hot herbal tea given before bed. If the air in the bedroom is kept moist, this can help prevent the child from waking with further attacks during the night. A very light diet is recommended, with plenty of fruit and vegetables, until the symptoms are completely clear. Slippery elm powder mixed with a pinch of ginger and cardamom, and honey to sweeten, and stirred into warm water, is soothing and nutritious.

EARACHE

Earache can be related to pain in the throat, gums, teeth or parotid glands (in mumps), which radiates to the ear. It can also be due to inflammation of the outer ear canal, and associated with swelling and an irritating discharge. Most commonly, however, especially in children under six, earache is caused by middle ear infection (otitis media). This may be either acute or chronic. Acute infections can occur as a sequel to other infections including colds, tonsillitis, measles or allergies.

Infection of the outer ear can be caused by an object stuck in the ear, a boil in the ear canal, scratching or fiddling with the ear (which often happens with a skin irritation such as eczema in or around the ears); or from chlorine in swimming pools, which can irritate the skin of children who swim frequently and who do not dry their ears properly.

Any discharge in the outer ear can be washed away gently with a warm infusion of antiseptic herbs, such as chamomile, elderflowers, golden seal (*Hydrastis canadensis*) or marigold, or a few drops of tincture can be used in warm water. One or two drops of warm olive oil with a few drops of essential oil of either chamomile or lavender (two drops to a teaspoon of oil) can be inserted into the ear canal before bed and plugged gently with a little cotton wool (Groppo et al 2002). Garlic oil can also be used but this may be rejected for social reasons. Tea tree oil may be preferable.

Otitis media: middle ear infection

Infection from the nose or throat can easily be carried, via the eustachian tube, into the middle ear and cause middle ear infection. Catarrh and swollen tonsils or lymph glands can block off the opening of the eustachian tube, creating stasis and a build-up of catarrh in the middle ear, and lead to infection. This may not be the whole story, as chiropractic adjustments can often help with drainage problems which lead to frequent acute or chronic ear infections. Some of the pathogenic micro-organisms that commonly cause otitis media include: *Haemophilus influenzae*; *Aspergillus* spp.; *Streptococcus pneumoniae* and *Moxaxella catarrhalis.*

Glue ear

This chronic condition of the middle ear is related to frequent upper respiratory infections – sinus, throat and middle ear infections – and is generally found where there are chronically enlarged tonsils, adenoids and lymph glands in the throat and neck area, which can block the eustachian tube and prevent normal drainage.

Treatment of acute middle ear infection

A recent trial of herbal eardrops in otitis media concludes that "herbal extracts have the potential to meet all of the requirements of appropriate medication that could be routinely used in the paediatric patient, namely in vitro bacterio-static and bacteriocidal activity against common pathogens, immunostimulation ability, antioxidant activity, and anti-inflammatory effects. They are also well-absorbed with good penetration into the tissue surrounding the tympanic membrane. They have been found to enhance local immunologic activity. Finally, herbal extracts are well-tolerated (owing to their long elimination time), easy to administer, and less expensive than the new antibiotics." Furthermore, this trial concluded that concomitant treatment with systemic antibiotics did

not increase healing time over eardrops alone (Sarrell et al 2003).

- As long as there is no pus in the ear and the drum has not perforated, a few drops of warmed oil can be dropped into each ear, and plugged with cotton wool. Oils can be chosen from the following.

- **Mullein oil:** This is made from yellow mullein flowers, picked in the summer when fresh, placed in a jar and covered in olive oil. This is left to macerate in sunlight for 2 weeks and then pressed. It has demulcent and anti-inflammatory properties, and helps to soothe pain and inflammation.

- **Garlic oil:** In laboratory tests, aqueous extracts of garlic and concentrated garlic oil have been shown to be more or as effective as several pharmaceutical preparations against *Aspergillus*, while demonstrating lower toxicity (Tillotson et al 2001, p. 417, Sarrell et al 2003).

- **St John's Wort oil:** This is made in the same way as mullein oil, using freshly picked yellow *Hypericum* flowers. It is useful for allaying pain and inflammation. A trial of 103 children with acute otitis media found drops of a herbal product containing garlic, mullein, marigold and St John's wort to be as effective as anaesthetic eardrops in the management of ear pain (Sarrell et al 2001). One or two drops of tincture of myrrh (*Commiphora molmol*) or golden seal (*Hydrastis canadensis*) can be added to oils to drop in the ears (Box 9.2).

Box 9.2   Recipe for eardrops

This recipe can be made up and kept in the medicine cupboard, for use when necessary.

15 drops golden seal (*Hydrastis canadensis*) tincture
5 drops myrrh (*Commiphora molmol*) tincture
15 drops eucalyptus oil
5 drops pasque flower (*Anemone pulsatilla*) tincture
15 drops lavender oil
Mix in 30 ml of olive oil or almond oil

Use 2 drops of the warmed mixture in each ear 3–6 times daily.

- **Essential oils:** Any of the following can be used, diluted (2 drops of essential oil to a teaspoon of olive oil): chamomile, eucalyptus, lemon, lavender or rosewood. These can also be massaged into the area around the ears, neck and throat. Hot compresses can be applied directly to the ears and neck area to ease the pain. Use a few drops of essential oil to a bowl of hot water. Repeat frequently as required. Foot baths can be used with the same mixture.

- A hot-water bottle, held against the painful ear, can also be soothing.

- Teas or tinctures can be given every 2 hours to help relax the child and soothe the pain, combined with remedies to resolve the infection and reduce the congestion: Antiseptic herbs include chamomile, echinacea, hyssop (*Hyssopus off.*), rosemary, thyme and peppermint; relaxant herbs include chamomile, passionflower and skullcap (*Scutellana laterifolia*). Herbs to reduce catarrhal congestion include ginger, elderflowers, plantain and ground ivy (*Nepeta hederacea*).

- If there is accompanying fever, limeflowers (*Tilia europea*) can be added to the prescription.

- Chamomile is particularly indicated in the treatment of earache as it has anti-inflammatory, antimicrobial and analgesic properties. It is recommended for children with heat and inflammation who tend to get irritable and "difficult" when unwell.

- Garlic capsules, one every 2 hours during the acute stage, can help resolve infection and catarrhal congestion. As the pain diminishes, until the child recovers completely, they can be given three times.

- Solid food is best avoided until the acute condition has cleared, but children need plenty to drink – water, diluted fruit juice, herbal teas, vegetable juice, but no milk produce.

- Dairy produce, wheat, red meats, sugar and refined foods are best omitted from the diet during acute infections. A light digestible diet will allow the energy of the body to be directed towards resolving infection.

Ayurvedic approach to ear problems

The ears are the province of ether and are ruled by *Vata*, and so are sensitive to pain. Soreness, irritation and inflammation in the outer ear can be treated with 10 drops of neem oil in a base of sesame oil. One or two drops of sesame oil rubbed into the external ear daily is considered to be preventative. Inflammation of the ear with pus is known as *Putikarna*.

Ear infections tend to be complications of colds and other *Kapha* problems associated with catarrhal congestion. However, other *doshas* can be involved. *Vata* symptoms involve intense pain associated with fear and anxiety, *Pitta* with burning, pain, heat and irritability, *Kapha* with congestion and mucus and greater tolerance of pain.

General treatments for reducing *Kapha* and for colds and catarrh can be applied to ear infections.

- A $\frac{1}{2}$ tsp of turmeric powder in hot water can be taken every 2 hours in acute infections and three times daily for chronic problems.
- A *Kapha* reducing diet is recommended, particularly avoiding dairy produce.
- Nirgundi (*Vitex negundo*) is the remedy of choice for external use in ear infections. The juice of the leaves is mixed with mustard oil and boiled. This medicated oil is dropped into the ear twice daily (Dash 1989).
- Alternatively bilva (bael fruit) root or a garlic clove is boiled with mustard oil and then filtered and used as ear drops.
- Ginger, garlic and onion are recommended in the diet.
- Other herbs recommended for the *doshas* involved:
  - *Vata*: Dashmula, bringaraj, ginger, asafoetida, lemon juice. For ear drops medicated oil of mullein or garlic
  - *Pitta*: mullein, echinacea, hops (*Humulus lupulus*), manjishta, bringaraj, fennel (*Foeniculum vulgare*)
  - *Kapha*: echinacea, hops, thyme, oregano (*Oreganum vulgare*), manjishta, Dashmula, bringaraj, ginger, asafoetida, lemon juice. Hot foot bath/ massage with mustard oil.

Treatment of recurrent middle ear infection and glue ear

It is important to treat the underlying conditions at the root of the problem and not solely the acute infections when they arise. Since chronic ear problems are largely related to throat, tonsil, nose, sinus and catarrhal problems, these need to be resolved, and the digestive and immune system strengthened through the use of herbs and diet (see p. 151, 160).

- Passive smoking has been found to be closely related to the incidence of glue ear. Affected children need to have plenty of fresh air and to be kept away from smoky or polluted atmospheres as far as possible.
- Ginger tea can be given daily to enhance digestion and clear phlegm.
- Mucus-forming foods are best avoided – milk produce, refined carbohydrates and excess wheat and sugar.

Children with recurrent upper respiratory and ear infections frequently suffer from chronic catarrh combined with chronically enlarged tonsils and cervical glands. In many cases this is related to an allergic response to milk produce or sometimes to wheat (see also Allergies, p. 186). A study of 153 children with earache concluded that 93.3% had allergies to foods or inhalants, and that an elimination diet gave a significant improvement (McMahan et al 1981). It is best to omit all milk produce from the diet, initially for 1–2 months, if the child suffers from these problems. During this time herbs can be given to help resolve the condition and, at the end of this period, the situation can be reassessed. Very often, within the first week or two, an infection arises, which represents the body's attempt to throw off toxins and preferably this should not be suppressed with antibiotics. After this there should be signs of improvement: infections should develop much less frequently and, should they arise, they are likely to be much milder. If positive change is observed after the first 2 months, the milk-free diet is best continued for a couple more months to give the child's immune system an opportunity to recover. If the child seems well after this (while continuing with the herbal treatment) small amounts of milk produce can gradually be introduced, goat's yoghurt initially,

once a week and slowly returned to the diet. Should an infection develop, milk produce should be avoided again until the symptoms are completely clear, and then re-introduced again, but this time more slowly. Milk produce may need to be kept to a minimum for the best part of a year, and other nutritionally comparable foodstuffs used to replace it to avoid compromising a child's nutrition.

- Garlic can be given every day, either in foods, as juice or in capsules, to enhance immunity to infection and as a decongestant.
- Drinks of lemon and honey or cider vinegar and honey will help to clear mucus and enhance immunity.
- Supplements of cod liver oil, 200–500 mg natural vitamin C and a children's multi-mineral and vitamin can be given daily (see Immune System, p. 152).

Herbal remedies need to be given during this time to enhance digestion and immunity and to clear catarrhal congestion in the nose, sinuses and throat. If the tonsils and lymph glands in the neck are inflamed or swollen, herbs can be added to the prescription for the lymphatic system (see Tonsillitis, p. 223).

- Herbs for the digestion – ginger, cinnamon (*Cinnamomum zeylanica*), fennel (*Foeniculum vulgare*), asafoetida, thyme.
- Herbs for the immune system – chamomile, echinacea, hyssop (*Hyssopus off.*), liquorice, peppermint and turmeric.
- Herbs to clear the catarrh – chamomile, elderflowers, eyebright (*Euphrasia off.*), thyme, yarrow and hyssop.
- Herbs for the tonsils and lymph glands – cleavers (*Galium aparine*) and marigold and burdock.

Choose one or two herbs from each group and combine them together as an infusion. Give a cupful three times daily.

Essential oils diluted in sesame oil (1–2 drops per 5 ml) can be massaged regularly around the nose, throat and ears, and steam inhalations can be given daily using chamomile, eucalyptus, lavender or rosewood. Hot compresses can be applied to the nose, ears and throat, and hand and foot baths can be given regularly using the same oils.

At the first sign of a cold, start to treat the ears with drops, and give the remedies for acute infections to help prevent the infection affecting the middle ear (see p. 227). The neck, throat and ears are best kept warm, and the child dressed up well to go outside in cold winter air.

COUGHS

A cough, nature's way of cleansing the air passageways, is a reflex response to anything that threatens to block the throat or bronchial tubes, whether it be an irritant inhaled from the atmosphere, a piece of food going down the wrong way or an infection causing irritation and phlegm. For this reason it may not be advisable to give cough mixtures which suppress the cough reflex, since they prevent this protective action by the body and may predispose to further infection.

Congestion, irritation and infection in the chest, as elsewhere in the respiratory tract, can be related to poor digestion, toxins in the bowel, poor elimination via other pathways (skin, bowels and urine), lowered vitality, poor diet, lack of fresh air and exercise, insufficient sleep or stress. When the vitality of a child is already lowered, it is easy for the child to become affected by changes in the weather, from warm to cold or from dry to damp, and to succumb to a cough or cold, and it will be blamed on the weather, or the child getting chilled, and the more long-term causes may be ignored. It is important to consider both when treating children. After immunizations, the child's immune system may be more vulnerable to infection and more prone to colds and coughs at this time, often coupled with a fever and malaise.

Emotional factors also play a considerable part (grief is the emotion which is traditionally connected to the lungs), and this can be related to moving from one school to another, one house to another, from loss of total attention once a baby brother or sister is born, or through parents arguing or divorcing, for example. If you feel that emotional stress plays a part, use supportive measures for the nervous system (see p. 246) even before any physical symptoms arise.

Mucus-producing foods are best kept to a minimum during the winter months, particularly cow's milk products, sugar and refined carbohydrates.

Should a cold or cough develop, omit these completely from the diet. Chronic catarrh that may be linked to an excess of these foods can provide a hospitable environment for micro-organisms that affect the respiratory tract. Adding mild spices to a child's diet may improve digestion, clear mucus and enhance immunity to infection (see also Immune System, p. 150).

The herbal treatment of coughs will depend entirely on the type of cough a child has.

1. A cough with a fever may accompany an infection, such as bronchitis or pneumonia.

2. A loose cough with catarrh. There may be catarrh in the nose or throat which starts watery but then thickens as the infection resolves. The child coughs up copious mucus and tends to be worse at night when lying down.

3. A dry, irritating or croupy cough which often accompanies laryngitis, croup and tracheitis. It often starts at night with coughing bouts, during which it is hard for the child to draw air. The coughing may make the throat or trachea sore and the child distressed or irritable. The irritation in the throat or chest which produces a dry cough may also be caused by mucus draining from the back of the nose during a cold, with catarrh or from infected sinuses, which trickles down and irritates the throat. Other factors to be considered include chemicals in the atmosphere (passive smoking, paint fumes, and so on), irritation in the digestive tract or nervousness causing constriction in the throat area. It may also be related to a need for more attention.

4. An intermittent, chronic cough can continue between acute infections. There may be associated lethargy or debility, poor appetite, thick phlegm in the chest, swollen neck glands, and a generally catarrhal condition.

Bronchitis

Acute bronchitis can develop from a cold or sore throat, or as a complication of measles (p. 183) and whooping cough (p. 234). Infection can either be viral or bacterial or more unusually, fungal. As the body rallies its defences to throw off the infection, the temperature rises and the child feels unwell.

Chronic bronchitis may develop after repeated bouts of acute bronchitis, by which time the child's vitality is lowered and resistance to infection is reduced. This requires examination of the child's constitution and background factors to lowered immunity including digestion and elimination, diet, exercise, allergies and the child's emotional environment. In chronic bronchitis there is a low-grade infection or inflammation of the bronchial tubes, causing intermittent coughing and general debility. A chronic cough, can also involve allergy to certain foods or environmental pollutants (see Allergies, p. 186).

Pneumonia

Pneumonia involves inflammation and infection of the lungs, usually by a virus or bacteria, sometimes a mycoplasma fungus. In children it occurs most often as a sequel to another respiratory infection such as a cold, flu or bronchitis. It may also be caused by the inhalation of irritant vapours or chemicals or by a foreign body, such as food or pus, which has carried pathogenic micro-organisms into the lungs. Pneumonia is an infection that indicates that the natural defences of the respiratory system are significantly compromised. The causes of lowered resistance include the effects of lifestyle – poor diet, weak digestion, lack of fresh air and exercise, pollution (from passive smoking, for example). It may also occur if a child is weakened by other pathology – cystic fibrosis, for instance – or poor nutrition as in malabsorption or if the lungs have been weakened by chronic problems, such as asthma, whooping cough or measles.

The alveoli of the lungs react like the rest of the respiratory system when irritated: they fill up with fluid, in this case exudate from the surrounding blood vessels. Now, instead of containing air, the affected alveoli are full of fluid, which reduces the available space in the lungs for breathing and exchange of oxygen and carbon dioxide. This causes shortness of air and produces breathing difficulties.

Herbal treatment of coughs

The herbal treatment of coughs is always aimed at assisting the homoeostatic mechanisms of the body. This includes helping the chest to clear itself of phlegm, inflammation and infection while,

at the same time, using herbs to enhance the immune system. It is important at the same time to address underlying imbalance contributing to lowered immunity, particularly diet, digestion and elimination.

Cough with fever

Bronchitis and pneumonia produce coughs with a fever, as the body tries to throw off the infection. The fever tends to be at its highest while the cough is still dry and harsh, and comes down as the child perspires and the cough becomes looser and more productive. Herbs can be used as an adjunct to antibiotic treatment should this be necessary.

Herbs to help the body's fight against infection and to resolve inflammation in the chest include echinacea, elecampane (*Inula helenium*), garlic, hyssop (*Hyssopus off.*) and thyme. One or two of these can be combined in a tea with diaphoretic herbs to bring down fever, such as chamomile, catnip (*Nepeta cataria*), elderflowers, hyssop, limeflowers (*Tilia europea*) and yarrow, and given every 2 hours. If the fever is high, use herbal teas separately to bring down the fever, and give them as frequently as you can (see Fever Management, p. 175).

To help loosen and expel mucus and to soothe irritated bronchial tubes, expectorant herbs can be given, such as coltsfoot (*Tussilago farfara*), slippery elm (*Ulmus fulva*), liquorice, marshmallow (*Althea off.*), white horehound (*Marrubium vulgare*) or mullein, which are soothing for a dry cough, or ginger, aniseed (*Pimpinella anisum*), elecampane, hyssop (*Hyssopus off.*) or thyme, which are more stimulating for a productive cough (Akoachere et al 2002). Elecampane root tea, with a small amount of ginger and liquorice and sweetened with honey, is pleasant tasting and I have found it generally effective for chest infections.

Garlic can be given as capsules every 2 hours, or as a honey, which is a useful way to give garlic to children. To make garlic honey cover four cloves of sliced or chopped garlic with 3 fl oz (100 ml) of runny honey. Leave overnight and then strain off the juice. Give in teaspoon (5 ml) doses several times a day. The honey itself has antimicrobial qualities.

Essential oils can be used for inhalations, baths, chest rubs, hand and foot baths and massage. Choose from eucalyptus, rosemary, lemon, lavender, pine and thyme, and dilute in a carrier oil such as sesame oil, 1–2 drops per 5 ml of carrier.

Catarrhal cough

Once a dry, irritating cough has become more loose and productive, expectoration of phlegm is required. A catarrhal cough can arise not only after a dry cough with fever but also with a cold, sore throat or influenza, which produces copious catarrh. Herbal treatment is aimed at clearing phlegm while enhancing the efforts of the immune system to fight off the infection.

Many herbs contain antimicrobial volatile oils and possess expectorant properties helping to loosen and expel phlegm. These include aniseed, rosemary, cinnamon, rose, ginger, hyssop and thyme, which can be taken in hot infusions, three to six cupfuls daily. Coltsfoot and horehound are also effective expectorants. Alternatively, thyme tea spiced with a little powdered ginger, cinnamon and cloves makes a stimulating and drying mixture. Garlic can be taken as capsules or in honey every 2 hours in the acute phase and three times daily until the cough has cleared.

Essential oils can be used for baths, inhalations, for massage to the throat, chest, back and feet, or used as hand and foot baths. Eucalyptus, ginger, lavender, pine, lemon or thyme are all suitable diluted in a base oil such as sesame.

Dry cough

A dry cough needs to be soothed and loosened by herbs with relaxing and demulcent properties, which also help to expel the loosened mucus. The following herbs can be taken in infusions or syrups: coltsfoot; slippery elm; linseed; liquorice; marshmallow; mullein or wild cherry bark (*Prunus serotina*).

If the child becomes distressed during the coughing bouts, it may make the cough worse. Relaxing herbs can be added to the prescription which will also help the child to relax and sleep at night, when a dry cough tends to be worse. Useful herbs include: chamomile, catmint (*Nepeta cataria*), cowslip flowers (*Primula vera*), lavender, melissa (*Melissa off.*) and limeflowers (*Tilia europea*).

As the cough improves it will begin to soften and the phlegm will become looser and easier to expel. You can now give the child expectorant herbs such as angelica (*Angelica archangelica*), aniseed, coltsfoot, elecampane, horehound, hyssop and thyme. To make thyme more palatable for small children, it can be given as a syrup. This is an effective remedy for relief of coughs, catarrh and sore throats. Take three handfuls of finely chopped thyme, cover them with runny honey and leave to macerate for a few hours. Alternatively, infuse one handful of chopped thyme in one cup of boiling water, until cool. Strain and add honey. This should be kept in a refrigerator and consumed within a few days. Give 1 tsp (5 ml) of either three or four times daily.

Another useful recipe for dry coughs is to add $\frac{1}{2}$–1 tsp (2.5–5 ml) of a mixture of aniseed, coltsfoot, horehound, mullein and wild cherry to each cup of boiling water. Give this three to six times daily. Sweeten with honey if preferred.

Any of the above herbs can be used as strong infusions to add to bath water, especially for babies and small children, who will find it difficult to drink infusions. They can also be used for hand and foot baths, and as hot compresses applied to the chest and throat.

Essential oils can also be used in the bath, for hand and foot baths, steam inhalations, vaporizers and massage to chest, back or feet. Chamomile, eucalyptus, lemon, rosemary, lavender, pine and thyme are all applicable. Dry, croupy coughs respond well to steam and to humid atmospheres.

Frequent drinks of lemon and honey can also be given, to soothe the tickly cough. Garlic capsules, juice or honey can be given regularly three times a day until the child is completely recovered.

Chronic coughs

If a child's vitality and resistance is lowered, chronic coughs can linger after an acute infection. This is more likely if a child has not rested sufficiently or if the acute infection was not treated correctly, or after antibiotics. Alternatively, it can develop after immunizations, notably whooping cough and polio. In any chronic condition the underlying causes of lowered vitality always require investigation, whether it is caused by weak digestion, poor diet, insufficient elimination of toxins, fresh air and exercise, emotional problems or overuse of antibiotics. It could also be related to pollution or allergy (see Immune System, p. 187) (McElroy and Miller 2003).

Herbal treatment needs to include remedies to enhance the digestion and the immune system, such as echinacea, garlic, rosemary, thyme and turmeric as well as general tonics for convalescence, including ashwagandha, cat's claw (*Uncaria tomentosa*), marshmallow (*Althea off.*), astragalus (*Astragalus membranaceus*), burdock, liquorice, marigold and nettles. Resistant mucus can be expelled with the help of expectorant herbs such as aniseed, coltsfoot, elecampane, horehound, hyssop, liquorice, mullein and thyme. This may aggravate a chronic intermittent cough temporarily, but it becomes more productive and indicates that the child is more able to throw off the illness. Coltsfoot tea is considered the remedy of choice for chronic cough, as it contains bitter tonics as well as soothing and expectorant properties.

Hot lemon and honey drinks can be given regularly through the day. Supplements of garlic capsules, vitamin C and hemp seed oil can be taken to help the immune system. In acute infections, one or two garlic capsules and 100 mg vitamin C (chewable for children) can be taken every 2–3 hours; in chronic conditions, give three times daily. In either instance 1 tsp (5 ml) of hemp seed oil can be taken daily.

Blackcurrant tea can be effective for sore throats, coughs and catarrh.

Dilute essential oils can be used in baths, hand and foot baths, for inhalations, vaporizers, and chest massage. Choose from eucalyptus, lavender, rosemary, rose, lemon, pine and thyme.

A useful recipe to help ease bronchial congestion is onion syrup (Kim 1997). Slice an onion into a small bowl and drizzle honey over it. Cover and leave to stand over-night. The child can be given a teaspoon in acute infections every 2 hours and in chronic coughs two or three times a day.

Ayurvedic approach

Coughs can be *Vata* type, *Pitta* type and *Kapha* type. They come in stages: first *Vata* type, then *Vata* and *Kapha* and when *Pitta* is involved there is accompanying infection.

Causes (*Nidana*)

According to Ayurveda a cough can be caused by *Vata* blocking *Vata*, for example dust, unwanted particles or something else causing constriction or obstruction of *Prana* and *Udana Vayu*. *Vata* derangement is caused by, for example, suppression of natural urges such as sneezing (which deranges *Udana* and *Prana vayu*), excess dry foods, irregular eating, fasting, overwork, exhaustion, stress, worry, fear, grief and dry cold weather.

The function of *Udana Vayu* is to exhale. The body has to collect energy to clear the obstruction, hence the cough. Secondary *doshas* can be involved and obstruct *Vata*. *Kapha* as phlegm can be involved, as symptoms occur in the chest which is the main *Kapha* site.

Pathogenesis (*Samprapti*)

Low digestive fire and *ama* causes *Sama Kapha* and disturbed *Vata*. This leads to constriction and drying in the mouth, throat and respiratory tract. *Sama* blocks *Udana Vayu* and *Vata* starts overworking to clear the obstruction. *Vata* comes up in bouts with force and friction causing coughing as it rushes against the vocal cords. The direction of *Prana Vayu* is changed though not as much as in asthma. Instead of coming in it comes out. Coughing should not be suppressed as it is a natural urge. Also when downward movement of *Apana Vata* is obstructed, as in constipation/wind, it begins to move upward to the chest and throat and eventually to the head. This affects the eyes, back, chest, ribs and eventually comes out of the mouth as a cough.

Prodromal signs include throat irritation, loss of taste and appetite, erratic/slow digestion, tickly cough, lethargy, insomnia and anxiety which indicate accumulation of *Sama Kapha* and derangement of *Vata*.

Signs and symptoms (*Rupa*)

- *Vata* type: as *chaya*/accumulation of *Vata* increases into *prakopa*/aggravation, dryness is produced in the chest, throat, mouth, ribs, heart and head and results in a dry cough with violent bouts. There might also be mental agitation, pain or loss of voice.
- *Pitta* type: bitter taste in the mouth, fever, dizziness, vomiting, thirst, hoarseness, acidity, continuous coughing and yellow phlegm.
- *Kapha* type: mild pain in chest and head, heaviness, throat coughing, debility, runny nose, vomiting, loss of appetite and taste, thick, sticky white or clear mucus is expelled.

Vata type cough

In treatment of *Vata* type cough, *Vata* is reduced using ghee, oil enemas, a wholesome diet with basmati rice, whole wheat, barley gruel with bilva, ginger, Dashmul (see Appendix p. 304), chitrak (*Plumbago zeylanicum*), jaggery and black salt, warm and moist vegetables and sesame oil.

Ghee is mixed with *Vata* reducing herbs and formulae. These include ashwagandha, ginger, pippali, liquorice, calamus (*Acorus calamus*), chitrak, Dashmul, kapikachu (*Mucuna pruriens*), bala, guduchi, Triphala, Trikatu, gokshura (*Tribulus terrestris*) and shatavari. These herbs promote digestion and relieve coughs. Raw honey and sugar cane can be mixed with the herbs chosen and barley. Ghee should be taken before meals unless there is upper body dryness. For a *Vata* cough with phlegm: ginger, pippali, asafoetida, barley powder with ghee can be used.

Other therapies include massage and oil fomentations. For constipation and gas retention digestive herbs and bowel-cleansing herbs or enemas are recommended.

Other useful formulae

- Sitopaladi churna: Contains sugar, vamshalochan (Bamboo), pippali, cardamom, and cinnamon; 3–6 g in a teaspoon of honey and a little warm water to be taken am and pm.
- Talisadi churna can also be used in the same dose (see Asthma, p. 236).
- Eladi gutika: Contains cardamom, cinnamon, pippali, sugar candy, liquorice, grapes (*Vitis vinifera*).
- Khajoor (*Phoenix dactilifera*) is recommended for chronic and dry cough; 1–4 tablets to be sucked slowly.

Pitta type cough

The traditional approach to treating *Pitta* would involve purgation using, for example, castor oil. To clear phlegm, Ayurvedic doctors administer emetics with ghee, liquorice and sugar cane. However, in the West we use expectorants to clear phlegm. After the *doshas* are cleansed, the child is put on *Pitta* reducing foods and liquids, i.e. those with cooling and sweet properties (see p. 158). Expectorants and *Pitta* reducing herbs can be used, including: lotus seeds (*Nelumbo nucifera*), pippali, musta (*Cyperus rotundus*), liquorice, fresh ginger, amalaki, sandalwood, bibhitaki, vamsha lochana (*Bambusa bambos*), gokshura, mixed with ghee, sugar cane and honey. For thick phlegm, dry and cooling foods and drinks are recommended. Neem and honey are added to the above herbs. Grape juice mixed with sugar cane, sugar cane water and milk is traditionally used in India.

Kapha type cough

In India, in the treatment of *Kapha* type cough, Ayurvedic doctors first administer an emetic if the child is strong, with barley and pungent herbs such as pippali. Here again expectorants are used in the West. Then castor oil is given as a purgative. Foods eaten by the child should be light, including vegetable soup, pippali, and a little ghee, sesame oil, mustard oil, honey and bilva fruit. Herbs including sandalwood, vasak (*Adhatoda vasica*), tulsi, apamarga (*Achyranthes aspera*), amalaki, musta, haritaki, calamus, bala, chitrak, punarnava (*Boerhavia diffusa*), amlavetasa (*Garcinia pedunculata*), bibhitaki, gokshura, ginger and black pepper mixed with raw honey are recommended.

Useful formulae

- Trikatu, taken with honey or hot water
- Lavangadi vati: contains cloves, black pepper
- Khadira (*Acacia catechu*) is prescribed for bronchitis, cough and phlegm.

Kapha/Vata type cough

Herbs used include pippali, ginger, musta, haritaki, amalaki, made with honey and ghee.

Kapha/Pitta type cough

Pitta reducing herbs, i.e. bitters such as guduchi, chiretta (*Swertia chireta*) are recommended as well as vasak, turmeric, vamsha lochana, cardamom and honey.

Whooping cough

A child will be prone to pertussis infection if tired or run down, particularly if this is due to recurrent respiratory infections, with coughs, or if there is a history of asthma. A robust child should throw off whooping cough more easily than a child whose immunity is compromised. If there is weakness in the chest and a tendency to chronic catarrh, or congestion in the digestive tract, with a history of constipation, diarrhoea or tendency to tummy upsets, a child may be more susceptible and find the infection harder to fight off. It is important to work preventatively, to support the immune system, resolve tendencies to infection, catarrh or digestive disturbances as they arise, so that a child is able to withstand infection, by whooping cough or other respiratory infections, as best as possible (see Immune System, p. 150). Infusions of antiseptic and decongestant herbs such as echinacea, coltsfoot, elderflowers, elecampane and thyme can be given as preventative medicine three times daily. These will help to strengthen the chest and clear phlegm as well as any digestive congestion. Garlic and vitamin C are useful supplements.

Although whooping cough can be a very distressing illness for both parents and children, the more reassuring aspect is that the onset is gradual. At the first signs of possible infection herbal treatment can be started immediately. There are from 10 days to 2 weeks to treat the child, before the coughing becomes more serious, and the whooping begins.

Herbal treatment of whooping cough

At the first signs of a cold or slight cough, infusions of sundew, coltsfoot, elecampane, and thyme can be given, sweetened with liquorice, and/or honey if necessary. Up to 4–6 cups a day is recommended.

Sundew (*Drosera rotundifolia*) is an effective herb against a number of infecting organisms (*Streptococcus*, *Staphylococcus* and *Pneumococcus*) as well as whooping cough. It contains a substance called plumbagin, which appears to be responsible for much of its beneficial effect. It also has a relaxing effect on the muscles in the bronchi, preventing spasm in a coughing bout. It is best used in small doses, and its effect has been confirmed to be most effective in whooping cough, especially when used with thyme.

Elecampane (*Inula helenium*) is a specific for irritating coughs in children, and particularly useful where there is profuse mucus as in whooping cough. It is relaxing to the bronchial muscles while, at the same time, stimulating the expulsion of mucus. It has an antibacterial action and is used effectively in bronchitis and pneumonia as well as whooping cough (Cantrell et al 1999).

Coltsfoot (*Tussilago farfara*) relaxes and soothes the chest. With a demulcent and a gentle expectorant action, it helps to loosen and expel the mucus. It is a particularly good remedy for persistent coughs.

The volatile oils in thyme have an antiseptic action, which helps to resolve infection. Thyme is also a relaxant, reducing spasm in the bronchii while, at the same time, its expectorant action helps to loosen and expel mucus. Thyme can be used for any cough with spasm, combined with other herbs or simply as thyme tea or syrup (see p. 55).

If they are treated properly at the onset, the symptoms of whooping cough can be prevented from worsening to the point where the distressing coughing begins. If, however, serious coughing sets in, the same herbs can still be used, every hour or so, and one or both of the following herbs can be added to the prescription: wild cherry bark (*Prunus serotina*) (this has a powerful sedative action on the cough reflex, which is vital in the whooping stage) and wild lettuce (*Lactuca villosa*). A sedative and muscle relaxant, wild lettuce is especially useful where there is much fear and panic (it may be useful for parents as well). Tension will only aggravate the spasm in the bronchi, so it is most important that the child is kept as relaxed as possible. Red clover (*Trifolium pratense*) helps to relax bronchial spasm while, at the same time, it stimulates expectoration.

Herbs can be given in the following ways:

- Teas – to be taken as often as possible, sweetened with liquorice, honey or aniseed.

- Tinctures – easier because they are more concentrated. Between five and ten drops of a prescription can be given in thyme syrup or a drink every 2 hours. If the condition becomes more serious, they can be given every hour if necessary.

- Hand and foot baths – using teas or tinctures, diluted in water, these can be administered two or four times daily.

- Inhalations or baths using strong infusions or tinctures in hot water.

- Essential oils – choose from basil, cypress, eucalyptus, lavender, marjoram or thyme and use them as inhalations, in vaporizers, diluted in massage oils for the chest, feet or abdomen. A few drops can be put on the pillow at night, on a damp towel on the radiator or used in a plant spray to spray the room.

● Compresses – teas, tinctures or oils in warm water can be applied frequently to the chest.

Garlic, with its antiseptic action in the chest, is useful in the treatment of whooping cough. It relaxes the muscle in the bronchial tubes and helps expectoration. It can be given in capsules or juice, or in the following recipe:

Chop three heads of garlic and pour over $\frac{1}{2}$ pint (300 ml) of boiling water. Cover. Leave to macerate for a day. Strain. Give 1 tbsp (20 ml) every one or two hours. Store in a refrigerator and use within 3–4 days.

Slippery elm (*Ulmus fulva*) food, made into a gruel and given three times daily, is also useful as it relaxes and soothes the chest, while being light, nutritious and easy to digest.

A child with whooping cough should eat only a light diet, with no milk products, no sugar, no starchy foods and plenty of soups, grated vegetables, fresh fruit, chicken or fish. Supplements of hemp seed oil (1 tsp/5 ml) daily, vitamin C (200 mg three times daily) and garlic juice, honey or capsules (every 2 hours) can be given.

It is important for the child to rest as much as possible to give the body a chance to rally its defences. Chamomile tea will help a child rest and sleep. Exertion can bring on coughing and deplete the child's energy, so the child needs to be kept calm. Parental reassurance during coughing fits will probably be needed, as fear and panic will only serve to aggravate breathlessness and coughing.

If the child vomits after coughing, once the coughing bout has stopped, herb teas sweetened with honey can be given to prevent dehydration. Fresh air is always beneficial in the room, while chemicals and cigarette smoke may further aggravate coughing.

ASTHMA

Asthma is not normally found in children under 2 years of age, although other respiratory disturbances cause wheezing, both in infants and older children: bronchiolitis in infants causes wheezing and trouble with breathing in and out when the bronchioles become inflamed and blocked. Children

with croup wheeze, but it is characterized by trouble breathing in and not out as in asthma (see p. 238).

Asthmatic bronchitis affects children mostly between the ages of two and six years. Wheezing is accompanied by a fever, dry cough and some difficulty breathing, and it is caused by constriction of bronchi and bronchioles, as a result of an allergic response to infection in the bronchi or to the mucus it produces. It normally occurs in children younger than those who normally develop classic asthma, it tends to develop in allergic children and always occurs as a result of infection. Thus it requires treatment for the infection as well as the accompanying allergic response.

Obstruction of the airways by either spasm, hyper-responsiveness of the bronchial tubes, inflammation or swelling of the respiratory mucosa is certainly on the increase and can be triggered by a variety of different factors, which may act separately or in combination. Many asthmatics are allergic to pollen, house dust, animal fur and a variety of foods, and may also be prone to other allergic reactions, such as eczema and hayfever. A recent review suggests that "food allergy should be considered in any child with asthma" (Roberts and Lack 2003) (for background causes of allergic asthma see Allergies, p. 186).

Asthma can be set off by a smoky or cold, foggy atmosphere. Certain household chemicals can also cause irritation of the bronchial mucosa and predispose to spasm. Any respiratory infection (cough, cold or influenza, for example) can irritate the bronchial tubes and cause them to constrict.

An asthmatic child may well have a tendency to chronic catarrh or repeated respiratory infections, which weaken the lungs. Emotional factors can often play a part. Children with asthma may be being "suffocated" by an over-protective parent, or there may be nervousness, hypersensitivity, disharmony in the family or the surroundings, particularly insecurity, causing constriction in the chest. When asthma has been set off, the anxiety that this may cause, and distress, if the attack is severe, may serve as an aggravating factor in itself. Recent research confirms the link between anxiety, depressive symptoms and asthma (Kovacs et al 2003), also suggesting the use of inhaled corticosteroids is associated with a negative effect on patients' mental health (Bonala et al 2003).

Inheritance can be another factor, predisposing the child to asthma or eczema. Digestive disturbances may also be implicated as they can cause irritation of the vagus nerve, which feeds the stomach and the bronchial tubes, causing the constriction of muscles in the chest.

The most important line of treatment is to prevent attacks and, preferably, to resolve the chronic problem. This necessitates constitutional treatment of the child. In an allergic child it is important to attempt to discover which substances the child is allergic to or irritated by and the background causes of allergy. Although there may be a variety of possible allergens: foods, pollen, animal dander, feathers, plants, moulds or the housedust mite, for example, it is an uphill struggle to prevent contact with these, and food is by far the easiest area to work with. If the offending foods can be found and omitted from the diet, it takes a considerable strain off a debilitated immune system, which then has a greater ability to resist sensitivity to other substances, such as animal dander or the house-dust mite.

The most common food allergens implicated are milk produce, wheat, eggs, oranges and artificial colourings, flavourings and preservatives (particularly sulphur). While examining the diet for possible allergens and making necessary changes, the child can be treated with herbs, combining herbs to improve the function of the digestive and immune system and to decrease the allergic tendency, with herbs specifically to relax the bronchial tubes and expel the mucus. It is not enough simply to remove the offending allergic substances, even if the asthma improves, for the allergic tendency will remain, only to focus its attention later on some other food that is eaten regularly. Research has suggested that a low salt diet can ease the severity and frequency of asthma attacks and that yoga (Vedanthan et al 1998), swimming and singing can encourage the use of respiratory muscles, which can be trained to overcome moderate restriction in the width of the air passages in chronic asthma. Other research has shown swimming to decrease the severity of asthma symptoms (Rosimini 2003).

Herbal treatment of asthma

It may take a few months or even a year to treat asthma effectively with herbs, so it is important to be patient and not give up too easily. During this time, if the child already uses inhalers or other medication, herbs can be used in conjunction with these. As the condition improves, the child should be able to use inhalers or steroids less and hopefully they can gradually be withdrawn.

- Herbs for the digestive and immune systems, such as chamomile, garlic, liquorice, yarrow and propolis can be combined with herbs to relax the bronchi and expel the mucus, such as coltsfoot, grindelia (*Grindelia camporum*), hyssop (*Hyssopus off.*), lungwort (*Pulmonaria off.*), mullein, sundew and thyme, and soothing herbs to relieve irritation in the chest like comfrey leaf (*Symphytum off.*), marshmallow (*Althea off.*), mullein and plantain.

- Research on patients with chronic airways obstruction has indicated that essential oil inhalations have a positive effect on mucus clearance but this is not advised during acute attacks (Hasani et al 2003).

- When asthma is aggravated by a respiratory infection, thyme, garlic, echinacea, liquorice, balm of gilead (*Populus gileadensis*) and hyssop, with their antimicrobial, antispasmodic and expectorant properties, will help resolve infection as well as relax the airways.

- Ginkgo (*Ginkgo biloba*) leaf extracts have been shown to benefit children's asthma (Keville 1996). A small trial with Ginkgo shows promising results in improving the clinical symptoms of asthma. The herb appears to work by a number of mechanisms, notably as a platelet-activating factor antagonist (Mahmoud et al 2000). Liquorice is a very interesting herb in this context. It has soothing and expectorant properties, and helps to support the adrenal glands, providing a natural counterpart to cortisone and helping to reduce the effects of stress and allergic reactions. This is particularly useful for children using cortisone inhalers or oral steroids when seeking to find a herbal alternative. It may be possible to withdraw the use of steroid medicines/inhalers gradually over a period of time (Shibata et al 1996).

Herbs that support the nervous system, help to relax the child and counter stress and tension can be added. These include chamomile, hops (*Humulus lupulus*), lemon balm, limeflowers (*Tilia europea*), skullcap (*Scutellaria laterifolia*) and vervain (*Verbena off.*). During an asthma attack, hot foot baths can be made using infusions of these herbs. Hot compresses can also be applied frequently to the chest.

- A useful remedy for asthma, which may be used in these different ways, is an infusion of equal parts of chamomile, coltsfoot, elecampane and thyme. Add two parts of this infusion to one part ginger and liquorice decoction. Give $\frac{1}{2}$ tsp (2–3 ml) every 15–60 minutes, depending on the severity of the attack.

- Thyme tea alone can be excellent for children to strengthen the respiratory system and relieve mild asthma.

- There are several powerful herbs for asthma, such as the schedule three herbs ephedra (*Ephedra sinica*), lobelia (*Lobelia inflata*), and jimson weed (*Datura stramonium*). These are frequently used by professional herbalists, although I do not use them in my practice. Lobelia, also known as Indian tobacco or asthma weed, has antispasmodic properties and has long been used in the treatment of bronchial asthma. It contains lobeline, an alkaloid that has a nicotine-like effect on the central nervous system. Ephedra, a herb native to China where it is known as Ma Huang, is another specific for asthma. It contains the alkaloid ephedrine, well known for its slimming effects and frequently used for increasing metabolism in slimming preparations. It also acts as a bronchodilator and an expectorant.

General advice in the treatment of asthma

Herbal teas can be sipped during an asthma attack, but food is best avoided until the chest has settled down. The following foods are useful preventatively however to counter the problem generally: pure, unrefined sunflower seed oil (which contains inulin helpful in the treatment of asthma); foods rich in vitamin A – carrots, spinach, peas, beetroot, fish liver oils, watercress, apricots; foods rich in calcium; garlic for the immune system; vitamin C containing foods to stimulate the expulsion of mucus from the chest and enhance the immune system; drinks of lemon and honey to help clear the mucus.

Asthma can be aggravated by faulty breathing. Breathing exercises taught properly and practised regularly by the child can improve lung function, as well as help calm emotional stress – breathing has a direct connection to feelings and state of mind.

Abdominal breathing is easily learned and is simple to practise with an asthmatic child. As one slowly breathes in, the abdomen should expand outwards and, as one breathes out, it relaxes down again. If one uses the abdomen instead of the top part of the lungs, breathing will be more relaxed, and, if one counts while breathing, control over the breath can be gained. Begin by breathing in for three seconds and out for three seconds. If the child finds this easy, gradually increase the time it takes to breathe in and out. Because the difficulty with asthmatics is with breathing out, shape the mouth as if to whistle and blow the breath out as slowly as possible. Research has shown that Buteyko breathing technique (mimics pranayama) can improve symptoms and reduce bronchodilator use (Cooper et al 2003). Both meditation (Wilson et al 1975) and hypnotherapy have also shown positive effects in small trials (Hackman et al 2000).

The fact that coughs and colds often bring on an attack and, if frequent, can actually weaken the lungs and predispose to asthma, means they need to be treated at their onset. If a child has frequent colds or other respiratory infections, this will require further investigation and remedial measures taken to enhance their immunity (see Immune System, p. 150). The child's diet should be analysed and potential allergens like milk, wheat and eggs should be kept to a minimum. If there is a history of asthma or allergies in the family, or if there is a tendency to wheezing during respiratory infections or to frequent coughs and colds, herbal teas can be given regularly as a preventative. Chamomile, coltsfoot, elecampane and thyme in hot infusions can be given sweetened with honey, two or three times daily.

If a child suffers from other allergies, it is important that they are treated constitutionally (see Allergies, p. 186). Plenty of fresh air and gentle outdoor exercise should be part of the child's daily routine. All exercise should be gentle; vigorous exercise, especially in cold air, can bring on an attack. An asthmatic child needs to be encouraged to take plenty of rest and relaxation. Over-stimulation and frightening or over-exciting games or television programmes are best kept to a minimum. Emotional stresses and strains within the family may be better discussed openly, so that any exaggerated fears may be dispelled and there is an opportunity for mutual support.

Ayurvedic approach to asthma

The Sanskrit term used in Ayurvedic medicine for asthma is *shvasa* meaning difficult breathing. It is caused by *Kapha* blocking *Vata*. *Kapha* forms first and therefore is the primary *dosha* that requires treatment. As in other health problems, a child's constitutional *dosha* can predispose them to asthma. *Vata* type children who tend to be nervous, shy, fearful and insecure may be more prone to asthma while the influence of the *Kapha* stage of life may contribute to the accumulation of mucus in the chest which serves to block the bronchii.

Bronchial asthma (*tamaka shvasa*) is classified predominantly as being caused by a disturbance of *Vata* which causes bronchospasms. Coughing, fever, allergies, diarrhoea owing to indigestion, vomiting, cold, dry weather, smoke, breeze, drinking very cold water, and a high *Vata* diet, can all lead to *Vata* derangement. Aggravated *Vata* begins to move upwards in the *pranavaha srotas*, the respiratory channel, aggravating *Kapha* and making it difficult to breathe. Eating *abishyandhi* food (wet, viscous and sticky food like yoghurt, pork and salt) and low digestive fire lead to the accumulation of *ama* (toxins) in the body. *Vata* is also obstructed by *Kapha* accumulating in the stomach (the origin site of *Kapha*), rising up into the chest and causing breathing difficulties. *Kapha* becomes *sama* (i.e. mixed with *ama*) sticky, and thick and creates congestion. When movement of *Vata* is obstructed by *Sama Kapha*, it spreads in all directions and disturbs the channels of respiration and *prana*.

Prodromal signs (*Purvarupa rupa*)
These include pain or heaviness in the throat and chest, poor appetite, astringent taste in the mouth and abdominal rumbling. Once symptoms manifest there may be a crackly cough, loss of taste or appetite, runny nose, dry mouth and thirst and difficulty breathing, particularly lying down. The child may desire warm things. Breathing tends to be worse on cloudy days, after drinking cold water, from cold breezes or direct wind and when eating *Kapha* increasing foods. Another form of asthma is associated with *Pitta* and involves fever and infection and tends to improve with cool drinks, cool foods and cool air.

Specific *dosha* symptoms
- *Vata*: dry cough, wheezing, dry skin, thirst, constipation, anxiety, the child desires warm liquids. Attacks happen mainly at dawn or dusk.
- *Pitta*: wheezing, coughing with yellow phlegm, sweating, irritability, fever, the child desires cold air. Attacks occur mainly at noon or midnight.
- *Kapha*: wheezing and coughing with excess clear or white phlegm, rattling chest sounds. Attacks occur mainly in morning and evening.

Pathogenesis (*Samprapti*)
Low digestive fire causes accumulation of *ama* and affects *Kapha* in the chest area causing *Sama Kapha* and creating congestion. *Prana* and *Udana Vayu* become aggravated by high *Vata* diet, etc., leading to dryness, and constriction in the bronchi and bronchioles, in the channels that carry *Prana* in the body. There is no place for *Prana* to go down and *Udana* to go up. Constipation disturbs *Apana Vayu* which controls the movement of all the other *Vayus*.

Ayurvedic approach to treatment of asthma

The aim of treatment is to clear *Kapha* from the lungs through therapeutic emesis, or expectorants, then to treat the *Vata* derangement.

Treatment of *Kapha*: *Kapha Shamana*

- Pippali churna and honey
- Liquorice in small amounts as an expectorant, rather than therapeutic vomiting (has antimicrobial properties active against *Staph. aureus* and *Candida albicans*)
- Turmeric
- Boswellia (*Boswellia serrata*).

A randomized controlled trial using boswellia gum was carried out on 40 patients who had bronchial asthma for between 3 and 15 years. They were given 300 mg three times daily over a period of 6 weeks and it was reported that 70% of them showed significant improvement indicated by "disappearance of physical symptoms and signs such as dyspnoea, rochi, number of attacks … as well as decrease in eosinophilic count" (Tillotson et al 2001, p. 415).

Tylophora asthmatica or *Tylophora indica* are used to treat accumulation of mucus in the chest. Several studies have been done on the treatment of asthma using *Tylophora asthmatica* (Williamson 2002, p. 61). Other research has been carried out into the anti-asthmatic effects of anthrapachaka leaf (*Tylophora indica*) and its anti-allergic properties, 10–15 drops of the tincture can be given once a day for no more than 7–10 days per month for effects lasting up to a month after stopping (Tillotson et al 2001). He states that excessive amounts can cause nausea and vomiting but it is certainly a herb that deserves more attention.

Useful formulae

- **Talisadi churna** contains: long and black pepper, ginger, cardamom, cinnamon, talispatra (*Abies webbiana*), Vamshe lochana (*Bambusa bambos*) and sugar and helps expectoration by liquifying phlegm.
- **Sitopaladi**
- Ayurvedic physicians also use: **Kanakasava**: contains *Datura alba*, liquorice, pippali, ginger, draksha (*Vitis vinifera*) dhataki (*Woodfordia fruticosa*), honey. It acts as an expectorant.
- **Vasasva** contains: vasak (*Adhatoda vasica*), jaggery, dhataki (*Woodfordia fructicosa*), cinnamon, cardamom, kankola (*Piper cubebs*), ginger, long and black pepper, and tagar (*Valeriana wallichii*). Clears phlegm in coughs and asthma.

Garlic is also used for its antimicrobial, decongestant properties, and to reduce *Kapha*. It is active against *Staphylococcus, Candida, E. coli, influenza type B and herpes simplex* 1. Cinnamon also helps to clear *Kapha* from the stomach and lungs.

For asthma associated with *Pitta*, ghee, vasak, vamsha lochana, ginger, pippali and brahmi are used.

For *Vata* ghee and pippali, vamsha lochana, guggul (*Commiphora mukul*) lemon or lime juice and ashwagandha are commonly prescribed. Castor oil purgation is used to clear *Vata* from the bowels. Narayan oil is applied to the chest. Enemas are considered the quickest way to relieve *Vata*.

Treatment for all doshas

- Tridoshic herbs include haritaki, bala and saffron.
- After attacks it is advisable to strengthen lungs with tonics like Chyawan prash (which is a jam prepared mainly from amalaki (*Emblica officinalis*)), ashwagandha, bala haritaki and brahmi, to prevent further attacks.
- A *Kapha* reducing diet is recommended to help reduce mucus production, followed by *Vata* pacifying diet.
- Yoga is recommended, particularly the fish, bow, plough, half wheel, cobra and palm tree postures. Those who practise yoga postures in combination with relaxation and breathing exercises have been shown to have less asthma attacks probably because of the calming effect that yoga has on mind and body and this helps to balance *Vata* and reduce constriction in the bronchi (Wilson et al 1975).
- Pranayama (breathing exercises) may also be helpful. According to Ayurveda, *Pitta* types should do left nostril breathing, inhaling through the left nostril and exhaling through the right. *Kapha* children should do right nostril breathing and *Vata* types alternate nostril breathing. Research has demonstrated that pranayama may help asthma sufferers if practised regularly (Williamson 2002, p. 62).

HAYFEVER (ALLERGIC RHINITIS)

Strictly speaking, hayfever is an allergic reaction to grass pollen, which usually occurs at its worst in May, June and July, often a stressful time for children as it is exam time. The term was originally related to symptoms caused by dust when haymaking and now includes a variety of seasonal allergic reactions due to pollen or some other airborne substance. Although most of the symptoms of over-sensitivity of the respiratory mucosa caused by hayfever are more annoying than serious, hayfever can trigger an asthma attack in a susceptible child. Hayfever rarely occurs before the age of five, and children tend to be worse affected during adolescence. Very often, these are children with an existing allergic tendency, who perhaps exchange a former allergic reaction, such as eczema, for hayfever (see Allergies, p. 186). There may be an inherited disposition to allergies and/or hayfever, or it may be that weak digestion, poor diet or low general health has rendered the immune system and respiratory tract over-susceptible to pollen. Hayfever often occurs in children who have a tendency to chronic catarrh or frequent respiratory infections, as the mucous membranes are already irritated.

It appears that hayfever has become widespread only in the last century, during which time the consumption of sugar has increased dramatically. It could be that the detrimental effect sugar has on immunity is related to an increased incidence of allergies in children and adults alike. Allergic rhinitis is a major challenge to health professionals. A large number of the world's population, including approximately 40 million Americans, suffer from allergic rhinitis.

Wheat is a member of the grass family. If wheat is removed from the diet during the hayfever season, the allergic symptoms can very often be reduced, if not eliminated. It appears that when wheat is removed from the diet, the body is better able to cope with the extra exposure to grass-related substances during the hayfever season. I have seen this work well countless times, and it is well worth the effort. It is also a good idea to cut out cow's milk produce, sugar and refined carbohydrates at the same time.

There is a way of desensitizing a child before the hayfever season to prevent the allergic reaction to pollen, using honey, and especially the wax capping on honeycombs. For 2–4 months before the hayfever season, give a dessertspoonful or two (10–20 ml) of honeycomb, bee pollen or honey with each meal. Local honey will contain the type of pollens in the surrounding countryside to which the child is likely to be exposed, so this is best. This preventative treatment often works well.

Herbs can be given to enhance immunity and general health for a few months before the hayfever season begins, to enable the child to cope with the high levels of pollen when they come (the Immune System, p. 150). Useful herbs include golden rod (*Solidago virgaurea*), plantain, ground ivy (*Nepeta hederacea*), echinacea, garlic, ginseng and liquorice, which can be continued throughout the hayfever season. Golden rod has anti-inflammatory and astringent properties. Ground ivy has been used for centuries for its anti-inflammatory, antiseptic and astringent actions which have been borne out by recent research (Mascolo 1987).

Ayurvedic approach

According to Ayurveda, hayfever is caused by toxins/*ama* in the body and the main approach to treatment is removal of impurities from the blood. According to Vasant Lad hayfever is a *Kapha* problem as it affects the respiratory tract and the lungs, which are ruled by *Kapha*. However once the heat rises in spring and *Pitta* is increasing, the phlegm is liquefied and the mucous membranes of the respiratory tract become irritated and inflamed, giving rise to sensitivity to pollen and the resultant *Pitta* and *Kapha* symptoms of inflammation, redness, sneezing, running nose and eyes and a tendency to wheezing. However, David Frawley (2000, p. 169) states that hayfever is a condition of autoimmune derangement and relates it more to *Vata* derangement as *Vata* types are the most sensitive. Dr Vinod Verma (1995, p. 226) recommends taking turmeric daily for a year to remove toxins and to enhance resistance to allergens. A traditional formula known as Mahamanjista, the main constituent of which is manjishta (*Rubia cordifolia*), is also recommended as it is one of the most popular Ayurvedic formulae for cleansing the blood. Daily practice of *jalnetti* is also advised which may be possible for older children. This is the administration of warm salty water through alternate nostrils using a netty pot. It helps to open blocked passages and melt and clear excess *Kapha*.

As with other symptoms Ayurvedic medicine classifies hayfever according to the dominant *dosha* revealed by the symptoms.

- *Vata* type characterized by scanty phlegm, dry cough, tendency to headaches, insomnia, constipation, wind, restlessness and anxiety.
- *Pitta* type involves red, burning eyes, inflamed mucosa with runny nose and eyes, thirst, feeling of heat, and tendency to loose stools and skin rashes.
- *Kapha* types are prone to abundant white phlegm, feeling dull, congested, heavy and lethargic. The appetite will be low and bowels sluggish.

Herbal treatment of hayfever

- The following herbal remedies can be given, which help to reduce hayfever symptoms as well as to support the immune system: chamomile, echinacea, elderflowers, euphorbia (*Euphorbia pilulifera*), eyebright (*Euphrasia off.*), marshmallow (*Althea off.*) and liquorice. These can be taken in hot infusion, three to six times daily depending on the severity of the hayfever.

- Butterbur (*Petasites hybridus*) (Lee et al 2003) and stinging nettle (Mittman 1990) have both been tested on a small scale on patients with allergic rhinitis and both show some efficacy. Research indicates that nettle acts as a potent anti-inflammatory, with mechanisms of action including inhibition of biosynthesis of arachidonic acid metabolites and reduction in the release of pro-inflammatory cytokines (Obertreis et al 1996, Mills and Bone 2000).

- *Ephedra sinica* is a specific for hayfever. It is one of the Schedule 3 herbs the use of which is restricted to the professional herbalist, because it is toxic in large quantities. A useful prescription for hayfever is equal parts of echinacea, ephedra, eyebright and euphorbia tincture $\frac{1}{4} - \frac{1}{2}$ tsp 3–6 times daily.

- If the mucus is particularly persistent, elderflower and ginger tea and honey may well help.

- Garlic, either as juice, perles or honey, is helpful and can be taken every 2 hours if necessary.

- Steam inhalations of chamomile – using strong tea or two drops of essential oil in a bowl of hot water – can help reduce the allergic response and tone the mucous membranes. Inhalations can be done two or three times a day in conjunction with herbal teas.

- Taking honey or honeycomb can be continued throughout the hayfever season.

Because allergic reactions, including hayfever, are related to a complex range of background causes and not only the offending allergens, it is always necessary to assess each individual child's constitution and lifestyle.

Ayurvedic treatment of hayfever

A novel, botanical formulation (Aller-7) has been developed for treatment of allergic rhinitis using a combination of extracts from seven medicinal plants including amalaki, ginger and long pepper, which have a proven history of efficacy and health benefits.

Vasant Lad (lecture notes 1991) recommends chewing grains of bee pollen before the spring to prevent hayfever, as well as taking tea made from equal parts of liquorice, long pepper, and lemon grass three times a day. For wheezing he recommends boiling a $\frac{1}{2}$ tsp of liquorice root in a cup of water for 5 minutes and before giving it to the child to add 5 drops of mahanaryan oil or $\frac{1}{4}$ tsp of ghee. This can be sipped every 15–30 minutes. Should it cause vomiting this is beneficial as it eliminates *Kapha* from the stomach and clears congestion and wheezing rapidly.

David Frawley recommends strengthening the immune system and the lungs prior to the hayfever season using dietary recommendations for one's *dosha* and taking tonic herbs such as ashwagandha and bala as well as Chayawan prash (Frawley 2000, p. 269).

All types of hayfever require treatment using herbs to reduce congestion and reduce the sensitivity of the mucous membranes. Holy basil is a popular remedy and can be taken as an infusion with honey.

- For *Vata*: calamus (*Acorus calamus*), ginger and liquorice tea. Ginger paste applied to the head (see headaches/pain). Calamus ghee inserted into the nostrils is used by Ayurvedic doctors.
- For *Pitta*: coriander leaf juice and tea, chamomile tea, gotu kola, ghee or gotu kola oil inserted into the nostrils. Sandalwood paste applied to the head, bitter and cleansing herbs such as amalaki and guduchi are recommended. For red itchy eyes Triphala ghee is used, applied to the eyelids. Triphala decoction and chamomile tea also makes good washes for the eyes.
- For *Kapha*: Trikatu, ginger tea, ginger and liquorice tea/powder with honey, cinnamon tea, cloves, calamus, are given as well as nasal administration of calamus ghee.

References

Achterrath-Iuckermann U, Kunde R, Flaskamp E, et al 1980 Planta Med; 39: 38–50

Akoachere JF, Ndip RN, Chenwi EB, Ndip LM, Njock TE, Anong DN 2002 Antibacterial effect of *Zingiber officinale* and *Garcinia kola* on respiratory tract pathogens. East Afr Med J 79(11): 588–592

Andrianova IV, Sobenin IA, Sereda EV, Borodina LI, Studenikin MI 2003 Effect of long-acting garlic tablets "allicor" on the incidence of acute respiratory viral infections in children. Ter Arkh 75(3): 53–56

Avallone R, Zanoli P, Puia G, et al 2000 Pharmacological profile of apigenin, a flavonoid isolated from *Matricaria Chamomilla* 1. Biochem Pharmacol 59(11): 1387–1394

Bauer R 2002 New knowledge regarding the effect and effectiveness of *Echinacea purpurea* extracts. Wien Med Wochenschr 152(15–16): 407–411

Bonala SB, Pina D, Silverman BA, et al 2003 Asthma severity, psychiatric morbidity, and quality of life: correlation with inhaled corticosteroid dose. J Asthma 40(6): 691–699

Bosio K, Avanzini C, D'Avolio A, Ozino O, Savoia D 2000 In vitro activity of propolis against *Streptococcus pyogenes*. Lett Appl Microbiol 31(2): 174–177

Cantrell CL, Abate L, Fronczek FR, Franzblau SG, Quijano L, Fischer NH 1999 Antimycobacterial eudesmanolides from *Inula helenium* and *Rudbeckia subtomentosa*. Planta Med 65(4): 351–355

Carle R, Isaac O 1987 Z Phytother 8: 67–77

Cooper S, Oborne J, Newton S, et al 2003 Effect of two breathing exercises (Buteyko and pranay*Ama*) in asthma: a randomised controlled trial. Thorax 58(8): 674–679

Crisan I, Ziharia CN, Popovici F, et al 1995 Natural propolis extract NIVCRISOL in the treatment of acute and chronic rhinopharyngitis in children. Rom J Virol Jul–Dec; 46(3–4): 115–133

Dash B 1989 Ayurvedic Cures for Common Diseases. Kind, Delhi, India, p.170

de Jongste JC, Shields MD 2003 Cough. 2: Chronic cough in children. Thorax 58(11): 998–1003

Donovan P 1988 Bowel toxemia, permeability and disease: new information to support an old concept. In Pizzorno JE, Murray MT (eds) A Textbook of Natural Medicine. John Bastyr College Publications, WA

Frawley D 2000 Ayurvedic Healing. Lotus Press, Wisconsin, p. 203

Gordon SB, Read RC 2002 Macrophage defenses against respiratory tract infections. Br Med Bull 61: 45–61

Groppo FC, Ramacciato JC, Simoes RP, Florio FM, Sartoratto A 2002 Antimicrobial activity of garlic, tea tree oil, and chlorhexidine against oral microorganisms. Int Dent J 52(6): 433–437

Hackman RM, Stern JS, Gershwin ME 2000 Hypnosis and asthma: a critical review. J Asthma 37(1): 1–15

Hasani A, Pavia D, Toms N, et al 2003 Effect of aromatics on lung mucociliary clearance in patients with chronic airways obstruction. J Altern Complement Med 9(2): 243–249

Hwang BY, Roberts SK, Chadwick LR, Wu CD, Kinghorn AD 2003 Antimicrobial constituents from goldenseal (the rhizomes of *Hydrastis canadensis*) against selected oral pathogens. Planta Med 69(7): 623–627

Iacono G, Cavataio F, Montalto G et al 1998 Persistent cow's milk protein intolerance in infants: the changing faces of the same disease. Clin Exp Allergy Jul; 28(7): 817–823

Keville K 1996 Herbs for Health and Healing. Rodale Press Inc, Emmaus, Pennsylvania

Kim JH 1997 Anti-bacterial action of onion (*Allium cepa* L.) extracts against oral pathogenic bacteria. J Nihon Univ Sch Dent 39(3): 136–141

Kovacs M, Stauder A, Szedmak S 2003 Severity of allergic complaints: the importance of depressed mood. J Psychosom Res 54(6): 549–557

Lad V 1998 The Complete Book of Ayurvedic Home Remedies. Piatkus, London, p. 249

Lad V (lecture notes 1991)

Lee DK, Carstairs IJ, Haggart K, et al 2003 Butterbur, a herbal remedy, attenuates adenosine monophosphate induced nasal responsiveness in seasonal allergic rhinitis. Clin Exp Allergy 33(7): 882–886

Mahmoud F, Abul H, Onadeko B, et al 2000 In vitro effects of Ginkgolide B on lymphocyte activation in atopic asthma: comparison with cyclosporin A. Jpn J Pharmacol 83(3): 241–245

Mantle F 2004 Complementary and Alternative Medicine for Child and Adolescent Care. Butterworth-Heinemann, London, pp. 51, 53

Mascolo N 1987 Biological screening of Italian medicinal plants for anti-inflammatory activity. Phytotherapy Research 1: 28–31

McElroy BH, Miller SP 2003 An open-label, single-center, phase IV clinical study of the effectiveness of zinc gluconate glycine lozenges (Cold-Eeze) in reducing the duration and symptoms of the common cold in school-aged subjects. Am J Ther 10(5): 324–329

McMahan JT, Calenoff E, Croft DJ, et al 1981 Chronic otitis media with effusion and allergy: modified RAST analysis of 119 cases. Otol/Head Neck Surg 89: 427–431

Mills S, Bone K 2000 Principles and Practice of Phytotherapy. Churchill Livingstone, London

Mittman P 1990 Randomized, double-blind study of freeze-dried Urtica dioica in the treatment of allergic rhinitis. Planta Med 56(1): 44–47

Obertreis B, Giller K, Teucher T, et al 1996 Anti-inflammatory effect of Urtica dioica folia extract in comparison to caffeic malic acid. Arzneimittelforschung 46(1): 52–56

Petersen M, Simmonds MS 2003 Rosmarinic Acid. Phytochemistry Jan; 62(2): 121–125

Phadke PS 2001 Home Doctor. Silverdale Books, Leicester, England, p. 93

Prusek W, Jankowski A, Radomska G, et al 1987 Immunostimulation in recurrent respiratory tract infections therapy in children. Arch Immunol Ther Exp (Warsz) 35(3): 289–302

Rau E 2000 Treatment of acute tonsillitis with a fixed-combination herbal preparation. Adv Ther 17(4): 197–203

Roberts G, Lack G 2003 Food allergy and asthma – what is the link? Paediatr Respir Rev 4(3): 205–212

Rosimini C 2003 Benefits of swim training for children and adolescents with asthma. J Am Acad Nurse Pract 15(6): 247–252

Safayhi H, Sabieraj J, Sailer ER, Ammon HP 1994 Chamazulene: an antioxidant-type inhibitor of leukotriene B4 formation. Planta Med 60(5): 410–413

Sarrell EM, Mandelberg A, Cohen HA 2001 Efficacy of naturopathic extracts in the management of ear pain associated with acute otitis media. Arch Pediatr Adolesc Med Jul; 155(7): 766–769

Sarrell EM, Cohen HA, Kahan E 2003 Naturopathic treatment for ear pain in children. Pediatrics 111(5 Pt 1): 574–579

Shibata T, Morimoto T, Suzuki A, et al 1996 The effect of Shakuyaku-kanzo-to on prostaglandin production in human uterine myometrium. Nippon Sanka Fujinka Gakkai Zasshi 48(5): 321–327

Tillotson AK, Tillotson NH, Robert A Jr 2001 The One Earth Herbal Sourcebook. Kensington Publishing Corps, New York

Vedanthan PK, Kesavalu LN, Murthy KC, et al 1998 Clinical study of yoga techniques in university students with asthma: a controlled study. Allergy Asthma Proc 19(1): 3–9

Verma V 1995 Ayurveda: A Way of Life. Samuel Weiser Inc., Maine, p. 226

Williamson E 2002 Major Herbs of Ayurveda. Churchill Livingstone, London, p. 62

Wilson AF, Honsberger R, Chiu JT, Novey HS 1975 Transcendental meditation and asthma. Respiration 32(1): 74–80

Zakay-Rones Z, Varsano N, Zlotnik M, et al 1995 Inhibition of several strains of influenza virus in vitro and reduction of symptoms by an elderberry extract (Sambucus nigra L.) during an outbreak of influenza B Panama. J Altern Complement Med 1(4): 361–369

Chapter 10

The nervous system

CHAPTER CONTENTS

Our nervous system clearly illustrates the relationship between mind and body. It is an amazing system of communication involving neuronal signalling by which the brain and the nerve cells can send messages via neurotransmitters across synapses from one nerve cell to another or to a collection of muscle fibres. To date we know of approximately 300 substances that act as neurotransmitters including endorphins, neuropeptides, adrenaline (epinephrine), noradrenaline (norepinephrine) and acetylcholine. Composed of neurones and nerve fibres, comprising the brain and spinal cord, the peripheral nerves and the autonomic nervous system, the nervous system is part of the physical body. Yet as well as controlling physical activities and sensations it expresses our thoughts and emotions … there is really little difference between mind and body except that which we have created. Just as physical symptoms can affect the way we think and feel, and create psychological problems, so thoughts and emotions have a direct effect on the physical body and can create physiological illness. Negative thoughts and feelings can diminish energy and vitality and reduce resistance, and can be expressed as disease in the body. Harmonious thoughts and feelings affect the chemical composition of the tissues and secretions of the body in a variety of beneficial ways and thereby help to promote good health. A large 20 year follow-up study of 22,461 Finnish adults found clear correlations between life dissatisfaction and mortality in men (though curiously not in women), suggesting that part of the effect is mediated via adverse health behaviour (Koivumaa-Honkanen et al 2000). It is of course difficult to untangle cause and effect, but happiness does indeed seem to promote health!

Treatment of disharmony in the body that addresses root emotional causes can be sought through a psychological approach, counselling or psychotherapy, for instance, and disharmony in the mind can be treated by physical means, including taking regular exercise, practising yoga, and through nourishing the nervous system as a tissue, through herbs and diet. Using herbal nervines and a nutritious diet, the function of the nervous system can be enhanced and in this way the behaviour of a "difficult" or unhappy child can radically change. There are many herbal medicines that have the ability to act on the nervous system. They contain molecules with pieces that resemble neurotransmitters found in the chemical messaging system. Some herbs stimulate receptor sites and act as agonists, while others are able to attach to receptor sites and block chemical reactions acting as antagonists.

THE ROLE OF DIET

Diet, the mind, and the emotions also have an interdependent relationship. How we feel psychologically affects what we eat, how it is digested, absorbed and assimilated, and how the body uses it. When we are stressed or unhappy the sympathetic nervous system inhibits the flow of digestive juices and thereby impairs digestion and absorption. In Ayurvedic terms this means diminishing digestive fire (*agni*). When relaxed our digestive juices flow more freely and we are more likely to derive the nourishment from the food we eat as it is better digested and absorbed. In turn our nutrition affects our psychological health.

There are certain nutrients which are vital to production of neurotransmitters and normal function of the nervous system of which we need an adequate supply at all times. These include essential fatty acids, vitamins C, B, and E, calcium, magnesium and zinc. Unless they are in plentiful supply during times of stress a deficiency may arise, further exacerbating any stress-related problems. Children vary widely in their psychological composition, and so also in their nutritional requirements. The greater the demands that stress imposes on our energy and physical processes, the greater the need for nutrients to support them.

Generally a healthy diet, with plenty of organic fruit and vegetables, nuts and seeds, whole grains and foods containing protein and essential fatty acids, should provide most of the necessary nutrients to support the nervous system. Those more highly tuned children who naturally require more of certain nutrients than others, more easily become deficient, and subsequently prone to stress, anxiety, irritability and psychological problems. Attention to diet and supplementation can prove beneficial, especially during stressful periods in a child's life.

A diet high in sugar, refined carbohydrates, junk foods and carbonated drinks may cause a deficiency of magnesium, calcium and B vitamins, which can predispose to symptoms such as insomnia, anxiety, agitation, nightmares, fatigue, poor appetite, bowel problems, depression and recurrent infections. Vitamin B3 may be deficient in children with a low protein diet, predisposing to irritability, fatigue, anxiety, headaches, insomnia, poor memory, emotional instability and skin problems. Vitamin B6 deficiency can cause anxiety, depression and personality changes. Vitamin B12 deficiency can give rise to depression, fatigue, nervousness and anxiety. It may occur during stressful periods because gastric acidity, necessary for proper B12 absorption, can be reduced by tension and anxiety.

Vitamin C has been researched widely for its ability to enhance resistance to stress and its use in the treatment of nervous and mental problems. It has been found for example that some schizophrenics can require up to 70,000 mg of vitamin C before their body reaches saturation, while others may only need 4000 mg. Emotional stress and strain causes the body to use much more ascorbic acid.

Deficiencies of essential fatty acids have been related to a variety of different nervous problems including learning problems and ADD. Children can obtain essential fatty acids from eating nuts and seeds and fatty fish and from supplements such as hemp seed oil and flaxseed oil. (For more on EFAs, see Immune System, p. 151).

Zinc deficiency has been shown to be related to depression, irritability, mood swings, tearfulness, sullenness, as well as schizoid behaviour. There is some research to indicate that zinc supplementation can aid motor development, increase vigour and increase playfulness in low-birthweight infants for example (Bhatnagar and Taneja 2001). High copper can upset zinc balance in the body, and has been associated with irritability and mood swings. Calcium and magnesium are essential for proper relaxation of nerve tissue. Deficiencies can cause cramps, muscle tension and twitching, headaches, poor appetite, debility, tiredness, anxiety, panic attacks, hyperactivity, insomnia and depression. Iron deficiency is linked to lethargy, tiredness, depression, anxiety and poor concentration.

In order to maintain a healthy nervous system, refined carbohydrates including white bread and pasta, white sugar, polished rice, and junk food should all be avoided. Not only do they compromise good nutrition but also contribute to constipation, giving rise to a toxic system, which can predispose to a range of illnesses. According to Ayurveda, toxins (ama) are the first cause of disease. Stress tends to cause a craving for sugar, the consumption of which can in turn further exacerbate stress. High consumption of sugar and refined carbohydrates, squashes and most soft drinks can upset sugar balance. When blood sugar rises children will experience a surge of energy but it then drops and they can feel weak, anxious or irritable, and crave something sweet to eat again.

The liver should regulate the amount of sugar going into the bloodstream but if under stress it will fail to do so efficiently, causing peaks and troughs in blood sugar levels. A high protein diet, the use of drugs and pollutants in food can also limit its efficiency. Hypoglycaemia imposes stress on the body because it is interpreted by the body as a danger signal. The adrenal glands respond to this by secreting adrenaline (epinephrine), putting into action the "fight or flight" mechanism. This has the effect of mobilizing glucose stores from the liver to raise the blood sugar, but it can also give rise to fear, palpitations, shakiness, cold and clammy hands, breathlessness and mood changes including irritability and anxiety. These mood swings seem to aggravate any existing stress and decrease the ability to cope with it. They make extra demands on the adrenal glands, increase the amount of adrenaline in the system and serve to deplete vital energy. They could also contribute to stress-related illness. Caffeinated drinks such as cocoa, cola drinks, chocolate, tea and coffee should be avoided, as caffeine is well known to exacerbate the effects of stress by potentiating adrenaline. It also causes loss of vitamins B and C.

When trying to understand why some children are more prone to hypoglycaemia than others, the role of the pancreas must also be considered. The pancreas secretes insulin, which causes sugar in the blood to enter the body's cells, and also glucagons, which help to regulate the release of stored sugar from the liver into the bloodstream. Stress may be a major factor in the regulation of both insulin and glucagon secretion from the pancreas, and resultant imbalances of blood sugar. However, regular consumption of refined sugar may also cause the pancreas to function erratically, causing poor sugar control, which becomes even worse under stress. In this way a vicious circle is created, and under even minimal stress children can fly off the handle for no apparent reason, be overly sensitive, or over-react to stress. Within Ayurvedic constitutional classifications, *Vata* and particularly *Pitta* type children are more likely to react badly to sugar and be prone to hypoglycaemia. With their highly active nervous systems *Vata* children burn up a lot of energy and with their erratic appetites they may not eat enough on a regular basis. *Pitta* types have a high metabolism and tend to crave sugar, and need to eat regularly to maintain their high energy levels.

DEALING WITH STRESS

Stress is a natural response to pressure, and seen positively it can bring out the best in some children, provided that it is interspersed with sufficient periods of calm. Tension or anxiety is a normal response to a difficult or challenging situation, which should settle once the problem is resolved. However, through extreme or long-term stress it may become habitual, although the original causes of it have passed. Resistance to stress can be impaired not only through poor nutrition but also through trauma, long-term allergies and digestive problems. Further stress-related physical problems may develop, such as stomach and bowel problems, allergies and skin problems. During times of pressure, when nutritional demands increase, essential fatty acids, vitamins B, C, and E, and minerals calcium, magnesium and zinc to support the nervous system can be increased through diet or supplementation and this will help to prevent the development of stress-related health problems.

Herbs can be given to provide additional support. Herbal tonics have the ability to nourish the nervous system and increase resilience to stress. They can be effective also when a child is tired and run down and the nervous system depleted. The herbs I tend to use include vervain (*Verbena off.*), rosemary, lemon balm, skullcap (*Scutellaria laterifolia*), wild oats (*Avena sativa*) and ginseng. The effect of both Korean ginseng (*Panax ginseng*) and American ginseng (*Eleuthrococcus senticosus*) on stress and well-being has been well documented. Both appear to have a paradoxical effect of either increasing or decreasing the stress response. This property, known as an adaptogenic action is believed to be due to ginseng's effect on the hypothalamic–pituitary–adrenal axis, increasing plasma corticotropin and corticosteroid levels (Nocerino et al 2000, Gaffney et al 2001).

Recent research in healthy subjects supports the anxiolytic properties of skullcap (*Scutellaria lateriflora*) (Wolfson and Hoffmann 2003). This action may be mediated by binding of the compounds baicalein and baicalin to the benzodiazepine site of the GABAA receptor (Hui et al 2000).

Chamomile, limeflower (*Tilia europea*), valerian (*Valeriana off.*), hops (*Humulus lupulus*) or passion flower (*Passiflora incarnata*) all have relaxant properties and can be given to calm nerves and relax tense muscles. A trial on 22 healthy subjects indicated an increase in positive mood ratings on exposure to chamomile oil (Roberts and Williams 1992) whilst other trials suggest that apigenin, a flavonoid found in chamomile, acts as a central benzodiazepine receptor ligand (Viola et al 1995). A double-blind randomized trial of the effect of passion flower (*Passiflora incarnata*) compared to oxezapam in patients with general anxiety disorder, concluded that *Passiflora* was as effective as the drug (Akhondzadeh et al 2001).

To help stress-related digestive problems and enhance resistance to stress and allergy, teas of lemon balm, chamomile, lavender or limeflower can be given to children instead of fruit juices and squashes, which are often high in sugar and additives and can actually disturb behaviour and exacerbate feelings of stress. Hot herbal baths and massage using relaxing essential oils of lavender, rose, chamomile or geranium can be very relaxing and soothing for a tense child. Inhalations of frankincense oil will calm and deepen breathing.

Ayurvedic approach

The three gunas

Everything in creation, according to Ayurveda, is pervaded by three prime qualities or *gunas*, known as *Sattva*, *Rajas* and *Tamas* and we can clearly observe the effects of these qualities in the different mental and emotional states that we perennially experience.

Sattva is the principle of love, light, harmony and perception. Being *Sattvic* is the balanced state to which many of us aspire, with clarity of mind, intelligence and wisdom, tranquillity, compassion and love. When people are in a *Sattvic* state they radiate light, joy and happiness. From *Sattva* comes the clarity or peace of mind and understanding through which we are able to perceive the truth and really experience the world through our five senses. Health of mind and body is maintained by *Sattvic* living.

Rajas is the quality of energy, action, movement and turbulence, which activates all movement, whether it is the movement of ideas in the mind or instructions to the body to spring out of bed in the morning. The three biological *doshas*, *Vata*, *Pitta* and *Kapha*, also arise primarily through *Rajas* as they are mobile or vital energies. In the mind *Rajas* provokes thought and mental activity, and is responsible for inspiration and creativity but in excess it can cause restlessness, agitation, passion, aggression, anger, over competitiveness and over-ambition. It is said to give rise to self-motivated or self-seeking action that leads to unhappiness, with a tendency to be constantly on the look out for new stimuli and challenges, seeking fulfilment in the outer world and not at peace with ourselves. In a *Rajasic* state we can dissipate our energy through excess activity and once tired and depressed *Tamas* takes over.

Tamas is the quality of darkness, inertia, stability and dullness. Heavy, and solid, it engenders calmness, steadiness and groundedness, "solid as a rock". In the body it produces inactivity, and enables us to sleep. An excess of *Tamas* in the mind can obstruct movement causing laziness, lethargy, attachment, irrationality, stubbornness, confusion, depression and delusion. We may feel dull-minded and drowsy, with little motivation to do anything, we may struggle to see things clearly and our minds can be filled with doubts and negative thoughts. According to Ayurveda, it is excess *Tamas* that is responsible for ignorance and our inability to perceive our true inner selves.

Although an interaction of all three *gunas* is necessary, when *Sattva* predominates it makes for the correct balance of all three gunas. When *Sattva*, *Rajas* and *Tamas* act together in unity, this balance is known as "pure *Sattva*". By eating a healthy diet, and living a harmonious lifestyle with love, wisdom and other *Sattvic* attributes, we can experience inner peace and a sense of joy and fulfilment. When *Rajas* or *Tamas* are excessive they make for ill health and unhappiness and yet in balance they can still be seen positively. *Tamas* enables necessary rest, relaxation and recovery from activity, so that we can replenish our energy. We need *Rajas* as well to survive in the world for we cannot spend all day doing nothing in a state of bliss! Also *Rajas* can be used to convert *Tamas* into *Sattva*.

Foods for the mind

In Ayurveda, food, like everything else in creation, falls into the same categories (Table 10.1). There are *Sattvic*, *Rajasic* and *Tamasic* foods which have the ability to increase these qualities within us when we eat them.

Sattvic foods

These are the best-quality foods that help to enhance health and strength, energy and vitality, and lay the foundations for a *Sattvic* state of mind. *Sattvic* foods are fresh, light, juicy, sweet, nourishing, energy-giving and tasty. They are easy to digest and so do not tax our energy through the process of digestion. They include fresh vegetables, including carrots, sweet potatoes, beetroot, turnips, seasonal fruits like sweet oranges, apples, grapes, dates, bananas, and mangoes, coconut, coconut milk, salads, mung beans, chick peas, lentils, sprouted beans, yoghurt, lassi, fresh milk (4 hours after milking it becomes *Rajasic*), butter, ghee, grains such as rice, rye, barley, sunflower seeds, pumpkin seeds, hazelnuts, almonds, almond milk, rice, raw cane sugar and honey. Rock salt, black pepper and lemons are also *Sattvic*. Fresh, organic cow's milk is considered most *Sattvic* and it is normally boiled before being consumed as this makes it more digestible. It should never be drunk cold, straight from the fridge nor mixed with tastes that conflict with it, such as sour, pungent and salty, but taken with other sweet foods like grains, sweet fruits and cereals. Milk and ghee build up *ojas*.

Rajasic foods

These are medium-quality foods, often high in protein and carbohydrate. They tend to be stimulating

Table 10.1 Categories of foods for the mind

	Sattvic	Rajasic	Tamasic		Sattvic	Rajasic	Tamasic
Grains	Rice	Millet	Wheat	Herbs and	Coriander	Bay leaves	
	Tapioca	Buckwheat	Bread	spices	Cumin	Black pepper	
	Blue corn	Corn	(more than	(contd)	Fennel	Cinnamon	
	Rye		8 hrs old)		Fenugreek	Cloves	
	Barley				seeds	Fenugreek	
	Rice milk				Rose	leaves	
					Saffron	Ginger	
Nuts and	Coconut		Peanuts			Mint	
seeds	Coconut milk						
	Almonds						
	Almond milk			Meat	None	Fish	Beef
	Hazelnuts					Shrimps	Lamb
	Pumpkin seeds					Chicken	Pork
	Sunflower seeds						
				Condiments	Black pepper	Sea salt	
Fruit	Mangoes	Sour apples	Avocado		Rock salt		
	Pears	Guavas	Watermelon				
	Pomegranate	Sour fruits	Apricots	Sweeteners	Honey		White sugar
	Peaches	Bananas	Plums		Raw cane sugar		
	Figs	Berries		Dairy	Fresh milk	Eggs	Hard cheese
	Sweet oranges	Currants			Fresh yoghurt	Homogenized	Dried milk
	Lemons				Lassi	milk	
	Sweet grapes				Butter	Sour milk	
	Dates				Ghee	Sour cream	
	Sweet apples					Cheese	
Vegetables	Carrots	Potato	Mushrooms	Others		Fried food	Old stale food
	Sweet potatoes	Tomatoes	Garlic			Salted bread	Preservatives
	Beetroot	Cauliflower	Onion			Sweets	Overcooked
	Lettuce	Broccoli	Pumpkin			Biscuits	food
	Sprouts	Spinach				Salted crisps	Frozen food
	Turnips					Chips	Dried food
						Pickles	Fizzy drinks
Beans	Mung	Red lentils	Black			Chutneys	Peanuts
	Yellow lentils	Aduki	Pinto			Tea	Sweets
	Kidney	Toor dhal	Urad dhal			Coffee	Chocolate
	Lima					Alcohol	Crisps
	Chick peas						Ice cream
	Sprouted beans						Popcorn
Herbs and	Anise	Chillies	Flax seeds				Alcohol
spices	Cardamom	Asafoetida	Turmeric				Old bread

and capable of generating high levels of energy. They taste bitter, sour, salty, pungent, and have hot and dry qualities. They include meat, cheese, eggs, fish, hot, spicy and fried foods, pickles, potatoes and other root vegetables, pasteurized milk, sweets, biscuits, sea salt, salted bread, tea and coffee.

Sattvic foods become *Rajasic* if they are fried in oil and pungent spices, or overcooked. Foods that are hotter or colder than body temperature are said to be *Rajasic*. We need such foods to enable us to carry out our activities and responsibilities and keep pace with the changing world, but excessive intake of these foods is said to create restlessness, excitement, agitation, anger, jealousy, deceit, egoism and over high energy.

Tamasic foods

These are low-quality devitalized foods and include unpalatable over-cooked, tinned, dried, processed, frozen and junk foods as well as left-over food that has been "spoiled", i.e. cooked and left too long to go off. *Tamasic* foods use a lot of energy to be digested. They include sweets, fizzy drinks, snacks like crisps, chocolate, ice cream, popcorn, excessive alcohol, and all foods containing preservatives. Meat, onions, garlic, peanuts and dried milk are considered *Tamasic*, as is bread that is more than 8 hours old. Hot and cold foods taken together, and incompatible food combinations like milk and vinegar, radishes and honey, bread and bananas, produce *Tamas*. *Tamasic* foods are best avoided as much as possible for they can damage health and impair mental function. In children they are said to predispose to behavioural problems like hyperactivity.

There are many other influences that also increase *Sattva*. As well as consuming pure food and water, Ayurvedic philosophy advocates that we need to avoid obvious toxins like pesticides, we should get adequate sleep so that we can be in a good state of mind, we should spend time outside in nature, walking in the sunshine, sitting by water, listening to the waves or to birds singing or the wind rustling in the trees, to purify the senses. We should have a balance of activity and rest and relaxation and allow time to reflect before acting or speaking. We need to be in loving, nurturing relationships, to be kind and tolerant, avoiding anger and criticism and pointing out peoples' faults, rather we should go out of our way to make others feel better.

Ayurveda is primarily *Sattvic*, advocating a way of life with love, faith, peace, non-violence and other *Sattvic* virtues.

The mental forms of the *Doshas*: *Prana*, *Tejas* and *Ojas*

These are the more subtle forms of the three *doshas* which exert their influence in the mind. They fulfil

similar functions as their three counterparts in the brain, but on a more subtle level.

The mental form of *Vata* is called *Prana*. It promotes mental adaptability, the ability to communicate, and coordinate ideas in the mind. It gives us the will to live, to grow and heal ourselves. It is our basic life force. Too much *Prana* causes loss of mental control, as the life force loses its connection with the brain and body, leading to loss of sensory and motor coordination, and predisposing to learning and behavioural problems such as ADHD. Children with excess *Prana* might feel ungrounded, stressed, perhaps alienated, with a poor sense of identity. Anxiety, insomnia and palpitations can occur. Too little *Prana* causes lack of mental energy, enthusiasm and curiosity. Our life force and healing energy is diminished and receptivity and creativity inhibited. The mind and senses can be dull and heavy, we lose motivation, and our attitudes can become conservative and rigid.

The mental form of *Pitta* is called *Tejas*, the fire of the mind. *Tejas* promotes intelligence, reason, passion to learn, self-discipline and perception. It is the basic clarity of mind. Too much *Tejas* can cause an overly critical and discriminating mind, headache, burning sensations in head and eyes, doubt, anger, irritability and enmity. Children with excess *Tejas* can be hard to please, prone to temper tantrums, often nothing can satisfy or placate them. Too little *Tejas* can cause an inability to inquire or discern, uncritically accepting things and losing the power to learn from our experiences. Children tend to be passive and impressionable and may come under the influence of others as they can lack purpose and lose direction.

The mental form of *Kapha* is *Ojas*, the essential vital fluid of the body in subtle form in the mind.

Ojas promotes mental strength, contentment, patience, fortitude, calm and the capacity for good memory and sustained concentration. It is our basic mental and psychological stability and endurance in life. *Ojas* is essentially our peace of mind. Excess *Ojas* causes heaviness and dullness in the mind, as well as self-content that causes unwillingness to change or grow. Generally high *Ojas* is much less of a problem than excess *Prana* or *Tejas*, which are the main factor in mental disorders. High *Prana* dries out *Ojas* and high *Tejas* burns it up. Excess *Prana* and *Tejas* go along then with low

Ojas. When *Ojas* is low children may lack self-confidence, have difficulty concentrating, have poor memory and lack faith. It prevents consistency in their thoughts and balance in their emotions. Nervous exhaustion or mental problems are likely.

Prana, Tejas and *Ojas* control *Vata, Pitta* and *Kapha* in the body. *Tejas* is the light of perception, *Prana* allows us to coordinate our perceptions and *Ojas* allows us to stabilize them. According to Ayurveda, factors that balance them include meditation, prayer, self-study, deep sleep and relaxation. *Prana* particularly is strengthened by time spent in nature. Attributes like faith, love, receptivity, compassion and understanding are also important. Factors that imbalance them include the use of drugs, excess exposure to mass media influences, TV or computers, over-stimulation through, for example, strong sensations like overly bright colours, loud noise, excess or pretended emotions (Athique 1998).

We can observe the effect that disturbance of the three *doshas* has on *Prana, Tejas* and *Ojas* through mental and emotional disturbances commonly experienced by children. When *Vata* is high, children are likely to be restless, nervous, insecure, anxious and fearful. They can develop phobias as well as sleeping problems and nightmares. They are likely to be more fearful at night in the dark and their fears can be set off by frightening images, TV programmes, stories and so on. *Pitta* children tend to be energetic and hot headed. They are likely to be aggravated at times of pressure such as before exams, interviews and competitions, because they are highly competitive and fear failure. They generally react with moodiness, resentment, irritability, anger and temper tantrums. They have a tendency to suppress their emotions until the point that their anger explodes. Crying and expression of emotions is very important for *Pitta* types for the release of tension and stress. *Kapha* children are generally more placid and resilient, slower to react emotionally. Under stress they tend to become lethargic, withdrawn, tired and lacking in motivation. They might eat more and comfort eating is likely. They put on weight easily and are reluctant to take exercise. They can sit for hours doing seemingly very little, perhaps watching TV.

Ayurvedic treatment for the nervous system

There are many beneficial Ayurvedic herbs for the nervous system.

- Ashwagandha is one of the herbs I use most in my practice. It is the main herb for balancing *Vata*, and it is *Vata* that is behind most nervous problems. It is a nourishing nerve tonic, calming an agitated mind, enhancing resilience to stress and promoting energy as well as good sleep.
- Gotu kola is an excellent herb for promoting brain function, for poor concentration and for calming an agitated mind. It is one of the best herbs for *Pitta* although it can be used for all constitutions. An oil prepared from coconut oil and gotu kola can be massaged on to the soles of the feet and the head to calm the mind and promote relaxation.
- Brahmi (*Bacopa monnieri*) is similarly one of the best brain tonics, which enhances concentration, memory and mental clarity. It pacifies *Vata*, and is used in the treatment of epilepsy, depression and hyperactivity. It also clears *Tamas* from the mind.
- Sandalwood is considered a brain tonic, to lift the spirits and is particularly indicated for *Pitta* children. It is used in mental debility, irritability and poor concentration through an agitated or restless mind.
- Shatavari is indicated for *Pitta* and *Vata* problems. It acts as a brain tonic, promotes energy and vitality and helps to relieve pain.
- Bringaraj is a calming remedy for *Vata* and *Pitta* disorders, such as headaches and anxiety.
- Liquorice is used as an adaptogen, supporting the adrenals and increasing resilience to stress.
- Bala is used as a tonic to the nervous system and for *Vata* disorders generally.
- Jatamansi (*Nardostachys jatamansi*) is a good sedative and brain tonic, enhancing concentration and memory. It is one of the best herbs for stress related headaches (however it is on the CITES list of endangered species and needs to be obtained from sustainable sources).
- Vacha is a well-known brain tonic, which is used to clear *Tamas* from the mind and enhance intellectual function.

BEHAVIOURAL PROBLEMS

There are a variety of factors that require consideration in behavioural problems, which can be attributed to both emotional and physical causes.

Almost any kind of physical problem can affect a child's behaviour, and this is easily demonstrated by a change of mood during acute infections, when a child is more likely to cry or feel insecure and clingy. Low-grade digestive problems may play a part. Loose, smelly stools may indicate an inflammatory problem, chronic infection or a malabsorption problem, and can deplete the child nutritionally and predispose to lowered vitality and poor health. Constipation will cause an accumulation of wastes and toxins in the body and this affects the state of mind, contributing to lethargy and irritability. Worms can disturb bowel function and are often associated with irritability and moodiness, lethargy and poor sleep. There is evidence to suggest a link between impaired intestinal permeability and autism (White 2003).

Junk food and foods containing artificial additives (particularly tartrazine and aspartame) can all have significant effects on a child's temperament. Refined sugar products (soft drinks, sweets, biscuits, cakes, honey, dried fruits and fruit juice) are all leading causes of hyperactive or disruptive behaviour. A sugar "challenge" of a high carbohydrate breakfast (i.e. sugared cereal, milk and orange juice) has been shown to reduce the attention span of both normal and hyperactive children (Minsky 2002, p. 53).

A frequent cause of behavioural changes in children is food intolerance or allergy. Common allergens such as chocolate and milk produce, can cause a variety of disturbances, ranging from insomnia to temper tantrums, aggression and black moods. Gluten, eggs, yeast, salicylates and corn may act similarly. Allergic reactions to foods can be mild or extreme. They can primarily affect the brain tissues, causing a cerebral allergy and possibly even causing psychotic behaviour. If a child becomes lethargic, irritable, depressed or difficult, and immediately feels better after eating a certain food, such as sugar, chocolate or milk, this could indicate the implicated food, or it could indicate hypoglycaemia. Suspected foods should be omitted from the diet for several months while the background causes of the allergy are treated.

Nutritional deficiencies can disrupt the nervous system and these can be created by a diet that is high in sugar and refined foods and low in vegetables and fruit and unrefined oils. Such diets tend to be lacking in B complex vitamins, vitamins C and E, essential fatty acids and a wide range of minerals and trace elements, including calcium, magnesium, zinc and manganese, all of which are vital to normal brain function. These nutritional deficiencies can also predispose to food allergies.

Hypoglycaemia can also cause mood swings and erratic behaviour, evident when a child is moody and irritable, pale or dark round the eyes until eating, after which they recover. A major cause of low blood sugar is the over-consumption of sugar and refined carbohydrates. It can often occur in children with allergies.

Attention deficit disorder (ADD) and attention deficit hyperactivity disorder (ADHD) involve problems related to attention and concentration and often restlessness, distraction, sleeplessness, tantrums and disruptive behaviour, and frequently an inability to cope with school. A recent review suggests that diet modification should play a major role in the management of ADHD but is relatively neglected. ADHD has been linked to food sensitivities, fatty acid deficiencies, food additives and excess refined sugar (Schnoll et al 2003).

Heavy metal toxicity and lead from car fumes, for instance, can affect behaviour. Lack of fresh air and exercise, over-exposure to polluted smoky atmospheres and excess exposure to noise, computers or television can all create problems.

Birth trauma could also be implicated. If the birth was long, difficult or traumatic, oxygen was short or drugs were used, these could all affect the baby. The passage through the birth canal can affect the central nervous system, and this is best detected by a cranial osteopath, whose work can have a significant effect on a child that has been difficult since birth.

Experts in the field have found that lack of physical touch and expressions of affection and of parents sharing sufficient "quality time" with their children can contribute to a variety of behavioural problems. If parents and teachers do not help children to channel their energy in positive ways and encourage quiet and calming pastimes like listening to music and reading, there may be a tendency for them to be hyperactive (Minsky 2002). It is possible that a "difficult" child is unconsciously picking up and reflecting stresses within the family unit. Often a child can feel responsible for emotional problems experienced by their parents. The changes in life that children almost inevitably experience can prove difficult for some. The transition from being an only child to being the sibling can be challenging. Aggression in a young child may reflect jealousy and aggression towards the newborn baby, the overt expression of which the child knows is not permissible. Other difficult periods may be connected with starting at play school, or moving house or school, realizing that homework is here to stay or moving into adolescence.

Treatment of behavioural problems

The child's daily diet needs to provide all the nutrients the nervous system needs to be able to function normally (see p. 249). During times of stress the body will metabolize these nutrients faster than normal, so supplementation may be necessary. A multi-mineral and -vitamin tablet, with extra vitamin C tablets and plenty of fruit and vegetables, nuts and seeds and unrefined oils in the diet, with no junk food and very little sugar, would be helpful.

Nourishing nervine and adaptogen herbs will support a stressed or depleted nervous system, enhancing resilience to stress. Good examples of these, vervain (*Verbena off.*), rose and skullcap (*Scurtellaria laterifolia*) can be given as teas or tinctures three times daily. Oats (*Avena sativa*) are rich in nutrients for the nervous system, and have a tonic nervine action. They can be taken as a decoction or tincture three times daily, or eaten as porridge. For tense, anxious children and those prone to temper tantrums, chamomile, limeflower (*Tilia europea*) tulsi, rose, skullcap and liquorice used regularly can make a significant difference.

Herbs that have a gentle action on the liver and pancreas can be included in prescriptions when there is low blood sugar, allergy or heavy metal toxicity. They may prove helpful particularly for children with anger, irritability or depression.

Dandelion root, burdock, vervain and rosemary can be combined with peppermint to disguise the bitter taste and make the prescription more palatable.

Dilute essential oils of ylang ylang, tulsi, sandalwood, lemon balm, rosemary, lavender and chamomile can be used for baths, massages and inhalations. Massage is especially beneficial for comforting restless, anxious or tense children. Using sesame oil as a base is particularly therapeutic (see p. 84).

Some of the ways in which mental and emotional disturbances are reflected through the body include:

* Digestive problems – constipation, diarrhoea, wind, stomach pain, colic, nausea and vomiting.
* Lowered resistance to infections, producing recurrent illness, allergies (e.g. asthma, hayfever, eczema), skin problems such as boils and eczema, irritable coughs and insomnia.

Where stress is seen to be a contributory factor in any of these problems, herbs can be given to support the child's nervous system in addition to other herbs used for specific symptoms involved.

Other supportive measures for children include: breathing exercises, relaxation exercises, physical exercise (such as gym, games, martial arts, yoga, bicycling, dance), music and relaxation tapes, and sharing of creative or constructive activities between parents and children (painting, crafts, singing, walking, story telling). Singing is of particular interest, as it helps with control of breath and encourages correct abdominal breathing, which is very calming. Repetitive chants are fun and children often love them.

Support through herbs, diet and other measures chosen for children may be equally valuable for parents of difficult children, who naturally may become exhausted and depleted, especially when there are long-term sleeping problems.

ATTENTION DEFICIT DISORDER (ADD) AND ATTENTION DEFICIT HYPERACTIVITY DISORDER (ADHD)

ADD and ADHD are often related to food intolerance, particularly to certain food colourings and flavourings, dairy produce (notably casein), salicylates, wheat or gluten, corn, chocolate, caffeine in cola drinks, eggs and citrus fruits, especially oranges. There is often a relationship between a history of allergies, such as asthma, eczema, hayfever or migraine, in the family. A variety of other physical symptoms may accompany ADHD which serve as indicators of nutritional deficiency and/or food allergy. These include: dry skin, cradle cap or dandruff, dry, cracked lips, skin rashes, bed-wetting, frequent headaches, aching legs, fussy eating or poor appetite, excess dribbling, sweating or thirst, frequent infections and low resistance, catarrhal congestion, sweet cravings, bloating wind, diarrhoea or constipation.

It is essential that the daily diet provides adequate amounts of amino acids, vitamins and minerals, for the body to manufacture neurotransmitters and brain chemicals such as dopamine, serotonin and noradrenaline (norepinephrine). Trials comparing B vitamins to treatment with Ritalin found that B vitamins were more effective, safer and far less expensive (Minsky 2002).

Nutritional deficiencies are common in ADHD (Kidd 2000). Deficiencies in iron, zinc, B vitamins, magnesium, essential fatty acids, caused by lack of fresh fruit and vegetables, whole grains and unrefined oils in the diet, and aggravated by excess sugar and refined foods, are quite common, and can affect brain function, making the child more vulnerable to the adverse effects of toxic metals.

Magnesium is particularly important. It is essential to the metabolism of vitamin B6 and helps to prevent allergic responses. Deficiency can lead to tension and irritability, muscle tightness and spasm, poor physical endurance and lack of sleep. Lower than normal blood levels have been found in people with ADHD (Kozielec and Starobrat-Hermelin 1997).

Deficiency of essential fatty acids occurs widely in children and can be responsible for poor brain responses. A review found that a subgroup of ADHD subjects with symptoms similar to EFA deficiency demonstrated significantly low plasma arachidonic acid and docosahexaenoic acid levels than control subjects (Burgess et al 2000).

Safflower and sunflower oil are rich in DHA (docosahexaenoic acid), which is particularly important for normal cognitive function and may be helpful in ADHD. It is a nutrient that is incorporated into baby formulae for this very reason.

Fatty fish including salmon, sardines, tuna and mackerel are also good sources of DHA and other essential fatty acids.

Many children suffering from ADHD crave carbohydrates and can take some persuading to eat less sugar and simple carbohydrates and more protein, but the positive effects of changing the diet, including increased energy and better emotional control, should soon pay off. Fruit juices, once considered a healthy alternative to sugar and additive laden squashes, are high in natural sugar and most of them contain salicylates. The American Pediatric Association recommends that babies should not be given fruit juices, and that a maximum of 6 oz be given to children up to six, and 8–12 oz for children between 7 and 18 (Minsky 2002).

Impaired glucose metabolism may be a major contributory factor, caused by excessive intake of simple carbohydrates and nutrient poor junk foods, which lack, in particular, magnesium and zinc (which are essential to carbohydrate metabolism).

Pollution can have some effect. Inhaling or ingesting toxic metals, such as lead, cadmium and aluminium, may affect brain function, as may organic solvents in, for example, felt-tip pens, cleaning fluids and aerosol sprays. According to the US Congress and The Office of Technology Assessment "The National Academy of Sciences recently reported (in 1990) that 12 percent of the 63 million children under the age of 18 in the US suffer from one or more mental disorders and it identified exposure to toxic substances before or after birth as one of the several risk factors" (Neurotoxicity: Identifying and Controlling Poisons of the Nervous system, US Government Printing Office 1990). Heavy metal contamination from, for example, lead in house paint, old pipework, or mercury from amalgam fillings can also be to blame. Artificial lighting, strong magnetic fields and noise pollution from television, CD players, computers and videos can contribute to hyperactive behaviour. A study showed that when fluorescent lighting was removed from classrooms there was a major improvement in hyperactivity (Minsky 2002).

The consumption of alcohol, smoking and toxaemia during pregnancy, birth difficulties or antenatal lack of oxygen can also result in hyperactivity. Maternal smoking during pregnancy is linked with increased risk of offspring ADHD symptoms (Thapar et al 2003). Research suggests that passive smoking is responsible not only for much respiratory illness in children (Tamim et al 2003) but also for hyperactive behaviour.

Emotional stress can contribute to ADHD by further depleting the nervous system and by increasing the body's use of vital nutrients, contributing to vitamin, mineral and trace element deficiencies.

Systemic *Candida albicans* may also be a factor worth consideration. A disturbance of gut flora can occur due to poor digestion, lowered resistance, over-prescription of antibiotics or nutritional deficiencies, particularly of iron and zinc. If a child does not respond to dietary improvements, avoidance of possible allergens and dietary supplements, further investigations into candida could be worthwhile (see p. 185).

Treatment of attention deficit disorder and attention deficit hyperactivity disorder

- First and foremost a nutritious diet is a necessity. It is well worth eliminating suspect food allergens and sugar from the diet for an initial period of a month. Supplements of necessary vitamins and minerals, including: a multi-mineral and -vitamin tablet, B complex, zinc tablets (5–10 mg daily), vitamin C tablets (500 mg daily) and evening primrose oil (500 mg capsule daily), will not only correct nutritional deficiencies, but also promote the excretion of toxic metals. B complex is vital to the normal function of the nervous system but requires magnesium to ensure adequate absorption. A recent trial comparing Ritalin to dietary supplement treatment in 20 children concluded that food supplements may be of equivalent efficacy to Ritalin (Harding et al 2003).

- To avoid hypoglycaemia it is vital for children to have regular meals. It is worth checking how much a fussy eater has during school meals. (If you suspect candida, follow the advice on p. 185).

- Certain herbs can aid the elimination of heavy metals, including red clover (*Trifolium pratense*), coriander leaf, kelp (*Fucus versicolor*) and nettles, which can be combined with nervine herbs.

- Tonics to the nervous system include skullcap (*Scutellaria laterifolia*), vervain (*Verbena off.*) and wild oats (*Avena sativa*), and liquorice will support the adrenal glands. (See also Herbs in general treatment of behavioural problems, p. 254).

- To aid sleep, mildly sedative herbs such as chamomile, catnip (*Nepeta cataria*), cowslip (*Primula veris*), hops (*Humulus lupulus*) and limeflowers (*Tilia europea*) can be given singly or together. They can also be added in strong infusions to bath water or given as tea before bed and again during the night should the child awake.

Ayurvedic approach

ADD and ADHD are most likely to be *Vata* and *Vata/Pitta* disorders respectively. In children with poor mental performance, slowness, sluggishness and slow digestion, it can be related to *Kapha*. *Vata* problems will be exacerbated by noise, lots of change and movement, disruption of routine, over-stimulation for example by too much TV or family stress. ADHD can be aggravated by bright lights, heat, over-stimulation, and hypoglycaemia, indicating high *Pitta*.

Ayurvedic treatment

- For a restless, nervy, and easily distracted child, use nourishing *Vata* reducing herbs such as ashwagandha, bala, wild oats, gotu kola and shatavari.

- Chyawan prash could also prove beneficial (see Appendix p. 304).

- In India doctors used *Acorus calamus* as a brain tonic and for memory problems.

- Shilajit and liquorice help to strengthen the adrenals and are good supportive remedies for the nervous system.

- If a child is angry and aggressive use *Pitta* calming herbs such as sandalwood, gotu kola, chamomile, coriander, shatavari and bringaraj.

- Bacopa, gotu kola, shilajit and guduchi can improve memory and concentration (Tillotson et al 2001, p. 343). Maharishi Ayurved produces a syrup called MA 674 containing many of these herbs.

- Yoga and meditation can be helpful in management of a range of nervous problems. More yoga classes are being held in schools as the benefits are becoming more widely accepted. Vasant Lad recommends yoga asanas that can help children to relax and relieve stress. Camel, cobra, bow, bridge and spinal twist are all recommended (Lad 1999).

- Breathing exercises have a soothing effect. Moon breathing (this through left nostril only) for 5–10 minutes is suggested.

INSOMNIA

There are many different causes of sleep disturbance including ADHD, allergies, hypoglycaemia, nutritional deficiencies, emotional stress, anxiety and fear, candida, over-stimulation, e.g. TV or computer games, over-tiredness, physical problems such as skin rashes, digestive problems, asthma or catarrh causing difficulty breathing, acute infections, coughs, colds, fevers, and headaches (see the relevant sections for more specific treatment of these).

Similarly according to Ayurveda there are numerous causes of insomnia (*anidra*). These include: disturbance of any sort, mental upset, digestive problems, pain, fever, restlessness, noise, over-tiredness, acute headache, sudden weather changes, over or inadequate covering of the body, extreme heat or intense cold, humidity, sweating, persistent coughing as well as disturbance of one of the *doshas*. Generally speaking however, insomnia is a *Vata* problem. It is said to be aggravated by wind and constipation, which disturbs *Apana Vata* which then affects the other *Vata*s in the body.

Treatment of insomnia

Ascertaining the underlying cause is the first step towards effective treatment.

- Good nutrition is vital, with plenty of whole foods and fruit, vegetables, nuts and seeds. Junk foods and drinks such as cocoa, chocolate, cola drinks, tea or coffee and fruit squashes (especially ones containing sugar or aspartame) should be avoided.

- Hot drinks of yeast extract will help to boost the B vitamins in the body, and fresh fruit will increase vitamin C, both of which are needed by the nervous system to ensure proper relaxation.

- The last meal of the day is best eaten at least 2 hours before bedtime, as the process of digestion can prevent complete rest.

- Foods containing plenty of calcium, such as parsley, watercress, dried figs, sesame seeds and tahini, may be helpful as they promote relaxation.

- A warm herbal bath before bed with strong infusions or dilute essential oils of limeflower, clary sage, lavender, chamomile, neroli or rose will relax tense muscles and calm an overactive mind.

- Limeflower (*Tilia europea*) makes a relaxing remedy that is pleasant tasting when taken as a tea. It relieves anxiety, calms restless and excitable children and relaxes muscle tension and thereby aids sleep. Taken in hot infusion, limeflowers have a decongestant action, helpful for clearing catarrhal congestion, while the mucilage has a soothing action, relieving irritating, harsh coughs and sore throats, all of which can contribute to sleep problems.

- A cup of tea or 1–2 tsp of tincture (diluted in a little warm water) of limeflower, lavender, chamomile, catnip (*Nepeta cataria*), lemon balm or hops (*Humulus lupulus*) can be given before bed.

- Herb pillows have traditionally been used for sleep problems. Suitable herbs include chamomile, catnip, hops, lavender, lemon balm, limeflowers (*Tilia europea*), orange blossom (*Citrus aurantium*) and sweet woodruff (*Galium odoratum*).

- In a randomized double-blind, controlled clinical trial, a valerian/hops (*Valeriana off./Humulus lupulus*) mixture was as effective as benzodiazepines for non-chronic and non-psychiatric sleep disorders. This herbal mixture also had the advantage of lacking the withdrawal symptoms of benzodiazepine treatment (Schmitz and Jackel 1998).

- For a persistent problem try teas or tinctures of passionflower (*Passiflora incarnata*), wild lettuce (*Lactuca virosa*), wild oats (*Avena sativa*) or skullcap (*Scutellaria laterifolia*) with a little liquorice, before bed. This can be repeated if the child wakes during the night.

• Passionflower is one of the best tranquillizing herbs for chronic insomnia, whether from tension or exhaustion, and relieves many stress-related symptoms. Being both sedative and antispasmodic, it relaxes spasm and tension in the muscles, calms the nerves and lessens pain. Trials have suggested the flavonoids apigenin and chrysin both may mediate anxiolytic effect by means of their action as benzodiazepine receptor ligands (Viola et al 1995, Wolfman et al 1994). Apigenin is also well known for its anti-spasmodic and anti-inflammatory properties (Wren 1988). Passionflower exerts its beneficial effects on the nervous system by improving circulation and nutrition to the nerves. Its cooling properties help relieve symptoms related to excess heat in the system. Its relaxing effects in the chest soothe irritating and nervous coughs, and relieve spasm. It also relieves painful spasm in the gut.

• Giving nervine herbs during the day to a child with insomnia is very helpful as it helps to relax accumulating tension and aid sleep at night. Chamomile, limeflower and skullcap can be given three times daily. Wild oats can be taken in decoction or tincture once daily in the morning. Catnip taken in infusion, or added to bath water, or in a sleep pillow, is particularly useful. Catnip is a tranquillizing herb, helpful for allaying restlessness and anxiety and fear and for preventing nightmares.

• The above herbs can be given nightly until the child develops a good sleeping pattern, after which the dose can gradually be reduced. During this time wild oats, skullcap, vervain and rosemary can be given three times daily if a child becomes run down from poor sleep. Over-tiredness can create a vicious circle and predispose further to insomnia.

• Tapes of stories or soothing music along with relaxation exercises and deep breathing are all helpful in promoting good sleep.

Ayurvedic treatment of insomnia

• According to Ayurveda, drinking warm milk before bed promotes peaceful sleep. Adding ground almonds and a pinch of cardamom or

---

Box 10.1   A traditional sleep recipe

Brahmi (*Bacopa monnieri*) 500 mg
Vacha (*Acorus calamus*) 500 mg
Amla (*Emblica off.*) 1 g
Shankapushpi (*Convolvulus pluricaulis*) 500 mg
Take $\frac{1}{4}-\frac{1}{2}$ tsp three times daily with water or milk

---

nutmeg will help nourish the nervous system and settle the digestion before bed.

• In India a nutmeg paste is used around the eyes and on the forehead to promote sleep. A salve made of nutmeg and ghee applied to the eyelids is also said to induce sleep.

• A dose of $\frac{1}{4}-\frac{1}{2}$ tsp ashwagandha powder taken with raw sugar and ghee at night is traditionally used (Dastur 1983). Ashwagandha is an excellent sedative and nourishing to a depleted nervous system. It is particularly recommended for all problems associated with excess *Vata*.

• A decoction of amalaki, musta (*Cyperus rotundus*), guduchi, brahmi and jatamansi (*Nardostachys jatamansi*) is given for insomnia of any origin.

• Simple brahmi tea has a relaxing effect, calming an agitated mind, and can be given before bed. Equally well it can be mixed in equal parts with bringaraj, jatamansi and shankapushpi (*Convolvulus pluricaulis*). Steep $\frac{1}{4}-\frac{1}{2}$ teaspoonful in $\frac{1}{2}$ cup of hot water for 10 minutes, sweeten with honey if required.

• Draksasava (2–8 tsp at night) is helpful. This is a mildly alcoholic preparation of grapes and spices, sweet and considered ideal for children.

• Amalaki and pomegranate juice is also used.

• A traditional recipe for sleep is shown in Box 10.1 and one of the author's recipes is shown in Box 10.2.

• Oil massage using sesame oil (see p. 84) at night, particularly to head, limbs and soles and instilling oil in ears has a relaxing and calming

Box 10.2   The author's sleep recipe

1 part gotu kola (*Centella asiatica*)
1 part jatamansi (*Nardostachys jatamansi*)
1 part shankapushpi (*Convolvulus pluricauls*)
1 part ashwagandha (*Withania somnifera*)
$\frac{1}{2}$ part cardamom (*Elettaria cardamomum*)
Give $\frac{1}{2}$ tsp of the powder mixture and heat it in
a little warm milk and sweeten with jaggery or
honey, morning and night.

effect, especially for *Vata* children. *Pitta* children are better with sunflower oil, coconut oil and jasmine oil. *Kapha* children can be massaged with corn oil. Massage followed by a warm shower or bath is particularly effective for promoting good sleep.

- Hair oil made from aloe vera juice (kumari) and sesame oil boiled together can be rubbed on the head before bed to calm the mind. Brahmi oil works well when massaged on the soles of the feet and the scalp at bedtime.

- Medicated nose drops (*nasya*) are popular in Ayurvedic medicine for sleeping problems and children respond particularly well to them. Brahmi (*Centella asiatica*) ghee or plain ghee is used; 2–4 drops in each nostril.

NIGHTMARES

Nightmares are common in children up to the age of 12 and tend to occur more in *Vata* predominant children. They are mainly related to fear and anxiety and other psychological stresses. Naturally they can follow exposure to frightening or violent images on TV or in books or disturbing events of the day. *Vata* children tend to be particularly sensitive and their nervous systems easily disturbed.

Nightmares can also be related to digestion, especially to eating too much too close to bedtime. Cheese has a reputation for causing nightmares, probably because it is hard to digest. According to Ayurveda, eating late can leave a residue of heavy food in the stomach at bedtime which blocks the flow of *prana* in the *majja dhatu* (nervous system) (Lad 2002). Children are best eating at least 2 hours prior to going to bed. Other physical causes of nightmares include enlarged adenoids, or catarrh restricting breathing and reducing oxygen to the brain. Lack of fresh air in a room may also be to blame. *Vata* children tend to sleep lightly which means that they are likely to spend more time in REM sleep than other children. They tend to be sensitive to the slightest noise, which can easily bring them into shallow sleep, the realm of nightmares.

Bed wetting is another cause of sleep disturbance, rousing children from a deep sleep. Having said that, nightmares can be experienced by all children and the subject matter of the nightmares can indicate which *dosha* is out of balance. The nightmares of *Vata* children tend to be active or hyperactive. They may have many different dreams in the same night, which are generally forgotten by morning. They dream of running, jumping, moving, travelling and flying and their dreams tend to be fearful, of being chased, attacked, falling from a height or being locked up. The nightmares of *Pitta* children tend to be violent, aggressive and active. They tend to involve school, studying, teachers, competing, failing an exam, coming last in a competition, humiliation, fire, war, fighting and maybe killing. The nightmares of a *Kapha* child tend to be more gentle, calm and romantic. They often involve water, the sea, swimming, gardens, flowers, trees, birds, eating sweets and possibly drowning.

To help prevent nightmares in children their environment needs to be as *Sattvic* as possible. Stories, poems, music, the decoration of their room, all need to feel harmonious to the child. An oil massage to the soles of the feet and the scalp before bed using sesame, brahmi or bringaraj oil will help to relax and reassure the child. Jatamansi (*Nardostachys jatamansi*) and shankapushpi (*Convolvulus pluricaulis*) tea can be given before bed, and a jatamansi sleep pillow will help to promote deep sleep.

In other cultures gypsies use a sprig of rosemary or mugwort (*Artemisia vulgaris*) against nightmares; in Greece basil is popular, and the Moroccans use sprigs of southernwood (*Artemisia abrotanum*).

References

Akhondzadeh S, Naghavi HR, Vazirian M, Shayeganpour A, Rashidi H, Khani M 2001 Passionflower in the treatment of generalized anxiety: a pilot double-blind randomized controlled trial with oxazepam. J Clin Pharm Ther 26(5): 363–367

Athique M 1998 Ayurvedic Anatomy and Physiology. College of Ayurveda, London

Bhatnagar S, Taneja S 2001 Zinc and cognitive development. Br J Nutr 85 (Suppl 2): S139–145

Burgess JR, Stevens L, Zhang W, Peck L 2000 Long-chain polyunsaturated fatty acids in children with attention-deficit hyperactivity disorder. Am J Clin Nutr 71(1 Suppl): 327S–330S

Dastur JF 1983 Everybody's Guide to Ayurvedic Medicine. DB Taraporevala Sons and Co. Private Ltd. Bombay, p. 218

Gaffney BT, Hugel HM, Rich PA 2001 *Panax ginseng* and *Eleutherococcus senticosus* may exaggerate an already existing biphasic response to stress via inhibition of enzymes which limit the binding of stress hormones to their receptors. Med Hypotheses 56(5): 567–572

Harding KL, Judah RD, Gant C 2003 Outcome-based comparison of Ritalin versus food-supplement treated children with AD/HD. Altern Med Rev 8(3): 319–330

Hui KM, Wang XH, Xue H 2000 Interaction of flavones from the roots of *Scutellaria baicalensis* with the benzodiazepine site. Planta Med 66(1): 91–93

Kidd PM 2000 Attention deficit/hyperactivity disorder (ADHD) in children: rationale for its integrative management. Altern Med Rev 5(5): 402–428

Koivumaa-Honkanen H, Honkanen R, Viinamaki H, Heikkila K, Kaprio J, Koskenvuo M 2000 Self-reported life satisfaction and 20-year mortality in healthy Finnish adults. Am J Epidemiol 152(10): 983–991

Kozielec T, Starobrat-Hermelin B 1997 Assessment of magnesium levels in children with attention deficit hyperactivity disorder (ADHD). Magnes Res 10(2): 143–148

Lad V 1999 The Complete Book of Ayurvedic Home Remedies. Judy Piatkus Limited, London

Lad V 2002 Textbook of Ayurveda. The Ayurvedic Press, Albuquerque, New Mexico

Minsky BC 2002 Our Children's Health. Vital Health Publishing, Connecticut

Nocerino E, Amato M, Izzo AA 2000 The aphrodisiac and adaptogenic properties of ginseng. Fitoterapia 71 (Suppl 1): S1–5

Roberts A, Williams JM 1992 The effect of olfactory stimulation on fluency, vividness of imagery and associated mood: a preliminary study. Br J Med Psychol 65 (Pt 2): 197–199

Schmitz M, Jackel M 1998 [Comparative study for assessing quality of life of patients with exogenous sleep disorders (temporary sleep onset and sleep interruption disorders) treated with a hops-valarian preparation and a benzodiazepine drug.] Wien Med Wochenschr 148(13): 291–298

Schnoll R, Burshteyn D, Cea-Aravena J 2003 Nutrition in the treatment of attention-deficit hyperactivity disorder: a neglected but important aspect. Appl Psychophysiol Biofeedback 28(1): 63–75

Tamim H, Musharrafieh U, El Roueiheb Z, Yunis K, Almawi WY 2003 Exposure of children to environmental tobacco smoke (ETS) and its association with respiratory ailments. J Asthma 40(5): 571–576

Thapar A, Fowler T, Rice F, et al 2003 Maternal smoking during pregnancy and attention deficit hyperactivity disorder symptoms in offspring. Am J Psychiatry 160(11): 1985–1989

Tillotson AK, Tillotson NH, Robert A Jr 2001 The One Earth Herbal Sourcebook. Kensington Publishing Corps, New York

US Congress and the Office of Technology Assessment 1990 Neurotoxicity: Identifying and controlling poisons of the nervous system. US Government Printing Office

Viola H, Wasowski C, Levi de Stein M et al 1995 Apigenin, a component of *Matricaria recutita* flowers, is a central benzodiazepine receptor-ligand with anxiolytic effects. Planta Med 61: 213–215

White JF 2003 Intestinal pathophysiology in autism. Exp Biol Med (Maywood) 228(6): 639–649

Wolfman C, Viola H, Paladini A et al 1994 Possible anxiolytic effects of chrysin, a central benzodiazepine receptor ligand isolated from passiflora coerulea. Pharmacol Biochem Behav Jan; 47(1): 1–4

Wolfson P, Hoffmann DL 2003 An investigation into the efficacy of *Scutellaria lateriflora* in healthy volunteers. Altern Ther Health Med 9(2): 74–78

Wren RC 1988 Potter's New Cyclopedia of Botanical Drugs and Preparations. Daniel, London

Chapter 11

The urinary system

CARING FOR THE URINARY TRACT

The urinary system is an elaborate system of filtration that performs the vital task of producing and excreting urine. In so doing it cleanses the body of waste products and toxins and helps to maintain a constant internal environment by governing the water and chemical composition and the acid–alkali balance of the body. The Chinese consider that the kidneys are the seat of vital energy, known as kidney *Jing*, which promotes longevity and immunity. The urinary tract can fall prey to some of the ills of modern living in its eliminative work. Solvents, paint, synthetic fragrances and colours, preservatives and nitrogen waste from a high protein diet (Keville 1996) have to be passed out of the body via urine and all impose a strain on the kidneys and can contribute to urinary problems. To look after their kidneys, children need to be encouraged to drink plenty each day to assist the kidneys in their cleansing work, to flush through toxins and waste products of metabolism and to prevent them from causing irritation of the urinary tract along the way.

There are many herbs that exert their action on the urinary system and these can be used preventatively and therapeutically. Marshmallow (*Althea off.*), corn silk (*Zea mays*), comfrey leaf (*Symphytum officinale*) and oats (*Avena sativa*) all have a demulcent action in the urinary tract. Many of the aromatic herbs that are popular as herbal teas are rich in volatile oils that not only have antimicrobial properties, but also have diuretic action. Thus drinking chamomile, mint, lemon balm, fennel (*Foeniculum vulgare*), rosemary or thyme tea or adding them regularly to diet can work as preventative medicine in the urinary system. Cranberries and bilberries/blueberries are also valuable, helping to prevent pathogenic bacteria from adhering to the walls of the urinary tract and in this way helping to prevent infection. During any kind of infection or inflammatory process, the use of diuretic herbs to increase the flow of urine can help the body to throw off accumulated toxins and debris produced in the system from the immune system's fight against infection and inflammation. Such herbs include celery seed (*Apium graveolens*), cleavers (*Galium aparine*), dandelion leaf, corn silk (*Zea mays*), couch grass (*Agropyron repens*) and uva ursi (*Arctostaphylos uva ursi*).

Ayurvedic approach

Apana Vata is the main seat of *Vata* in the body and governs the function of the urinary system. Anything that disturbs *Vata* can contribute to an interruption of the urinary tract's excretory function and cause pain and is largely responsible for problems such as an irritable bladder and bed wetting in children. When urinary tract infections develop and symptoms present such as pain and burning when passing water, *Pitta* has also become involved.

According to Ayurveda the kidneys are weakened (and *Vata* disturbed) by drinking too much or too little water, drinking excessively cold and iced liquids, cold weather, too much change and travelling, excessive thinking or worry, overuse of antibiotics and not heeding the urge to urinate. Fear and fright damage the kidneys on a psychological level. The kidneys are particularly delicate in sensitive or traumatized children (i.e. *Vata* disturbances). If toxins accumulate in the body, they can lodge themselves in the kidneys and urinary tract, especially if the kidneys are weakened by the above factors, and cause problems such as dysuria and urinary tract infections.

The most popular Ayurvedic remedy for tonifying and strengthening the kidneys is shilajit, a special mineral pitch exuded by various rocks in India. It improves kidney and bladder function, and is said to have antimicrobial properties, to strengthen the nervous system, and help dissolve stones. It can be used for all *doshas* and is an important strengthening and rejuvenative herb. It is used particularly for dysuria, oedema and urinary tract infections.

Other popular remedies for the bladder are gokshura (*Tribulis terrestris*) which is often used with Triphala, purslane (*Portulaca oleracea*) and punarnava (*Boerhavia diffusa*). Ashwagandha regulates *Apana Vata* and makes a valuable adjunct to treatment.

URINARY TRACT INFECTIONS

Urinary tract infections can enter the body via the urethra, then pass into the bladder causing cystitis. From the bladder infection can pass along the ureters to the kidneys and cause pyelonephritis. Other serious kidney infections can develop as secondaries from other childhood infections such as streptococcal throat infection causing tonsillitis. Infections in babies may be related to structural abnormalities, but most often they are caused by *E. coli* bacteria from the bowel that creep round from the anus. Their journey is aided by wiping from back to front rather than vice versa after urination or a bowel movement. Urinary tract infections tend to affect girls more than boys due to their anatomical differences, in that the passage from the urethra to the bladder is much shorter in girls. Vaginal infections such as thrush can also be related to urinary tract infections.

To flush invading bacteria out of the urinary tract drinking plenty of water is always recommended. Herbal teas can be alternated with water and other fluids such as barley water. This can be made by simmering 4 oz/100 g of washed barley in 1 pint/600 ml of water until the barley is soft. This is then strained and a little lemon juice and honey added. Children can drink this lukewarm several times daily.

Treatment of urinary tract infections

- Herbs can also be given to soothe the irritated lining of the urinary tract and help overcome infection. Soothing diuretic herbs such as comfrey leaf (*Symphytum off.*), corn silk (*Zea mays*), marshmallow (*Althea off.*) and couch grass (*Agropyron repens*) given as lukewarm infusions/decoctions will relieve burning and pain on passing water. In acute infections these may need to be given every 2 hours throughout the day.

- These can be combined with anti-inflammatory and antiseptic herbs including fennel (*Foeniculum vulgare*), chamomile, horsetail (*Equisetum arvense*), uva ursi and yarrow.

- Certain herbs such as *Boerhavia* (Abo et al 1999) and uva ursi (*Arctostaphylos uva ursi*), commonly used in urinary tract infections have been proved through research to have antimicrobial properties. Uva ursi contains arbutin which has been found to be effective against *E. coli*, a common UTI pathogen (Siegers et al 2003).

- Infusions/decoctions of these herbs can also be used for hand and foot baths and can be effective used in a shallow bath for the child to sit in for about 10 minutes, two or three times a day.

- If there is accompanying fever and malaise, herbs can be added to teas and hand and foot baths for fever management such as boneset (*Eupatorium perfoliatum*) yarrow, chamomile, elderflowers and limeflowers (*Tilia europea*).

- Cranberry juice has received some attention as a treatment for urinary tract infections. Cochrane reviews indicate that there is evidence for its effectiveness in preventing urinary tract infection (Griffiths 2003). Cranberry juice, sweetened with passionfruit/apple juice (not sugar), can be given regularly to counteract infection. It does this in two ways: firstly by making the urine too acid for bacteria like *E. coli* to survive; secondly (as mentioned above) by stopping bacteria from adhering to the walls of the urinary tract. It may be difficult to drink sufficient amounts of cranberry juice to be an effective deterrent to infection (the normal recommended dose is 3–6 fl oz daily or $1\frac{1}{2}$ oz of the berries) and concentrated extracts in the form of tablets may prove more effective.

Should urinary problems start after a course or regular treatment with antibiotics giving probiotics containing *Lacto-acidophilus* to re-establish normal bacterial population of the gut may be a valuable adjunct to herbal treatment.

Ayurvedic approach

Dysuria or scanty, painful and difficult urination can occur with or without an accompanying infection. It can be caused by disturbance of any of the three *doshas*.

Vata type is characterized by severe pain in the lower back, rectum and urinary channel. Urination will be frequent but scanty, with strangury and sharp or colicky pain. There may be constipation, insomnia and other *Vata* symptoms including mental agitation.

Pitta type is characterized by yellow or strong-smelling urine, urination is frequent, often profuse, with burning. There may be fever, irritability and other *Pitta* symptoms.

Kapha type is characterized by pale or milky urine, feeling of heaviness in the lower abdomen and dull pain in the kidney area.

- For all three *doshas* barley water is generally recommended as well as $\frac{1}{2}$ tsp of gokshura powder with honey, twice daily. Gokshura (*Tribulis terrestris*) is considered the best general diuretic and its tonic properties to the kidneys prevent it from aggravating *Vata*.

- For *Vata* type: A *Vata* reducing diet is recommended and demulcent, diuretic herbs can be given to soothe irritated mucous membranes and enhance urination. These include gokshura, bala, purslane (*Portulaca oleracea*), fresh holy basil juice, and marshmallow root (*Althea off*.). Traditional formulas used in India include Gokshuradi guggul and Chandraprabha tablets, three times daily. An infusion (pour boiling water over herbs and leave to infuse for 4 hours) of sesame seeds and liquorice taken in small quantities sipped throughout the day has a soothing and relaxing effect. Rubbing sesame oil over the abdomen is also recommended.

- For *Pitta* type: A *Pitta* reducing diet is recommended avoiding spices, oils and sour fruit. Cooling diuretics such as gokshura, punarnava (*Boerhavia diffusa*), amalaki juice with raw sugar or sugarcane juice, and bringaraj root, sandalwood with rice water, honey and sugar (Dastur 1983, p. 263), decoction of raisins, juice of watermelon with a little raw sugar and cumin seeds are also used. Chandanadi is a popular formula, the main constituent of which is sandalwood (*Santalum album*). Gotu kola can be used to soothe pain.

- For *Kapha* type: An anti-*Kapha* diet is recommended, avoiding cold drinks, fruit juice, dairy products, oils and fats. Warming spices and diuretics are indicated such as cinnamon, juniper berries (*Juniperus communis*), coriander seed, celery seed (*Apium graveolens*) and fennel (*Foeniculum vulgare*). Formulas include trikatu and chandanadi.

IRRITABLE BLADDER

For an irritable bladder a paste is made in India from amalaki and saffron with rose water and applied over the pubic region (Dastur 1983, p. 269). A milk decoction of gokshura or shatavari and gokshura is also used. Gokshura guggul is also effective.

Ayurvedic treatment of urinary tract infections

- To relieve symptoms of urinary tract infections the main herb used is gokshura.
- Turmeric, shilajit, pomegranate (*Punica granatum*), amalaki, varuna (*Crataeva nurvala*) and guduchi can also provide relief.
- Tillotson quotes a clinical trial in India using varuna (*Crataeva nurvala*). Of 84 patients studied, with urinary tract infections accompanied by dysuria, 55% were cured, 40% showed improvement, with a 5% failure rate (Pramod 1982, cited by Tillotson et al 2001).

Pitta:

- Since acute infections are usually due to *Pitta*, to treat them effectively children need to follow an anti-*Pitta* diet, avoiding all spices (except coriander), and all nightshades particularly tomatoes.

- Guduchi is one of the main anti-*Pitta* herbs cooling heat and inflammation. One to two ounces of fresh juice is taken with honey or milk three times daily. In this instance I use $\frac{1}{2}$ tsp of the powder similarly.

- Sandalwood is also used for *Pitta* conditions with burning urination. It cools heat and has antimicrobial properties. It is often used as sandalwood compound (Chandanadi churna), which includes sandalwood, fennel, long pepper, long pepper root, black pepper and cloves. Its properties are diuretic, alterative, febrifuge and urinary antiseptic. It is generally taken in doses of 1–4 g, 2–3 times per day in water or warm milk.

- Amalaki with turmeric powder and honey can be taken in warm water.

- Triphala powder with ghee and honey will clear toxins and help resolve infection.

- Hot milk with ghee and raw sugar, and sandalwood powder with rice water and raw sugar followed by a drink of warm milk are reputed to bring fast relief in urinary problems such as cystitis.

- Rasayana churna is a powder containing guduchi, gokshura and amalaki which can be taken in warm water. I have used this in my practice with success on numerous occasions.

- Other useful remedies include shilajit, coriander, lemon grass (*Cymbopogon* spp.), fennel seed and punarnava (*Boerhavia diffusa*).

- Cranberry, coconut or pomegranate juice can be added to diet to soothe and flush out the urinary tract.

- Cucumber juice mixed with honey and fresh lime is a traditional home remedy for cystitis.

- Sandalwood powder mixed with 1tsp of celery seed in a glass of water.

- Half a glass of barley gruel with half a glass of buttermilk.

- The juice of half a lime.

These are all considered excellent diuretics to cool heat and inflammation.

Vata:

Vata urinary tract infections tend to be chronic, low grade and irregular.

- A *Vata* reducing diet should be followed.
- Herbs should be taken to tonify the kidneys such as ashwagandha, bala and shatavari along with mild diuretics such as lemon grass and/or coriander seed.
- Gokshura guggul is also used in *Vata* cases.

Kapha:

For *Kapha* treatment, a *Kapha* reducing diet is recommended avoiding dairy products and fats.

- Helpful herbs include cinnamon, juniper berries and parsley as tea.
- Anti-*Kapha* formulas such as trikatu can be taken along with shilajit.

BED WETTING

Bed wetting that occurs in a child older than 4 or 5 years who has already developed bladder control is frequently related to stress. It could be jealousy of a new baby, anxiety about moving house, changing school, trouble with schoolwork, teachers, peers, upset over family discord or anything else that causes stress, over-excitement, insecurity or unhappiness. A child who wets the bed will need plenty of reassurance from parents rather than reprimanding for something they cannot help and probably find humiliating. Fear of others outside the family being aware of the problem and of the social isolation this could mean becomes a stress in itself, which can exacerbate the problem.

If a child has never developed proper bladder control, it may be that nerves and muscles governing bladder function are not yet mature enough. Once a child is over 4 years and still wetting the bed regularly there may be underlying causes that require addressing. These include structural abnormality, diabetes, chronic urinary infection, dietary deficiency (particularly of calcium and magnesium), overuse of refined foods and sugar, over-sensitivity to food additives or chemicals in drinking water or food allergy. Some children tend to wet the bed more if they get cold, so parents need to ensure they are well covered at night in bed and put extra night clothes on them if they habitually kick off the bedcovers in their sleep.

Treatment of bed wetting

- Infusions of horsetail (*Equisetum arvense*) St John's wort (*Hypericum perforatum*) or corn silk (*Zea mays*) can be given through the day, to soothe an irritated bladder and to encourage normal nervous control of the bladder.

- A recent Cochrane Review indicates that tricyclic antidepressants such as imipramine are effective in treating nocturnal enuresis, though have a far higher rate of relapse compared to alarm type treatments (Glazener et al 2003). St John's Wort is an effective alternative to imipramine (Schulz 2002) and a well-established remedy for bed wetting and thus can offer a possible adjunct to treatment should behavioural and dietary measures not be effective.

- Other useful herbs include agrimony (*Agrimonia eupatoria*), American cranesbill (*Geranium maculatum*), herb Robert (*Geranium robertanum*), ladies mantle (*Alchemilla vulgaris*) and parsley.

- Plantain leaf tea or plantain leaf glycerite can be taken 2–3 times during the day as a general urinary tissue tonic.

- When bed wetting can be related to anxiety or stress, relaxing herbs like lemon balm, skullcap (*Scutellaria laterifolia*), vervain (*Verbena off.*) and wild oats (*Avena sativa*) can be added to the remedy.

- Hypericum oil can be massaged into the lower spine and abdomen when settling the child down for sleep.

- Chamomile oil can also be soothing; 2 drops of chamomile oil can be added to a teaspoon of St John's Wort oil.

- Broad-spectrum mineral deficiencies may be involved in bed wetting, including zinc, selenium and copper. Calcium and magnesium are essential for proper nerve and muscle function and it is worth giving a child mineral and trace element supplements before bed. Sesame seeds are high in calcium and may prove helpful.

- On a psychological level children benefit from encouragement and being rewarded for each dry bed. Parental or peer pressure on the child may only serve to aggravate the problem. Giving children drinks at night should obviously be avoided.

Ayurvedic approach

Herbs are given to balance *Vata*, to strengthen the nervous system and the urinary tract.

- Shilajit is a popular remedy. For children younger than 5 years, quarter of a gram is given twice daily, mixed with milk on an empty stomach. For children up to age 15, half a gram is given twice daily. A much-used Ayurvedic formula containing shilajit is Chandraprabha. Children of about 5 years are given half a tablet in the morning and another half in the evening on an empty stomach with half a cup of milk. Children over 10 years of age can take one full tablet, twice daily with milk.

- Sesame seeds (1tsp) are given to children to chew at night presumably for their calcium content but also because sesame is a major remedy used to balance *Vata*.

- A warm sesame oil massage at night followed by a warm bath can be effective in promoting good sleep and uninterrupted by enuresis.

References

Abo KA, Ashidi JS 1999 Antimicrobial screening of *Bridelia micrantha, Alchornea cordifolia* and *Boerhavia diffusa*. Afr J Med Med Sci 28(3–4): 167–169

Dastur JF 1983 Everybody's Guide to Ayurvedic Medicine. DB Taraporevala Sons & Co. Private Ltd, Bombay

Glazener CM, Evans JH, Peto RE 2003 Tricyclic and related drugs for nocturnal enuresis in children. Cochrane Database Syst Rev (3): CD002117

Griffiths P 2003 The role of cranberry juice in the treatment of urinary tract infections. Br J Community Nurs 8(12): 557–561

Keville K 1996 Herbs for Health and Healing. Rodale Press, Inc, Pennsylvania

Schulz V 2002 Clinical trials with hypericum extracts in patients with depression – results, comparisons, conclusions for therapy with antidepressant drugs. Phytomedicine 9(5): 468–474

Siegers C, Bodinet C, Ali SS, Siegers CP 2003 Bacterial deconjugation of arbutin by *Escherichia coli*. Phytomedicine 10 (Suppl 4): 58–60

Tillotson AK, Tillotson NH, Robert A Jr 2001 The One Earth Herbal Sourcebook. Kensington Publishing Corps, New York

Chapter **12**

The skin

CHAPTER CONTENTS

THE FUNCTIONS OF THE SKIN

The skin is wonderfully designed to fulfil many different functions. It affords protection to the body against infection, pollution, extremes of temperature and climate, sunlight and physical injury. Antiseptic substances are secreted by the skin to ward off potential pathogens, and beneficial bacteria on the skin act as a back up in defence, inhibiting any proliferation of unfavourable micro-organisms. When the weather is cold blood vessels in the skin constrict to keep the heat inside the body and when it is hot, blood vessels dilate to bring blood to the surface allowing the body to loose heat and maintain its optimum temperature.

With its several million sweat glands, the skin is also a major organ of excretion. Sweat contains water, mineral salts, nitrogenous wastes and other toxins and is similar in content to urine. Not only does the skin aid elimination of wastes and toxins, it also prevents the loss of vital body fluids and thereby helps the kidneys' work in maintaining the correct water and electrolyte balance in the body. This eliminative pathway can be used therapeutically when necessary. Herbal diaphoretics such as chamomile, catnip (*Nepeta cataria*), limeflowers (*Tilia europea*), yarrow, lemon balm (*Melissa officinalis*) and basil taken in warm infusion will increase perspiration by stimulating blood flow to the skin and thereby help to clear waste products from the body, as well as relieve fevers during infections.

Sweat also forms a protective acid mantle, which acts to inhibit the growth of harmful micro-organisms. If children do not regularly take sufficient exercise to produce a sweat, this can increase the burden on the other eliminative pathways, the lungs, bowels and kidneys. It is important to the health and balance of the skin that its mantle is not disturbed by overuse of creams, moisturizers, deodorants, perfumes and cosmetics that contain substances that could be harmful such as mineral oils, petroleum, nitrates, ammonia, artificial colours and fragrances. Biological washing powders can also cause problems.

As a sense organ, the skin is richly supplied with nerve endings, which carry messages to the brain about the environment, heat or cold, pleasure or pain. Not only this, but the skin also relays messages from inside out and reflects how we feel physically and emotionally. The pale pinched face of an anxious child, the rosy lustre of a happy care-free child, the glow on the cheeks of a healthy child and the sallow complexion of a sick child, can speak volumes about a patient before the consultation formally begins.

The many skin problems that are seen in children can reflect both their reaction to their outer environment and their inner state. Rashes and eczema for instance, may be related to contact with outside allergens, micro-organisms, chemicals, sunlight, pollutants, etc. or may be related to tension, anxiety, grief or fear. The skin's ability to deal with potential irritant factors depends to some extent on the nutrients brought to the skin by the underlying blood vessels and ultimately from the digestive tract. Deficiencies of minerals, vitamins, essential fatty acids and trace elements can impair the skin's natural defences and predispose to a variety of skin disorders. A healthy skin does not develop a fungal infection because its local immune mechanisms are able to inhibit fungal growth. On the other hand impaired skin function will prevent local defence mechanisms from resolving the infection without treatment. A healthy skin also depends on blood flow bringing nutrients to the skin and carrying away the waste products of metabolism. Poor circulation or a state of toxicity of the blood contributes significantly to skin problems.

AYURVEDIC PERSPECTIVE ON SKIN PROBLEMS

In the treatment of skin conditions I have found an Ayurvedic perspective of enormous help. If one can broadly categorize skin problems into three types, *Vata*, *Pitta* and *Kapha*, then the treatment is fairly straightforward and generally works well. It is not hard to see how most skin problems fall easily into these categories: dry, itchy, scaly skin, aggravated by cold and stress (*Vata*); hot inflammatory or infected conditions, aggravated by heat and heating foods, reflecting a state of heat and toxicity in the body (*Pitta*); and cool, itchy clammy, oozing skin problems aggravated by cold, damp weather and dairy products and sugar (*Kapha*). However, skin diseases tend to be more common in *Pitta* types as *Pitta* can overheat the blood and predispose to toxic conditions that are expressed through the skin. Factors causing *Pitta* skin problems include incorrect diet, overuse of sour, salty or pungent tastes, heavy, sweet or oily foods, over-exposure to the elements and overuse of cosmetics, perfumes, synthetic creams, etc.

Pitta skin conditions are accompanied by heat and often by infection and irritability. They are aggravated by heat and exposure to the sun and application of most oils. *Vata* skin problems are associated with distension, gas or constipation. They are aggravated by wind and dryness and relieved by the application of oils, especially sesame. *Kapha* skin problems are often accompanied by mucous congestion, lethargy and sluggish metabolism. They are aggravated by cold and damp and application of oils tends to aggravate (Frawley 2000, p. 219).

The skin relates to the plasma (*rasa dhatu*), and to the blood (*rakta dhatu*). Skin diseases, therefore, relate to the lungs and the liver (see *Dhatus*, p. 73). For this reason the use of expectorants and diaphoretics to cleanse the lungs, and alteratives and bitter tonics to cleanse the liver, are important in the treatment of skin conditions (Frawley 2000, p. 218).

For general treatment of skin problems, useful herbs include turmeric, barberry root bark (*Berberis vulgaris*), sandalwood and guggul for acute cases. For chronic cases, tonic herbs such as bala, liquorice root, shatavari and gokshura (*Tribulus terrestris*) are recommended, once diet and gently detoxifying herbs have been used and the tongue is clean. Turmeric with its effective anti-inflammatory action is one of the best herbs for all skin problems and has received much research for its multitude of properties. A key constituent, curcumin, has been shown to have anti-inflammatory, antibacterial and antioxidant effects (Araujo and Leon 2001) whilst combined curcuminoids appear to help protect epidermal skin cells from free radical stress (Bonte et al 1997). Being a polyphenol, the compound curcumin stabilizes collagen (Landis and Khalsa 1998, p. 342).

Turmeric is in fact good for all connective tissue. A number of trials have investigated using turmeric or its constituents in treating cancer – a small trial testing the effect of a curcumin ointment on 62 patients with external cancerous lesions reported promising results in reducing symptoms and some reduction in lesion size (Kuttan et al 1987). Turmeric can be used both orally and topically. It is used to enhance healing after surgery, it reduces adhesions and minimizes scar formation, possibly by reducing over-proliferation of fibroblasts (Phan et al 2003). It is particularly applicable in the treatment of inflammatory skin problems such as eczema and herpes since it reduces heat and cleanses the liver. It also has healing properties and acts as a good insecticidal remedy (see Scabies, p. 281).

Ghee is considered excellent for external use in skin problems such as rashes and burns. In India it is prepared by placing ghee in a copper vessel with half the amount of water to ghee. It is kept for a month, stirring occasionally with a copper spoon. Ghee prepared in this way is considered much more absorbable by the skin. Aloe vera gel is another beneficial application for most skin problems, as is the juice of coriander leaves. Saffron is a specific herb used in India for nourishing the skin and is taken internally as a milk decoction, 5–10 stigmas (threads) to one cup, and also used in external skin preparation (Frawley 2000) (not suitable for children under 2).

For treatment of *Pitta* skin problems: children should follow an anti-*Pitta* diet, avoiding possible allergens such as dairy produce, vegetables from the nightshade family, as well as oranges, peaches and strawberries. Drinking coconut juice is helpful along with coriander leaf juice.

Exposure to sun and heat is best avoided as far as possible. Useful oils for external application include coconut oil, brahmi, bhringaraj. Aloe vera gel and rosewater applied to the skin will cool heat. Bitter cleansing herbs such as burdock root, red clover (*Trifolium pratense*), guduchi, manjishta and laxative herbs such as dandelion root and Triphala can be helpful.

> For treatment of *Vata* skin problems: children should follow an anti-*Vata* diet. Laxative herbs and enema therapy are generally used, followed by *Vata* soothing herbs such as bala. Triphala powder mixed in warm water or 1–2 Triphala guggul capsules can be given before bed. Soothing oils such as sesame can be applied to the skin.
>
> For treatment of *Kapha* skin problems: children should follow an anti-*Kapha* diet, avoiding all heavy, greasy and oily food, particularly cheese and yoghurt. No oils should be used externally. Diuretic herbs such as dandelion leaf or root are useful. 1–2 Triphala guggul capsules can be given before bed. A formula called Gokshura guggul is also used with warm water or ginger tea (Frawley 2000). Neem oil used in ointments on the skin is often effective.

One of the first signs of skin problems is dryness and lack of lustre, which reflects an impairment of skin function. I have found that regular massage using oils as in the Ayurvedic tradition helps to keep the skin in good condition. Sesame oil is particularly indicated in dry skin and coconut oil for a tendency to heat and inflammation.

ECZEMA

The herbal preparations that are best suited to the treatment of eczema depend on the type of eczema involved. Atopic eczema can develop when a baby is a few months old, particularly around the time of the introduction of solid food, and may indicate a clear relationship to certain foods. Introducing solid food too early before a baby is 4 months can often be a contributory factor, as the immature digestion of the baby is not able to digest the food properly. It is common for this type of eczema to be followed by other atopic symptoms such as asthma and hayfever.

Atopic eczema can be triggered by a number of different foods, including dairy produce, eggs, wheat and citrus fruits (Schnyder and Pichler 1999). Other foods which often affect eczema include:

- tomatoes,
- blackcurrant,
- sugar,
- chocolate,
- food additives,
- yeast extract,
- pork,
- beef,
- nightshades and nuts.

It can also be triggered by external irritants such as biological washing powders, chlorine in swimming pools, perfumes, wool and animal dander. Emotional upset or stress of any kind can cause or aggravate the condition by further inhibiting proper digestion and affecting the efficiency of the immune system. An eruption of the skin may be a means of emotional expression. The emotional aspect in eczema is well documented; in one survey 40 eczema patients were investigated using a standard personality test and compared to normal controls. The paper concluded that eczema patients tend to have higher levels of anxiety and greater problems dealing with anger and hostility (White et al 1990).

Breast milk contains many substances vital to normal development and function of a child's immune system, including gamma linoleic acid. Breast-feeding is particularly important for babies with a family history of eczema, asthma or hayfever, as even one exposure to cow's milk formula can set off an allergic response. Recent studies continue to point out the critical nature of a patient's nutritional status in helping to determine important health outcomes in paediatrics. Recent data concerning the composition of breast milk and its adequacy to support infant growth in the first 6 months of life, as well as trials that support breast-feeding, show the importance of breast-feeding to delay or reduce the incidence of atopic diseases such as eczema, allergies, and asthma, concluding that eczema tends to occur more in bottle-fed babies or children than those who were breast-fed (Fulhan et al 2003).

The severity of problems in babies and children related to cow's milk produce, tends to be underestimated. Not only can it frequently cause skin problems but also inflammatory bowel problems and respiratory airway inflammation. When a child is fighting an infection such as a cold or cough, the extra workload of the immune system may cause the eczema to worsen. Vaccinations have a tendency to aggravate eczema as they put further stress upon the immune system.

Seborrhoeic eczema occurs in the areas of the skin richly supplied with sebaceous glands such as the scalp (particularly in small babies; see cradle cap, p. 144), as well as the eyelashes and eyelids, the external ear canal, around the ear, nose and groin. There can be small bubbles just beneath the skin that can burst to produce a weeping rash which then forms dry crusts, or there may be a dry, scaly red rash, which can be intensely itchy.

If the skin is particularly dry it can crack and bleed. In longstanding eczema there is often dry, scaly, hard and thickened skin. Scratching of the skin by the child can introduce infection such as *herpes* and *Staphylococcus* into broken skin causing further inflammation. Where eczema occurs in the nappy area it is particularly prone to secondary thrush infection.

The time of year can also affect eczema. A survey of 506 patients found that there was a tendency for deterioration in the condition in winter and improvement in summer (Imai et al 1997). Dry itchy eczema in particular can be worse in winter, perhaps due to the dryness of centrally heated houses, lack of circulation and air to the skin and heavy winter clothes. Those children who tend to feel the cold may have poor circulation to their skin. Their skin will not be so well nourished and healthy as the skin of children with good circulation. Children who tend to overheat may have a tendency to excrete more toxins via sweat through the skin. Their skin problems tend to be worse during hot weather.

Eczema can be related not only to inherited susceptibility but also to deficiencies of certain nutrients that are vital for the immune system. It may often be related to a disturbance of the metabolism of essential fatty acids (Horrobin 2000). This can be linked to over-consumption of saturated fats and refined oils, sugar and food additives which interfere with EFA metabolism and lack of the right balance of omega 6 and omega 3 fatty acids in the diet. Deficiencies of zinc, B vitamins, calcium and magnesium and beta carotene can also be involved.

When considering cause and treatment of eczema, as all skin disease, the importance of good diet, efficient digestion and elimination of wastes via the bowels is of prime importance. Atopic conditions can be related to disturbance of the gut flora or chronic intestinal infections. The use of antibiotics, feeding with formula milk or a history of gut infection may be implicated.

Treatment of eczema

When treating atopic eczema, identification of dietary allergens and their temporary removal from the child's diet allows time for underlying causes to be addressed. Once there is an improvement in the skin, the foods can gradually be reintroduced. Where there is a familial tendency to allergy, the digestive and immune systems will need to be treated on a long-term basis, particularly by providing nutritional support through a healthy diet. Supplements may be useful until the skin improves, including vitamins B and C, multi-vitamins and -minerals, and evening primrose oil (see Immune System, p. 150). The use of probiotics which helps to re-establish a normal bacterial population of the gut can often be helpful.

If there is evidence of stress/emotional upset this may require the help of family support, or counselling. A child with eczema may be calling out for more love and attention, or reassurance during times of change or upheaval. A child with bad eczema may be singled out or teased at school and this may aggravate the problem and ideally requires sensitive handling by parents and teachers alike. Herbs for the nervous system (see p. 252) may well be indicated here.

The herbs chosen in the treatment of a child will vary from one child to another and choice relies on the taking of a thorough case history to enable an understanding of underlying causes.

- Generally speaking the state of digestion and elimination is addressed using digestive or mild laxative herbs as applicable (see Digestive System, p. 209).

- Herbs to support the immune system and reduce inflammation including chamomile, echinacea, nettles, red clover (*Trifolium pratense*) and yarrow, can be combined with herbs to support the adrenal glands such as liquorice and wild yam (*Dioscorea villosa*) which are particularly helpful if trying to reduce the use of steroid creams.

- Herbs to cool heat and clear toxins either via liver, kidneys or bowels can be effective, particularly where signs of inflammation occur. Burdock, fumitory (*Fumaria off.*), rose, chamomile, chickweed (*Stellaria media*), coriander leaf, nettles, dandelion root and leaf, red clover (*Trifolium pratense*) and heartease (*Viola tricolor*) are all applicable. Chickweed is an excellent cooling remedy for hot inflammatory skin conditions such as eczema, heat rashes, urticaria, sunburn, boils and spots. Its soothing properties can be helpful in associated hot inflammatory problems such as gastritis, colitis, acid indigestion and irritable bowel syndrome. Its diuretic properties help to clear the skin by aiding elimination of toxins from the body via the kidneys.

- For eczema associated with stress or anxiety, herbs can be added to a prescription to support the nervous system such as lemon balm, chamomile, skullcap (*Scutellaria laterifolia*), vervain (*Verbena off.*) or wild oats (*Avena sativa*).

Herbs to treat eczema are better given as teas rather than as tinctures.

Local applications

External preparations can be applied to help resolve inflammation and infection and to restore normal skin function. A recent double-blind trial of liquorice gel found it effective for atopic dermatitis (Saeedi et al 2003), whilst a preparation "Kamillosan" containing chamomile has been found to be slightly superior to 0.5% hydrocortisone in treating medium-degree atopic eczema (Patzelt-Wenczler and Ponce-Poschl 2000).

To moisten dry skin sesame oil or almond oil with a few drops of essential oil of chamomile or neem oil can be applied where there is inflammation. Two drops of oil can be added to 5 ml of base oil to massage into the skin or as a bath oil. Evening primrose oil, vitamin E oil or aloe vera gel can also be applied.

Alan Tillotson recommends a combination of olive oil and aloe vera gel as an emollient as well as castor oil and witch hazel (Tillotson et al 2001).

If the skin is weeping or infected:

- Rosewater with a pinch of turmeric can be applied.
- A strong infusion of *Calendula* flowers can be used in the bath or applied as a compress or lotion several times daily to the affected area.

- Other herbs suitable for washes or compresses include burdock, chickweed (*Stellaria media*), golden seal (*Hydrastis canadensis*), elderflower, yellow dock root (*Rumex crispus*).
- Chickweed can be used in an infusion, as a lotion or made into ointments and creams.
- Aloe vera juice with a little turmeric powder is also very effective.
- Turmeric is an excellent anti-inflammatory remedy and has effective antimicrobial properties $\frac{1}{2}$ –1 tsp stirred into a cup of hot water can be used as a lotion 2–3 times daily.
- Distilled witch hazel is cooling and can be applied to unbroken skin to speed healing.

A variety of herbs can be incorporated into creams and ointments and applied to the skin. Water-based creams are better for hot/weeping eczema while more oily ointments will retain moisture in more dry, scaly and itchy skin. A simple cream can be made using aqueous cream or a natural cream base into which can be stirred a strong infusion (i.e. double normal strength) of any of the above herbs, or a few drops of chamomile or neem oil. Use 3–5 drops of essential oil per 50 ml of cream base and 1 ml of neem oil.

Sleeping can be a problem if the skin is particularly itchy because eczema often gets worse at night when a child is tired. If a child becomes tired and run down through lack of sleep, this will only make matters worse (see Herbs for the Nervous System, p. 252).

Ayurvedic approach to eczema

Eczema or "*vicharchika*", is a form of "*kushta*". It is primarily caused by aggravation of *Kapha* and secondary involvement of *Vata* and *Pitta*. In fact simultaneous excesses of all three *doshas* are involved in all forms of skin disease, but some *doshas* are predominant for each variety. The *dosha* that is predominant is balanced first and then the other *doshas* are treated afterwards.

- *Vata* type: The skin tends to be rough, dry, hard, itchy and scaly. There may be associated constipation, wind and distension. The skin is aggravated by cold, wind, dryness and stress.

- *Pitta* type: There tends to be burning, redness, oozing, swelling and infection, which can be associated with fever, irritability and a feeling of heat. The skin is aggravated by heat and oil.
- *Kapha* type: The skin tends to be cold, raised, sticky, oozing, swollen and itchy, and associated with a pale complexion. It is aggravated by cold, damp and oil.

For general treatment of eczema tepid decoctions of sariva (*Hemidesmus indicus*), turmeric, manjishta, gokshura (*Tribulus terrestris*), Triphala, bringharaj, gotu kola and sandalwood (*Santalum album*) are recommended for internal use. Useful formulae include: Triphala guggulu, nimbadi churna, manjishtarishta and sarivadiarishta.

Tea or juice of tulsi leaves can be taken internally and used externally to bathe the skin (Rai 2000, p. 93).

Local applications

- Neem oil (see p. 272).
- Karanja oil (from the seeds of *Pongamia pinnata*).
- The affected area can be cleaned daily with warm water boiled with neem bark. After this a paste of neem bark can be applied over it and allowed to dry, or neem oil can be used.
- Turmeric is an excellent remedy, either used externally on affected areas mixed with aloe vera gel and internally $\frac{1}{2}$ tsp of turmeric powder can be given twice daily in milk.
- If the child is constipated use $\frac{1}{2}$ tsp of Triphala powder in $\frac{1}{2}$ cup warm water at night.

Diet

Children with skin problems are advised to avoid sour and salty foods as well as dairy produce, yoghurt or curd. Bitter foods like bitter gourd and drumstick and neem flowers are recommended.

Vata type eczema

A *Vata* reducing diet and lifestyle is recommended (see Principles of Ayurveda, p. 63) as well as regular sesame oil massage. If a child is constipated castor oil laxative or enemas can be administered. Nourishing and cleansing herbs including: Triphala,

guggulu (*Commiphora mukul*), shatavari, and cardamom can be taken internally. A prescription containing chitrak (*Plumbago zeylanica*), guduchi, cardamom and punarnava (*Boerhavia diffusa*) mixed with $\frac{1}{4}$ yoghurt and $\frac{3}{4}$ water is also used.

Medicated ghee can be used internally and externally. Useful herbs for medicating the ghee include Triphala, musta (*Cyperus rotundus*), manjishta, gokshura, chitrak, neem, guduchi, cardamom, punarnava, and calamus root. Traditionally, decoctions of Trikatu and Triphala, mixed with cane sugar and sesame oil are taken for 1 month. These decoctions are also mixed with sesame oil and applied topically.

Pitta type eczema

A *Pitta* reducing diet and lifestyle is recommended as well as cleansing the bowels using Triphala powder or capsules given at night before bed. Nightshade foods, oranges, peaches and strawberries, sour and hot spicy foods are best avoided.

Recommended herbs for internal use include: gotu kola, chirata (*Swertia chireta*), aloe vera juice, manjishta and amalaki. Gotu kola is a herb I use frequently in the treatment of a range of different skin problems. By increasing the microcirculation to the skin it brings nutrients and carries away toxins and wastes and in this way helps resolve inflammation and improve skin function. Bitter and astringent herbs such as guduchi, kutki (*Picrorrhiza kurroa*), kushta (*Saussurea lappa*), musta (*Cyperus rotundus*), neem and sandalwood (*Santalum album*) are particularly indicated. The above bitter herbs can be mixed with ghee to be taken as medicated ghee paste. Sandalwood and barley decoction also cool *Pitta*.

Helpful therapies for external application include: coconut juice, aloe vera gel, coriander leaf juice, gotu kola oil and bringharaj oil. Sandalwood in oils, creams, or the powder made into a paste has a cooling anti-inflammatory effect. I use a cream that contains sandalwood, neem and turmeric which is effective. Baths with herbs of musta, bakuchi (*Psoralea corylifolia*) and the formula Triphala can be useful. For inflamed or hot, burning skin problems, application of a lotion containing a Triphala decoction mixed with sandalwood, pippali, turmeric, musta, red sandalwood, liquorice root, vatsaka (*Ashatoda vasika*) and ghee is also used.

Kapha type eczema

A *Kapha* reducing diet and lifestyle is recommended. In India emetic therapy is used as first treatment. In the West expectorant herbs such as thyme, elecampane (*Inula helenium*) or hyssop (*Hyssopus officinalis*) may be used instead. Heavy, greasy and oily foods including cheese, yoghurt and oil massage should be avoided. Useful herbs for internal use include: gokshura (*Tribulus terrestris*), guggulu (*Commiphora mukul*), Triphala, manjishta, ginger, chitrak (*Plumbago zeylanica*) guduchi, cardamom, kushta (*Saussurea lappa*) gotu kola and punarnava (*Boerhavia diffusa*).

Chitrak, guduchi, cardamom and punarnava mixed with $\frac{1}{4}$ yoghurt and $\frac{3}{4}$ water, are also used internally.

Decoctions of Trikatu, Triphala, cane sugar and sesame oil are taken internally for a month. These decoctions are also mixed with sesame oil and applied topically. Siddhartha (mustard) is said to be effective used externally for weeping eczema. It is often combined with snuhi (*Euphorbia nerifolia*) in the form of a paste along with internal administration of khadir (*Acacia catechu*).

URTICARIA/HIVES

The characteristic raised skin wheals are caused by an allergic response, generally triggered by certain foods or medicines such as citrus fruit, milk produce, strawberries, chocolate, tomatoes, fish (especially shellfish), foods high in salicylates, nuts, artificial colourings, aspirin and penicillin. Urticaria can sometimes result from contact with substances such as animal dander, pollen, chemicals, foodstuffs, plants, creams and insect stings.

Research has emphasized the importance of food as a major factor in the aetiopathogenesis of atopic dermatitis (Oehling et al 1997). Another food allergen study (looking into the prevalence of IgE antibodies which are a classic sign of food allergy) in patients with chronic urticaria found that it was linked to food allergies (Kaeser et al 1994). The effect of antigens remains dormant until heat, pressure or other stimuli excite a reaction. The underlying causes of urticaria may be related to the condition of the digestive tract. Disturbance of the bacterial flora or chronic intestinal infections can be implicated. In some cases

skin eruptions can appear and disappear within a few hours of exposure to the allergen, and it is quite clear which substance the child is reacting to. However, some children have frequent bouts of hives, which can last for 5–6 weeks and make it harder to identify the allergen for a swift resolution of the problem. For effective treatment of urticaria it is important to identify the allergen and remove it, but if the bout is longlasting there may be more than one substance involved or there may be an underlying bowel problem or systemic candidiasis, requiring thorough treatment of the digestive tract. The digestive tract is very much influenced by a child's emotional state and digestive function clearly inhibited by anxiety and stress. In a study of 236 patients with chronic urticaria, stress and other psychological factors were found to be an important primary cause (Murray and Pizzorna 2001).

Treatment of urticaria

- The first consideration in treatment is to address underlying problems relating to stress (see Nervous System, p. 246) and digestion (see Digestive System, p. 194). Herbs for the nervous system, include chamomile, lemon balm, skullcap (*Scutellaria laterifolia*) and vervain (*Verbena off.*) and useful digestive herbs include fennel (*Foeniculum vulgare*) chamomile, mint, thyme, turmeric, burdock and ginger.

- A warm herbal bath can help to relieve the itching and inflammation in an acute reaction, using a strong infusion of wild pansy (*Viola tricolor*) and fumitory (*Fumaria off.*) or burdock and chickweed (*Stellaria media*). The child can be soaked for half an hour.

- Alternatively, a strong decoction of equal parts of burdock root, fumitory, golden seal (*Hydrastis canadensis*) and yellow dock root (*Rumex crispus*) can be used. These herbs can be left to infuse until tepid and applied frequently as a compress to the affected parts, or used to sponge the skin.

- Many herbs, including nettle, chamomile, liquorice and turmeric have anti-inflammatory properties – nettle is one often used in urticaria. Research indicates that nettle has an anti-inflammatory action mediated by an inhibitory effect on NF-kappaB activation (Riehemann et al 1999).

- Herbs for internal use need to include herbs to aid elimination via the bowels and kidneys, such as burdock, dandelion leaves and root, fumitory, nettles, red clover (*Trifolium pratense*) and wild pansy.

- Rose, chickweed, liquorice root and elderflowers are also cooling and cleansing and help to clear heat from the skin.

- Boswellia (*Boswellia serrata*) and liquorice and chamomile are useful anti-inflammatories.

- Supplements of natural vitamin C, 200–500 mg, can be given every 2 hours to switch off the allergic reaction. Vitamin B5 (pantothenic acid) and vitamin E and zinc are also useful.

Ayurvedic approach

Urticaria is known as *Sheeta Pitta* (cold bile disease) in Ayurveda. It is said that disturbance of *Agni* and either or all of the *doshas* can be behind this problem. It is aggravated by drinking cold water after taking exercise, exposing the body to cold when it is hot, exposure to cold wind or mental excitement. The most probable cause is when *Pitta* is disturbed and *Kapha/Vata* aggravated. Another possible cause is said to be intestinal worms.

- Half to one teaspoon of turmeric, mixed with a glass of milk or water, can be given to clear heat and toxins 2–3 times per day. Turmeric has long been recognized in India as the best remedy for urticaria and regular use of turmeric in cooking is said to prevent attacks of urticaria (Murthy and Pandey 1998).

- Another famous herb for skin problems such as urticaria is khadira (*Acacia catechu*).

- Other remedies used include Triphala guggulu, Nimbadi churna (contains neem and other spices). Also Manjishtarishta (containing manjista).

- A tea made from tulsi leaves or the juice of the fresh leaves is given to purify the blood.

- Mint tea taken internally can help relieve the itching.

- If there is constipation $\frac{1}{2}$ tsp of Triphala or haritaki is given in lukewarm water at night. Alternatively, 5 drops of castor oil taken on an empty stomach (in $\frac{1}{2}$ cup of any vegetable or fruit juice, or in plain water) is considered beneficial for allergies affecting the gut, skin and nasal passages and for treatment of worms (see Digestive System, p. 210).

Local applications

- For local application use turmeric in sesame oil and massage over the affected area once or twice per day.

- Another topical application involves rubbing the affected parts with mustard oil mixed with powdered rock salt.

- In India daily application of crushed fresh tulsi leaves mixed with black clay is used or tulsi juice is applied over affected areas (Rai 2000, p. 93).

- Neem oil or the juice of the leaves mixed with ghee applied to the skin is also considered effective.

- Avoidance of sour and salty foods and a *Pitta* reducing diet is recommended. Bitter foods and herbs are particularly useful, i.e. drumsticks, kerela (bitter gourds) and aloe vera juice.

PRICKLY HEAT

An itchy and irritating skin condition, the rash is caused by exposure to sun and hot weather and is made worse by sweating, so it is important to keep the affected child covered but cool, out of the hot sun.

The use of certain chemicals in sun tan lotions may contribute to prickly heat, so investigation into natural-based lotions may prove worthwhile (see Sunburn, below).

Prickly heat can indicate a child's inability to cope with extra heat because of excess internal heat. This can, in some cases, be related to excess "heating of foods" in the diet, poor bowel function and toxicity. In my experience the removal of "heating foods", such as garlic, onions and spices, citrus fruits, strawberries, chocolate and cheese from the diet can often prevent or relieve the situation.

Treatment of prickly heat

- The skin can be cooled by bathing the child with tepid or cool water.

- For better effect you can add distilled rosewater or infusions of burdock root, chamomile, chickweed (*Stellaria media*) cleavers (*Galium aparine*) or *Calendula*.

- To clear heat and toxins from the system, teas can be given internally, including burdock root, chicory root (*Cichorium intybus*), chickweed, cleavers, chamomile, dandelion root, nettles or peppermint. These can be given warm not hot, singly or as a combination of herbs made to taste, 3–6 times daily.

- Cleavers is a common hedgerow weed and a good cooling remedy, clearing heat, inflammation and toxins from the system. It has a diuretic action, aiding elimination of wastes, and also acts to enhance the lymphatic system, promoting lymphatic drainage of toxins and wastes so that they can be excreted via the urinary system. These actions combine to make cleavers excellent for skin problems such as eczema, psoriasis, acne, prickly heat, boils and abscesses. It can be used for lymphatic problems, such as lymphatic congestion and swollen lymph glands. Its bitter properties stimulate liver function and enhance digestion and absorption. A cooling drink made of cleavers was traditionally given every spring to "clear the blood".

Ayurvedic approach

In Ayurveda prickly heat is known as a type of *pidaka*. Children with a *Pitta* type constitution are most likely to get this problem. Treatment relies on instigating a *Pitta* reducing diet, avoidance of heat and humidity. Herbs to reduce *Pitta* and clear heat and toxins include turmeric, mint, gotu kola, manjista, neem and sariva (*Hemidesmus indica*). Bathing the skin with an infusion of tulsi or neem leaves or a decoction of sandalwood can be helpful.

A traditional recipe for prickly heat is made from equal parts of sandalwood (*Santalum album*), coriander seeds, musta (*Cyprus rotundus*) root and khus-khus grass (*Vertiveria zizaniodies*) root powdered together with rosewater or cold water and rubbed on the body (Dastur 1983). Also the juice of purslane (*Portulaca oleracea*) is cooling and soothing and can be applied externally.

SUNBURN

Overexposure of the skin to ultraviolet radiation can cause an acute inflammatory reaction. In addition the use of chemical products in sun tan creams on the skin may all contribute to weakening of the cells in the skin and predispose to burning. According to Ayurveda children with a *Pitta* predominant constitution have sensitive skins and are more prone to sunburn.

Generally, sunburn involves first-degree burning of the skin, and this can be helped considerably by herbs and natural medicines. When burning is more severe there may be symptoms such as dizziness, nausea, blisters, over-sensitivity to light and peeling of the skin. Repeated burning of the skin can prematurely age the skin, cause wrinkles and predispose to skin cancer.

To avoid burning the skin neem oil can be applied. This is reported to have the ability to act as a sun block and thereby help to protect the skin (Lad 1999). This can be applied to the skin before and after showering or bathing. To make neem oil use 2–3 drops of pure neem oil in a teaspoon of sesame oil. In India it is recommended that children drink coconut water or coconut milk and follow a *Pitta* reducing regime in summer. Coconut oil can also be used for daily massage, before and after bathing.

Treatment of sunburn

- First, the affected skin needs to be bathed with cold or tepid water to reduce the heat and inflammation.

- Then any of the following applied: pure aloe vera gel, coconut oil, ghee, cool cow's or goat's milk, calendula ointment, chickweed ointment, the pulp of pulverized lettuce leaves, comfrey juice or ointment, cucumber juice, "hyperical" ointment, which is made from *Hypericum* (St John's wort) and *Calendula* (marigold), lavender oil or plain, natural yoghurt.

- A cooling paste of sandalwood and turmeric which is made from mixing equal parts of the powder with a little water can also be applied. This is very effective but note that it will stain the skin for a couple of days and it can also stain clothes.

SKIN INFECTIONS

When the defence mechanisms in the skin are impaired for any reason, the skin will be less resistant to infection by bacterial, fungal or viral organisms. Bacterial infections include abscesses, boils and impetigo. Viral infections include warts and verrucae and herpes. Fungal infections include athletes' foot (ringworm) and thrush. While it is important to distinguish one infection from another and to treat it accordingly, it is also necessary to consider the child constitutionally. The skin reflects a child's internal health and any skin condition requires examination of not only a child's nutritional status, but also to the general level of health, especially where there are recurrent skin infections or slow-healing infections.

Spots, boils and abscesses

Spots, boils and abscesses are local infections of the skin and hair follicles caused by staphylococcal and other bacteria. They are considered to result from a toxic state of the blood. The liver is the main detoxifying organ of the body and so treatment gener-ally involves supporting the liver in its cleansing work and enhancing other eliminative pathways via sweat, urine and faeces. Abscesses, boils and pimples should be left alone as squeezing or touching may push the infection further into the skin or introduce new infection. Boils and spots should be allowed to come to a head of their own accord but this can be encouraged. Repeated attacks of boils demand particular attention as they indicate lowered resistance to infection and a generally run-down state. This may be related to a poor diet, weak digestion, constipation, chronic bowel infection, a sedentary lifestyle, excessive fatty and junk foods and sugar. In some cases they can be a sign of more serious illness, such as diabetes mellitus.

Treatment of spots, boils and abscesses

Treatment needs to consist of external treatment to draw out toxins and pus, combined with internal remedies to clear the hot, congested state of the skin and factors underlying this.

Local applications

- Hot poultices can be applied to the affected area and left for 30–60 minutes, three times daily. They can be prepared from any of the following herbs: burdock (leaves or root), chickweed (*Stellaria media*), comfrey (*Symphytum off.*) (leaves or root), marshmallow (*Althea off.*) (leaves or root), plantain leaves and slippery elm powder (*Ulmus fulva*). Moisten the dried herbs and mash them in hot water (or mash and heat the fresh herbs). Add a few drops of essential oil of eucalyptus, lavender or thyme. Place it on a gauze pad and apply. Cover with a clean firm bandage or dressing. Remove between applications to allow air to the area, and to stop the skin becoming over-moist.

- Alternatively a paste of $\frac{1}{2}$ tsp each of ginger and turmeric powder mixed with a little water can be applied daily.

- A cooked onion as a hot poultice is a folk remedy reputed to be effective.

- Herbs need to be applied daily until the boil or abscess has discharged, pain has resolved and the boil has cleared. If the boil is particularly stubborn, it may require lancing.

Internal treatment

- General treatment of the digestive and immune systems should be followed (see Immune System, p. 150).

- Starting the day with ginger tea will help enliven the digestion and clear toxins.

- Echinacea or wild indigo (*Baptisia tinctoria*) will help resolve infection and clear toxins from the body. Dandelion, agrimony (*Agrimonia eupatoria*), burdock, cleavers (*Galium aparine*), nettles, chickweed (*Stellaria media*) and red clover (*Trifolium pratense*) can be used to clear heat and toxins.

- Yellow dock (*Rumex crispus*) or liquorice can be added to prescriptions if there is constipation.

- These herbs are all best taken in hot infusions/decoctions, flavoured with peppermint if desired; $\frac{1}{2}$–1 cupful should be taken three times daily.

- A diet rich in fresh fruit and vegetables will provide the raw materials for the immune system and avoiding excess fatty red meats, sugar, fats and refined carbohydrates will help prevent further problems.

Ayurvedic approach

Boils are considered to be caused by *ama* (toxins) and tend to be associated with excess *Pitta*. *Pitta* type boils are characterized by heat, redness and swelling and associated with thirst and other signs of high *Pitta* such as intolerance of heat and irritability. *Kapha* type boils tend to be large, with much pus and associated with feelings of heaviness, dullness, laziness and a tendency to phlegm. *Vata* type boils are smaller, hard, dry and more painful. They take some time to come to a head and may migrate to other areas in the body. Their underlying causes are windy, dry, cold weather, constipation, stress and other *Vata*-aggravating factors.

Generally spots, boils and abscesses are caused by excess *Pitta* increasing foods, particularly fatty, fried, salty or sweet foods. Overexposure to heat as in very hot baths, showers, saunas and hot sun can also contribute. *Pitta* emotions of anger, resentment, jealousy, over-competitiveness or suppression of emotions are considered to raise internal heat.

Ayurvedic treatment

For treatment of spots, boils and abscesses a *Pitta* reducing diet is recommended with plenty of fresh fruit and vegetables and avoidance of dairy produce, bread, sweets, fried and oily foods, stale and junk food and refined carbohydrates. Hot spices should be avoided but turmeric and coriander are recommended. Cooling herbs to reduce *Pitta* can be given to clear heat and toxins including rose, turmeric, guduchi, manjista, katuka (*Picrorrhiza kurroa*), barberry (*Berberis aristata*), neem, bringaraj, gotu kola and sariva (*Hemidesmus indica*). Aloe vera juice is recommended, with a little turmeric. Lemon grass and chamomile tea is easy to give to children as it tastes pleasant and helps to clear inflammation. Coriander leaf/seed can be added to food.

For *Vata* type boils, a *Vata* reducing diet is advised as well as mild laxatives to clear toxins from the bowel. Triphala, $\frac{1}{2}$ tsp in warm water at night, is recommended. Triphala guggulu combines myrrh with Triphala and is particularly

cleansing. Guggul (*Commiphora mukul*) is said to "scrape" *ama* out of the tissues.

For *Kapha* type boils, warming spices to rekindle the digestive fire and expectorant herbs to clear phlegm from the system are advised. Herbs such as long pepper, black pepper, ginger, cinnamon, angelica and cardamom can be combined with bitter herbs to clear *ama* such as neem, turmeric, katuka (*Picrorrhiza kurroa*) and guduchi. Triphala is also recommended.

A neem powder paste can be applied: mix neem powder with warm water and apply paste at the site of the boil. The affected area can also be washed with triphala tea. Boil 1 tsp of Triphala in 1 cup of water. Allow it to cool, wash the affected area and let it dry on the skin.

To bring the boil to a head: apply cooked onions as a poultice or apply a paste of ginger powder and turmeric powder ($\frac{1}{2}$ tsp each) directly to the boil. Alternatively: mix $\frac{1}{2}$ tsp each of red sandalwood and turmeric powder in warm water and apply the paste locally. (Sandalwood oil can also be applied to the forehead to cool *Pitta*.)

Impetigo

This highly contagious *staphylococcal* infection of the skin commonly affecting the area around the lips, nose and ears, can develop as a secondary infection complicating eczema, herpes, urticaria or scabies.

- Warm decoctions or dilute tinctures of echinacea, golden seal (*Hydrastis canadensis*), myrrh (*Commiphora molmol*), St John's wort (*Hypericum perforatum*), marigold or wild indigo (*Baptisia tinctoria*) can be used to bathe the affected area and then it should be gently patted dry with a paper towel.

- A few drops of essential oil of eucalyptus, lavender, tea tree or thyme can be added to a bowl of just boiled water (or a facial steamer) and used to steam the face.

- Internally, red clover (*Trifolium pratense*), echinacea, burdock, wild pansy (*Viola tricolor*), turmeric, *Calendula*, neem or wild indigo can be given as infusions/decoctions, flavoured with peppermint. Half to one cupful should be given three times daily.

Garlic and supplements of vitamin C (200–500 mg daily) will help the body to resolve the infection.

Warts and verrucae

The wart virus produces small hard growths made up of dead cells which may disappear spontaneously after weeks, months or even years but their departure can be hastened considerably by using herbs. Warts are particulary contagious where there is moisture, such as in bathrooms and around swimming pools. Infected children are best advised to dry their feet well after bathing and not to run around barefoot in such places to avoid infecting others.

According to Ayurveda, warts appear when *Vata* and *Kapha* disturbances combine on the skin. When *Vata* predominates, pain and roughness develop. When *Pitta* predominates, they look blackish-red. When *Kapha* predominates, they are greasy, knotty, and the same colour as the skin.

Treatment of warts

Several remedies can be applied directly to the wart including

- neat lemon juice,
- raw garlic juice,
- yellow juice from the fresh greater celandine plant (*Chelidonium majus*),
- white juice from dandelion stalks or unripe figs,
- tincture of thuja (*Thuja occidentalis*),
- inner sides of broad bean pods, oil of tea tree and
- fresh elderberry juice,
- turmeric powder in aloe vera juice can also be applied.

The chosen remedy should be applied once or twice daily until the wart disappears. My favourite remedy is greater celandine which I grow in the garden especially for this purpose as it is the fresh juice that works so well, better than an infusion or tincture of the plant. In general it takes 3 weeks of once daily applications for the wart to disappear.

Where there are crops of warts or the child has a history of recurring warts, constitutional treatment may be necessary. Internal treatment needs to include herbs to enhance resistance to infection as well as herbs for the digestion and liver and general cleansing of the system. Burdock, echinacea,

dandelion root, red clover (*Trifolium pratense*), neem, turmeric, heartsease (*Viola tricolor*), and peppermint can be given three times daily as teas or tinctures. Garlic and vitamin C supplements will boost immunity.

Herpes and cold sores

Cold sores are caused by the *herpes simplex* virus, which lives dormantly in the nerve endings of many children after an initial infection through oral contact. It can be reactivated when the child is run-down either by infection such as a cold or flu, a fever, pneumonia or due to poor diet, vitamin and mineral deficiencies or by other physical or emotional stress. Cold sores can also be activated by changes in skin temperature, exposure to hot sun, sunburn and equally to exposure to extremes of cold.

The infected child needs to be kept away from close contact with other babies or children during the initial and subsequent infection, especially those with other skin problems such as eczema or nappy rash as these can be further complicated by secondary herpes infections. It is also important to discourage children from scratching cold sores, which may irritate or itch, as this can introduce a secondary bacterial infection such as impetigo. If this occurs the cold sores will not clear as they should and will instead become red and inflamed with pus-filled centres.

According to Ayurveda herpes is essentially a *Pitta* disorder arising from disturbance of *Rakta dhatu*.

Treatment of cold sores

- Internal treatment is aimed at boosting immunity to the virus and clearing inflammation and toxicity using herbs such as echinacea, turmeric and wild indigo (*Baptisia tinctoria*), as well as enhancing the elimination of toxins using alterative herbs such as burdock, dandelion root, cleavers (*Galium aparine*), *Calendula*, peppermint, nettles, red clover and yellow dock (*Rumex crispus*).

- Liquorice has been shown to be active against the herpes virus (Pompei et al 1979) and can be added to chosen herbs.

> **Box 12.1   Recipe for cold sore cream**
>
> 10 drops tea tree oil/turmeric oil
> 10 drops lavender/rosemary oil
> 10 drops true melissa/lemon grass oil
> 10 ml rosewater
> Mix into 15 g unperfumed ointment or cream
>   base.
> Liquorice cream or paste can also be applied
>   topically to herpes sores.

- Supplements of vitamins C and B, zinc and cod liver oil will help boost immunity.

- Some amino acids can both stimulate and inhibit the activation of the herpes virus. Lysine helps to inhibit infection by controlling multiplication of the virus. In a survey of 1543 patients using lysine, 88% considered the supplement an effective treatment (Walsh et al 1983). Lysine is found in mung beans and beansprouts, brewer's yeast, chicken, lamb, dairy produce, eggs and in most fruit and vegetables. Arginine can help predispose to infection and foods rich in this amino acid should largely be avoided by a child who is prone to cold sores. These include peanuts, chocolate, carob, coffee, coconut, nuts, seeds, potatoes, sweetcorn, oats, wheat, rice, soya beans, lentils, peas and gelatine.

- The anti-herpes diet includes lots of fruit, especially citrus fruits, berries and kiwi fruit for their immune-enhancing antioxidant properties. Vitamin B rich foods such as meat, eggs and yoghurt promote healthy nerve function and can help to reduce the severity and frequency of attacks.

Local applications

- At the first sign of irritation creams prepared with herbs with antiviral effects can be applied and then reapplied every 2 hours afterwards until symptoms subside. Herbs that are effective against the herpes virus include: St John's wort (*Hypericum perforatum*), turmeric, melissa, calendula, and neem. A recent double-blind placebo-controlled trial of 66 patients with a history of recurrent herpes labialis found that a cream containing extract of *Melissa officinalis* resulted in a shortening of the healing period, prevention of spread and significant relief of subjective symptoms (Koytchev et al 1999).

- In Ayurvedic medicine aloe vera gel and turmeric are used as well as ghee medicated with neem or other *Pitta* reducing herbs such as haritaki, pomegranate (*Punica granatum*) and gotu kola. Gotu kola (*Centella asiatica*) has been shown, in an alcoholic extract, to be effective against herpes simplex (Zheng 1989). Tannins from the pericarp of *Punica* have been found to be effective against herpes (HSV-2) and to have a strong virucidal effect (Zhang et al 1995) and the fruit extract of haritaki has been shown to be effective against HSV-1 (Kurokawa et al 1995).

Tinea

This fungal infection can affect any area of the skin, and the nails, but most commonly affects the scalp, between the toes, and the groin, causing inflammation and intense itching. Tinea is highly contagious and can be highly resistant to treatment. Warm, moist conditions are ideal for the growth and spread of the infection, such as in/around swimming pools, changing rooms and bathrooms, or when sweating.

Treatment of tinea

- Herbs can be given to boost immunity, enhance digestion and clear toxins and infection. Cleavers (*Galium aparine*), burdock, dandelion root, echinacea, nettles, peppermint and red clover (*Trifolium pratense*) can be given as teas three times daily.

- Garlic or garlic supplements can also help the body to ward off the infection.

Local applications

- Many essential oils possess antifungal properties and make effective external applications. Undiluted oils of either lavender, lemon, tea tree, or a 20% dilution of thyme, neem or oregano can be applied three times daily on cotton wool.

- The essential oil of *Eucalyptus pauciflora* has been found to have potent antifungal activity against a number of human pathogenic fungi. A trial of 50 patients with either tinea pedis, tinea corporis or tinea cruris found that after 2 weeks of treatment 60% of patients had recovered completely whilst 40% showed significant improvement (Shahi et al 2000).

- Antimicrobial herbs can be applied to the affected areas either in the form of dilute tinctures or in a cream base. Echinacea, golden seal (*Hydrastis canadensis*), neem, wild indigo (*Baptisia tinctoria*), thyme, turmeric, myrrh (*Commiphora molmol*), marigold or thuja (*Thuja occidentalis*) are all suitable.

- Garlic, cinnamon, clove and tulsi also have antifungal properties and can be used in creams and washes.

- For athlete's foot, the feet can be bathed with decoctions or infusions of either agrimony (*Agrimonia eupatoria*), cinnamon, burdock, golden seal, *Calendula* or neem. The area needs to be dried thoroughly after soaking the feet for at least 5 minutes, especially between and underneath the toes.

- The affected area can be sealed off from the air to inhibit the infection by painting on either undiluted lemon juice or egg white repeatedly several times a day to form a glaze.

- Soaps are available containing neem and sandalwood and these can help back up treatment.

- I use a cream containing neem, sandalwood and turmeric which I generally find effective, but I tend to give internal treatments at the same time, particularly addressing low digestive fire and *ama* (see p. 197). Chronic intestinal infection with candida may be related to stubborn fungal infections on the skin and I find treatment of the digestion to be the best approach. Sugar and yeast-containing foods are best avoided.

Ayurvedic approach

In Ayurveda, ringworm is called *dadru* and children with *Kapha-Pitta* constitutions who tend to sweat a lot are more prone, especially to athlete's foot.

- Bathing with hot water boiled with vidanga (*Embelia ribes*) or neem leaves or applying a paste of neem leaves over the affected areas are popular treatments in India.

- A plaster of powdered mustard seed, turmeric, trikatu, with yoghurt and warm water, can be applied to the affected area.

- Alternatively a plaster made from neem, harataki, sesame and kantkari (*Solanum xanthocarpum*) is used.

- Sandalwood powder can be dusted on to the area.

- Aloe vera gel and turmeric powder (1 tsp gel to $\frac{1}{2}$ tsp powder) can be applied three times daily (socks should be worn in bed to avoid staining bed clothes).

- *Internally* turmeric, neem, chitrak (*Plumbago zeylanica*), ginger and Triphala are used to clear toxins.

- Bitter *Pitta* reducing herbs to clear heat and toxins can be given including guduchi, aloe vera juice, gotu kola, manjista and sariva (*Hemidesmus indica*). *Swertia chireta* is also recommended (Lad 1999). At night $\frac{1}{2}$ tsp of Triphala in warm water can be given.

PARASITIC INFECTIONS OF THE SKIN

Scabies

The tiny female mite burrows into the skin and lays eggs, causing an intensely itchy skin condition. Some children can develop an allergy to the mites and develop urticaria. Itching is aggravated by warmth and so tends to be worse when the child gets hot and in bed. Scabies is highly contagious and can be hard to eradicate, especially since it takes 6–8 weeks for the symptoms of intense itching to appear. It is best to treat all the family at once. When the eggs hatch they are passed from person to person by direct contact. To discourage the spread of the infection, clothing, bedding and towels need to be kept separate and pets may also need to be treated. Children need to be discouraged from scratching as this may introduce secondary infection into the skin.

Treatment of scabies

- A long hot bath at night followed by brisk drying will open up the pores and burrows. Essential oils (lavender, neem, rosemary or tea tree) can be applied immediately in a base of sesame oil.

- Alternatively an infusion/decoction or dilute tincture of wild indigo (*Baptisia tinctoria*), myrrh (*Commiphora molmol*), neem, echinacea, golden seal (*Hydrastis canadensis*) or turmeric can be applied on a cloth/flannel over the body.

- Clean nightclothes should then be put on and the child get into bed with clean sheets and ideally this should be repeated for the next two nights. All clothing, towels and bed linen need to be washed thoroughly on a hot wash, ironed afterwards when dry, and left for 3 weeks before using again.

- Internally cleavers (*Galium aparine*), dandelion root, echinacea, peppermint, burdock and red clover (*Trifolium pratense*) will help to clear toxins and infection which may predispose to lowered immunity on the skin.

Ayurvedic approach

In Ayurveda, scabies is known as *kachchhu*.

- Saffron (*Crocus sativus*) is the herb of choice in India. The petals of the flowers are used. They have a pungent and bitter taste. They can be applied in the form of an oil or given internally as a powder 1–2 g mixed in honey, twice daily. (not to be used in children under 2 years).

- The parts of the body affected by scabies should be washed daily with water boiled with neem leaves. Neem oil and soap can also be used.

- Sweet and sour foods should be avoided. Pickles, yoghurt and molasses are strictly prohibited. Other topical treatments include sandalwood oil, safflower seed oil, mustard or coconut oil boiled with garlic.

- In one study a combination of turmeric and neem applied topically eradicated scabies within 3–15 days in 97% of the subjects treated (Charles and Charles 1992). This formula is also traditional for ringworm.

- Sesame oil mixed with amalaki powder, ghee medicated with chitrak (*Plumbago zeylanica*) and finely powdered turmeric mixed with onion juice and a little water (Dastur 1983) are generally used in India.

Head lice

Head lice are endemic in school-age children and are fast becoming "super lice". Experience over the past decade has shown lice to be developing resistance to over-the-counter preparations to combat the problem and so a considerable amount of research has been developing into herbs as an alternative to such chemical preparations. Quassia (*Pricasma excelsa*), a herb native to the West Indies and Africa, is one of these herbs. Containing alkaloids, terpenoids and quassinoids, it is a food ingredient that is approved by the Council of Europe for use as a bitter in concentrates for beers, pastilles and lozenges (Bensky and Gamble 1986). It has traditionally been used by herbalists for digestive problems such as loss of appetite and indigestion. In the 1970s a clinical study was conducted at the Municipal Hospital in Copenhagen to test the efficacy of Quassia in a total of 454 people with either eggs, live lice or in contact with people with lice. After treatment with Quassia only three people still had lice but this may have been due to new infestation. No side effects were reported (Jansen et al 1978).

Treatment of head lice

- A solution of decocted quassia chips should be massaged well into the scalp, covering all the hair as well as the nape of the neck. This can be left on overnight and washed off the following morning. It can be used from time to time as a preventative, for example after the holidays when children are going back to the school, or attending gyms or pools.

- As an alternative one can use quassia with thyme and added lavender and tea tree oil to treat infestation and for regular preventative use.

- Head lice can also be treated effectively using essential oils in a base of olive oil which needs to be massaged into the hair and scalp at night, left on till morning and washed out thoroughly. A number of essential oils including thyme, tea tree, peppermint and rosemary have been shown to be effective in vitro against *Pediculus humanus* (Veal 1996). I have used a mixture of lavender, geranium, rosemary, eucalyptus and neem oil, 100 drops per 100 ml of sesame oil. Oil needs to be applied each night for five nights, repeated after a week for two nights and the problem should be solved.

- The child needs to sleep on a towel to prevent staining of bedclothes with oil. When the hair is covered with oil a nit comb can be used to comb through the hair thoroughly and remove the nits. Dipping the comb in hot vinegar will help to loosen the nits that tend to stick stubbornly to the hair.

- Interestingly there is an old-fashioned but effective remedy made with mint and vinegar to discourage head lice. Add 1 cup of vinegar just off the boil to 2 tsp dried mint leaves, cover and leave to cool. Strain and store in a well-sealed bottle. It can be used as a scalp rub/rinse for head lice, dry flaky skin and dandruff.

- Each time the hair is washed, plenty of conditioner should be applied and the hair combed through thoroughly with a nit comb to prevent re-infestation. Hairbrushes, combs and towels should be kept separately from other members of the family.

References

Araujo CC, Leon LL 2001 Biological activites of *Curcuma longa* L. Mem Inst Oswaldo Cruz 96(5): 723–728

Bensky D, Gamble A 1986 Chinese Herbal Medicine, Revised edition. Eastland Press, Vista, CA, USA

Bonte F, Noel-Hudson MS, Wepierre J, Meybeck A 1997 Protective effect of curcuminoids on epidermal skin cells under free oxygen radical stress. Planta Med 63(3): 265–266

Charles V, Charles SX 1992 The use and efficacy of *Azadirachta indica* ADR ('Neem') and *Curcuma longa* ('Turmeric') in scabies. A pilot study. Trop Geogr Med 44(1–2): 178–181

Dastur JF 1983 Everybody's Guide to Ayurvedic Medicine. DB Taraporevala Sons & Co. Private Ltd, Bombay

Frawley D 2000 Ayurvedic Healing. Passage Press, Salt Lake City

Fulhan J, Collier S, Duggan C 2003 Update on pediatric nutrition: breastfeeding, infant nutrition, and growth. Curr Opin Pediatr 15(3): 323–332

Horrobin DF 2000 Essential fatty acid metabolism and its modification in atopic eczema. Am J Clin Nutr Jan; 71 (1 Suppl): 367–372

Imai S, Takeuchi S, Mashiko T 1997 Seasonal changes in the course of atopic eczema. Hautzart 1987 38(10): 599–602

Jansen O, Nielsen AO, Bjerregaard P 1978 *Pediculosis capitis* treated with Quassia tincture. Acta Dermatovener (Stockholm) 58(6): 557–559

Kaeser P, Revelly ML, Frei PC 1994 Prevalence of IgE antibodies specific for food allergens in patients with chronic urticaria of unexplained etiology. Allergy 49(8): 626–629

Koytchev R, Alken RG, Dundarov S 1999 Balm mint extract (Lo-701) for topical treatment of recurring herpes labialis. Phytomedicine 6(4): 225–230

Kurokawa M, Nagasaka K, Hirabayashi T, et al 1995 Efficacy of traditional herbal medicines in combination with acyclovir against herpes simplex virus type I infection in vitro and in vivo. Antiviral Res 27(1–2): 19

Kuttan R, Sudheeran PC, Josph CD 1987 Turmeric and curcumin as topical agents in cancer therapy. Tumori 73(1): 29–31

Lad V 1999 The Complete Book of Ayurvedic Home Remedies. Judy Piatkus Limited, London

Landis R, Khalsa KPS 1998 Herbal Defence against Illness and Ageing. Thorsons, London, p. 342

Murray M, Pizzorna J 2001 Encyclopedia of Natural Medicine. Little, Brown and Company, London

Murthy NA, Pandey DP 1998 Ayurvedic Cure for Common Diseases. Orient Paperbacks, Delhi

Oehling A, Fernandez M, Cordoba H, et al 1997 Skin manifestations and immunological parameters in childhood food allergy. J Investig Allergol Clin Immunol 7(3): 155–159

Patzelt-Wenczler R, Ponce-Poschl E 2000 Proof of efficacy of Kamillosan(R) cream in atopic eczema. Eur J Med Res 5(4): 171–175

Phan TT, Sun L, Bay BH, et al. 2003 Dietary compounds inhibit proliferation and contraction of keloid and hypertrophic scar-derived fibroblasts in vitro: therapeutic implication for excessive scarring. J Trauma 54(6): 1212–1224

Pompei R, Flore O, Marccialis MA, et al 1979 Glycyrrhizic acid inhibits virus growth and inactivates virus particles. Nature 281(5733): 689–690

Rai Y 2000 Tulsi. Navneet Publications, India

Riehemann K, Behnke B, Schulze-Osthoff K 1999 Plant extracts from stinging nettle (*Urtica dioica*), an antirheumatic remedy, inhibit the proinflammatory transcription factor NF-kappaB. FEBS Lett 442(1): 89–94

Saeedi M, Morteza-Semnani K, Ghoreishi MR 2003 The treatment of atopic dermatitis with liquorice gel. J Dermatolog Treat 14(3): 153–157

Schnyder B, Pichler WJ 1999 Food intolerance and food allergy. Schweiz Med Wochenschr 129(24): 928–933

Shahi SK, Shukla AC, Bajaj AK, Banerjee U, Rimek D, Midgely G, Dikshit A 2000 Broad spectrum herbal therapy against superficial fungal infections. Skin Pharmacol Appl Skin Physiol 13(1): 60–64

Tillotson AK, Tillotson NH, Robert A Jr 2001 The One Earth Herbal Sourcebook. Kensington Publishing Corps, New York

Veal L 1996 The potential effectiveness of essential oils as a treatment for headlice, *Pediculus humanus capitis*. Complement Ther Nurs Midwifery 2(4): 97–101

Walsh DE, Griffith RS, Behforooz A 1983 Subjective response to lysine in the therapy of herpes simplex. J Antimicrob Chemother 12(5): 489–496

White A, Horne DJ, Varigos GA 1990 Psychological profile of the atopic eczema patient. Australas J Dermatol 31(1): 13–16

Zhang J, Zhan B, Yiao X, et al 1995 Antiviral activity of tannin from the pericarp of *Punica granatum* L. against genital Herpes virus *in vitro*. Chung Kuo Chung Yao Tsa Chih 20(9): 556

Zheng MS 1989 An experimental study of the anti-HSV-II action of 500 herbal drugs. J Trad Chinese Med 9: 113

Chapter **13**

The eyes

CHAPTER CONTENTS

THE FUNCTION OF THE EYES

As one of the sense organs, the eyes are intimately connected with the brain and can speak volumes about our state of mind. Positive and negative emotions like joy, excitement and happiness as well as fear, anxiety, anger, grief, and suffering can be reflected through the eyes, partly because they affect the facial muscles around the eyes. The expression in the eyes is one of the ways in which a parent first tells if their child is off-colour or unhappy.

Eyes have other functions. They are responsible for connecting us to light, which is responsible not only for vision but also influences our physical and mental well-being. Sunlight affects the secretion of endorphins that give us a feeling of well-being. During the winter months in the northern hemisphere, the many hours of darkness can predispose to seasonal affective disorder (SAD), and reduced resistance to infection, so it is important to encourage children to spend time playing or walking outside in the fresh air and sunlight, even on a dull day.

The production of tears and crying is another important function of the eyes. Tears produced when we cry contain endorphins, opiate-like substances, which help us to release tension and calm us down. In addition, tears are constantly washed in tiny amounts across the eyes to protect the eye from damage and to clear away debris.

The eyelids also protect the eyes. The inner and outer surfaces of each eye are covered with the delicate conjunctiva and tears produced by tear glands lubricate the conjunctiva and drain into the channels passing into the nose. The eyelids and conjunctiva are prone to various problems, which can be successfully treated using herbs.

CARE OF THE EYES

Elderberries, bilberries and blueberries (*Vaccinium* spp.) are rich in antioxidants, known as anthocyanosides, and help to protect the eyes. There has been a wide range of research on the properties of anthocyanosides. These compounds appear to help support repair and synthesis of new capillaries and thus have particular relevance in disorders of the retina (Boniface and Robert 1996). In a review of 30 trials *Vaccinium* anthocyanosides demonstrated promise for improving night vision though, as with much herbal research, better designed and larger trials are still required (Canter and Ernst 2004). A recent double-blind placebo-controlled trial of blackcurrant anthocyanosides concluded that they significantly helped reduce visual fatigue in video display terminal related eye strain (Nakaishi et al 2000). Anthocyanosides contain or boost the action of a molecule known as glutathione, a key antioxidant found in the aqueous humour and necessary for prevention of a variety of eye problems including cataracts in later life. Other herbs with a similar action include astragalus root (*Astragalus membranaceus*), milk thistle seed (*Cardus/Silybum marianus*), turmeric root, garlic and wheat sprouts.

Ayurvedic approach

According to the ancient Rishis of Ayurveda, our five senses are the gifts of the Gods of the five elements. The God of the Sky carries sound to our ears, the God of Air gives our skin the sensation of touch and feeling, the God of Fire draws the light of vision into our eyes, the God of Water brings taste to our tongues, the God of Earth brings smells to our nose (Tillotson et al 2001, p. 379).

One of the original branches of Ayurvedic medicine recorded in the Charaka Samhita, the earliest Ayurvedic textbook dating from around 2500 BC, is the *Shalakya Tantra*, the study of the mouth, eyes, ears, nose and throat. According to Ayurveda, observation of the eyes is very important as a diagnostic tool for imbalance elsewhere in the body. The eyes are mainly related to *Pitta* as they are concerned with light and perception, functions governed by *Pitta*. Radiation of light and heat is the province of *Pitta dosha* and according to Tillotson (Tillotson et al 2001, p. 382) "the eye captures within itself the fire of the universe, allowing perception of the constant and ever-changing flux of colors and shapes of objects ... because it captures fire and heat, the physical structure of the eyes requires immersing the cornea, lens and retina in the cooling aqueous and vitreous humors". This is why the eye is so sensitive to excess heat and light.

Pitta types certainly tend to be sensitive to heat and light and are more likely to need glasses than other *dosha* types (Frawley 2000, p. 312). When *Pitta* is disturbed it can weaken the eyes. Excess *Pitta* is indicated by pink, red or yellowish eyes with a burning sensation and photophobia. Most inflammatory diseases of the eyes such as conjunctivitis are considered to be *Pitta* problems.

An excess of *Kapha* can also have a negative effect on vision as it suppresses *Pitta*. Sinus congestion can also affect vision. When there is excess *Kapha* the eyes tend to be watery, mucousy or dull. Dryness or tremors of the eyes indicate *Vata* disturbance.

Ayurvedic treatment of eye problems

- In India there is an ancient practice of looking into the distance at the moon to benefit from its cooling rays and physicians recommend staring at a ghee lamp for 20 minutes a day to improve *tejas* or the lustre of the eyes and to promote good vision (Lad 1999, p. 172). To make a ghee lamp place a cotton wick in a small bowl and add ghee. Apply a little ghee to the end of the wick and light it. The lamp needs to be placed 2–3 feet away, any glasses removed and the patient needs to stare at the flame without blinking for 2–3 minutes.

- Ghee itself is considered to balance *Pitta* and to be the most important food for the eyes (Frawley 2000, p. 312). Taking 1–2 tsp twice daily is believed to improve eyesight. Apparently the older the ghee the better its properties.

- Triphala ghee is a special formula for the eyes which can be used to treat infectious conditions and also as a general tonic to the eyes.

- Triphala powder mixed with water is used as a wash for inflamed eyes. Boil $\frac{1}{2}$ tsp of Triphala in a cup of water for 3 minutes, cool it and strain through double or triple-folded cheesecloth or a paper coffee filter to clear all particles from the liquid. The eyes can then be washed (Lad 1999, p. 174).

- Chamomile and rose flowers are also suitable eye washes for pain, irritation or inflammation of the eyes. Chamomile infusion can be used in a sterilized eyebath or two drops of distilled rosewater can be put into each eye morning and night.

- Aloe vera gel or ghee can be applied to the eyelid.

- A paste of mung bean flour is used for soothing the eyes.

- Chyawan prash is an excellent tonic food for the eyes since amalaki is the main ingredient and is considered nourishing for the eyes.

- Amalaki juice with honey can also be used for conjunctivitis.

- In India an extract of darvi root (*Berberis asiatica*) is used dissolved in water to wash the eyes every 5–7 days. This is considered to help keep the duct system open and to cure and prevent conjunctivitis (Tillotson et al 2001, p. 383).

- Other anti-*Pitta* herbs are considered good for improving vision and prevention of eye problems. Common formulae include Sudarshan and Maha Sudarshan. These herbs include *Swertia chireta*, which cool and cleanse the eyes.

- Certain foods also have an affinity for eye tissue. The link between vitamin A and vision is well documented and there are certain carotenoids that are particularly beneficial. Lutein, zeaxanthin and lycopene all help to prevent eye disease (Tillotson et al 2001, p. 384). Spinach, kale and mustard green are high in lutein and zeaxanthin, while tomatoes, pink grapefruit, guava and watermelon are rich in lycopene. It is worth noting that cooking lycopene-rich foods like tomatoes in oil such as olive oil increases its bioavailability. An old recipe (Verma 1995, p. 218) to promote good vision and balance the *doshas*, recommended for children to take daily is: two medium-sized carrots grated and cooked in milk on a low heat for 15 minutes with five ground almonds and one ground cardamom.

- Crying is good for cleansing the eyes and chopping a raw onion is considered therapeutic as it increases lacrimation and thereby clears debris from the eyes. It is not considered beneficial to withhold the urge to cry. Not only can this, like suppression of other natural urges, disturb *Vata dosha*, but also it is said to impair the function of the lacrimal glands and may lead to dry eye problems.

Myopia or shortsightedness is known as *dristi dosha*. It is caused by the lens of the eye being overly convex or the ball of the eye being too long, so that rays of light are brought to focus before they reach the retina. Apart from blurred vision, myopia can cause watering of the eye due to strain, itching and a sensation of heaviness or burning in the eyes. Headaches and insomnia can also be related. According to Ayurveda factors that predispose to this problem include nervous debility, tendency to constipation and susceptibility to cold, which tend to predominate in *Vata* types.

- Giving Triphala at night before bed to cleanse the bowels is the first line of treatment. It can also be used to bathe the eyes and needs to be continued for a few months.
- The other medicine of choice is liquorice: $\frac{1}{4}$–$\frac{1}{2}$ tsp of the powder is mixed with $\frac{1}{4}$ tsp of ghee and $\frac{1}{2}$ tsp of honey and given twice daily on an empty stomach.
- If there is a susceptibility to cold or nasal congestion 2–3 drops of shadbindu oil can be inserted into each nostril daily (Murthy and Pandey 1998, p. 104).

CONJUNCTIVITIS

An inflammatory condition of the conjunctiva, which is caused either by infection by an adenovirus, injury to the eye from dirt, dust or pollution, a foreign body, or allergy. Conjunctivitis or "pink eye" is highly contagious and can occur among schoolchildren in epidemics. There may be associated cold symptoms, the conjunctiva becomes pink or red, it can feel sore and irritated and tends to be aggravated by bright light. The eyes may be watery, and a discharge can cause crusting and glueing up of the eyes and eyelashes in the morning after sleep. The eyelids tend to be swollen and the lymph nodes in front of the ear tender. If a child is prone to repeated attacks or chronic conjunctivitis it may be caused by irritation from chemicals in the environment or by food allergy, often to dairy produce or by an overgrowth *Candida* in the gut (see p. 185). Conjunctivitis also often accompanies hayfever.

BLEPHARITIS

This is inflammation of the eyelids, usually due to infection or allergy. The eyelids are red and swollen, and can feel irritated or sore. There may be a pus-like discharge causing sticking of the eyes and lashes after sleep, as in conjunctivitis.

Herbal treatment of conjunctivitis and blepharitis

Both conjunctivitis and blepharitis are treated similarly. Even if symptoms are confined to one eye it is always best to treat both eyes to prevent the spread of infection.

- When conjunctivitis occurs in young babies the best remedy is mother's milk. One drop in each eye should clear it quickly. Colostrum has been found to have half the in vitro activity of gentamicin against *Staphylococcus aureus* and *coliform* organisms – supporting its use as a first-line treatment (Ibhanesebhor and Otobo 1996).

- For older children, bathe the eyes three times a day with a herbal infusion prepared using previously boiled or distilled water, or alternatively use a decoction of chamomile, chickweed (*Stellaria media*), comfrey (*Symphytum officinale*), elderflowers, eyebright (*Euphrasia off.*), golden seal (*Hydrastis canadensis*), marigold, marshmallow (*Althea off.*), plantain, raspberry leaves (*Rubus off.*) or rosemary. The combination of anti-inflammatory and antibacterial effects of chamomile, make it an effective and gentle topical treatment (Carle and Isaac 1987).

- Golden seal is an American herb and an effective antiviral remedy with a long history of use by the Native Americans for treating infections and eye conditions. It contains an alkaloid, berberine, which has well-documented antimicrobial effects (Cernakova and Kostalova 2002). It is used in Germany as a treatment for hypersensitive eyes, inflammatory conditions of the eyelids, chronic and allergic conjunctivitis (Tillotson et al 2001, p. 397).

- A combination of chamomile, eyebright and marigold is an excellent recipe for sore, inflamed eyes, but any of the above herbs may be used singly or in combinations. Teabags of any of these can be soaked in boiling water, taken out when lukewarm and placed over the eye for 5–10 minutes – a different teabag should be used for each eye so as not to spread the infection.

- Distilled witch hazel or rosewater can also be beneficial combined with herbal infusions, decoctions or tinctures. For example, mix 10 drops of eyebright tincture in 3 tbsp (55 ml) of rosewater. A sterilized eye bath can be used by children who are old enough to manage it. For younger children, use cotton wool – separate pieces for each eye – to wipe the eyes from the outer part of the eye towards the nose.

It is always best to treat the child internally at the same time to enhance the immune system's ability to deal with infection, inflammation or allergy, and to treat the eyes specifically.

- Teas of chamomile, cleavers (*Galium aparine*), echinacea, elderflowers, eyebright or hyssop (*Hyssopus off.*), can be given three times daily, singly or in combination. Always make sure that eyebright forms part of the prescription.

For repeated bouts of conjunctivitis or blepharitis and suspected allergic response, it is important to isolate the allergen and remove it as far as possible.

- Use chamomile tea to bathe the eyes, and infusions of chamomile, yarrow or lemon balm internally three times a day.

- Recommend plenty of foods containing vitamins C, A and B and supplements of vitamin C and garlic. Whole milk, carrots, pumpkin, green leafy vegetables and tomatoes are all high in vitamin A. Green leafy vegetables, milk, almonds, citrus fruits and bananas are all rich in vitamin B2.

- As this infection is so contagious, good hygiene is vital to stop it from spreading to other members of the household. Separate towels should be used and all linen washed on a hot wash. (See also Allergies (p. 86), Candidiasis (p. 185), Hayfever (p. 240) and Treatment of Infections (p. 180).)

Ayurvedic approach to conjunctivitis

According to Ayurveda, causes of conjunctivitis include dust, smoke, cold or hot winds, over-straining the eyes, over-exposure to the sun or bright lights, fire, chemicals, gases, etc. and allergies. It tends to be associated with high *Pitta*.

To reduce *Pitta* the child is advised to avoid excess heat, such as sunbathing, saunas and very hot baths, to stay cool in the heat of summer and protect the eyes from the heat and glare of direct sunlight. It is also important to protect the eyes from sudden changes of temperature, excess cold, and wind, infection, dust, pollution and smoke. Prolonged concentrated work using the eyes such as reading, writing and close work like embroidery, especially in poor light, is contraindicated.

- A decoction of coriander seeds is recommended for burning eye symptoms and redness due to *Pitta* excess. The eyes can be washed 2–3 times daily with this decoction. One or two small cups of coriander seed tea can be taken per day to reduce *Pitta* (Verma 1995, p. 218).

- In India they use sandalwood (*Santalum album*) paste for its cooling effect to reduce *Pitta*. Sandalwood powder is mixed with a little warm water to make a paste, applied to the eyelids and forehead and left for a few minutes.

- Liquorice is considered to be an effective herb for promoting good eyesight and to cure problems related to excess *Pitta* and *Kapha*. Liquorice root decoction is also used for inflammatory eye problems and burning. The eyes can be washed with it 2–3 times per day (Verma 1995, p. 218).

- Other useful herbs include: Boswellia gum (*Boswellia serrata*), turmeric root, and shatavari.

- A turmeric solution can be made by stirring $\frac{1}{2}$ tsp of turmeric powder into $\frac{1}{4}$ cup of distilled warm water. This can be used to wash the outer eye and eyelid. This mixture can also be taken internally or added to drinks, soups or stews.

- Washing the eyes with rosewater can also be used.

- Triphala is very high in antioxidants and has a long history of effective use for a wide range of eye problems. It can be used as an eye wash and also internally, where it has mild laxative properties. $\frac{1}{2}$ tsp of the powder can be given in water 1–3 times daily (see also p. 287–288).

Dietary advice for conjunctivitis

Pitta

- *Pitta* reducing diet avoiding excessive amounts of pungent, sour and salty foods and increasing bitter, astringent and sweet-tasting foods is recommended (see p. 67).

- Ghee, mung beans, basmati rice, wheat, all sweet fruits and vegetables, and cool spices like coriander are recommended.
- Bathing in cool water is advised in India followed by a light massage with coconut oil or sandalwood oil (Ranade 1993, p. 55).

Kapha

- Taking garlic every day is considered good for eye problems related to excess *Kapha*. It is thought to be particularly for children as childhood is dominated by *Kapha*.
- For congestion around the eyes after a cold, use jalneti (see Sinus Congestion, p. 220) to remove accumulated *Kapha*.

STYES

An inflammation of a hair follicle of an eyelash can cause a stye, a pus-filled swelling on the eyelid, usually on the lower one, which generally comes to a head and bursts within four or five days. It may be a sign that a child is tired or run down and is more likely to occur if a child rubs or touches the eyes frequently and pulls eyelashes. It can be associated with a more general irritation of the eyelids or with blepharitis. A child with a stye needs to be discouraged from touching the affected eye, as this can cause spreading of the infection to the other eye.

Treatment of styes

- Eyebright (*Euphrasia off.*) has a long tradition of use for eye disorders in Europe and although modern herbalists may be more moderate in their claims about the power of eyebright than the ancients, it is still an excellent remedy for a variety of eye problems. Its astringent properties are good for relieving inflammatory eye infections such as styes, conjunctivitis, blepharitis, watery eye conditions and catarrh. It is particularly good for sore, itching eyes accompanied by a discharge, often seen in hayfever or measles, and for catarrhal conditions affecting the nose, throat, sinuses, ears, upper chest and causing sinusitis, headaches and coughs. It will also help those with oversensitive eyes, which

tend to run in cold and wind, or are irritated by smoky or stuffy atmospheres. It can be used either locally in lotions for the eyes or taken internally: 30 drops of the tincture in a glassful of rosewater makes an excellent eyewash. A cohort study of the efficacy of *Euphrasia* eye drops in conjunctivitis recently concluded that these drops could be used safely and effectively for various conjunctival conditions (Stoss et al 2000).

- If the stye is painful, a warm compress can be applied for a few minutes every two or three hours to soothe the discomfort and to help bring the stye to a head. An infusion or decoction of either burdock, chamomile, elderflowers, eyebright, golden seal (*Hydrastis canadensis*), marigold, marshmallow (*Althea off.*) or plantain can be used. Alternatively use 5 drops of tincture in $\frac{1}{2}$ a cup of equal parts of distilled water and rosewater or witch hazel.
- Infusions of either burdock, echinacea, eyebright and red clover (*Trifolium pratense*), sweetened with a little liquorice can be given internally, three times daily to help detoxify the system and increase resistance to infection.
- Garlic and vitamin C supplements are also recommended.

Ayurvedic approach

- According to Ayurveda, constipation is one of the common causes of *anjananamika* or styes. Therefore, $\frac{1}{2}$ tsp of Triphala powder in a little warm water at bedtime is given at the onset.
- A teaspoon of Triphala powder in a cup of water, left overnight, and squeezed and filtered the next morning, makes an excellent wash for the eyes (Dash 1989, p. 88).
- An infusion of tulsi, holy basil leaves, can also be used to wash the eyes.
- Sour foods and drinks are best avoided and bitter foods recommended.
- To reduce *Pitta*, exposure to the sun or extreme winds and rain is not advised until the eye has recovered.

References

Boniface R, Robert AM 1996 Effect of anthocyanins on human connective tissue metabolism in the human. Klin Monatsbl Augenheilkd 209(6): 368–372

Canter PH, Ernst E 2004 Anthocyanosides of *Vaccinium myrtillus* (Bilberry) for night vision – a systematic review of placebo-controlled trials. Surv Ophthalmol 49(1): 38–50

Carle R, Isaac O 1987 The combination of anti-inflammatory and anti-bacterial effects of chamomile, make it an effective and gentle topical treatment. Z Phytother 8: 67–77

Cernakova M, Kostalova D 2002 Antimicrobial activity of berberine – a constituent of *Mahonia aquifolium*. Folia Microbiol (Praha) 47(4): 375–378

Dash B 1989 Ayurvedic Cures for Common Diseases. Hind Pocket Books Ltd, Delhi

Frawley D 2000 Ayurvedic Healing. Passage Press, Salt Lake City, p. 312

Ibhanesebhor SE, Otobo ES 1996 In vitro activity of human milk against the causative organisms of ophthalmia neonatorum in Benin City, Nigeria. J Trop Pediatr 42(6): 327–329

Lad V 1999 The Complete Book of Ayurvedic Home Remedies. Judy Piatkus Limited, London, p. 172

Murthy NA, Pandey DP 1998 Ayurvedic Cure for Common Diseases. Orient Paperbacks, Delhi

Nakaishi H, Matsumoto H, Tominaga S, Hirayama M 2000 Effects of blackcurrant anthocyanoside intake on dark adaptation and VDT work-induced transient refractive alteration in healthy humans. Altern Med Rev 5(6): 553–562

Ranade S 1993 Natural Healing Through Ayurveda. Passage Press, Utah

Stoss M, Michels C, Peter E, et al 2000 Prospective cohort trial of Euphrasia single-dose eye drops in conjunctivitis. J Altern Complement Med 6(6): 499–508

Tillotson AK, Tillotson NH, Robert A Jr 2001 The One Earth Herbal Sourcebook. Kensington Publishing Corps, New York, p. 379

Verma V 1995 Ayurveda: A Way of Life. Samuel Weiser Inc, Maine

Williamson E 2002 Major Herbs of Ayurveda. Churchill Livingstone, London

Appendix 1

Index of herbs

Ayurvedic name	Latin name	English name
Ajwan/Adjwan	*Trachyspermum ammi*	Bishops weed
Ajamoda/Ajmoda	*Carum roxburghianum*	
Amalaki/Amla	*Emblica officinalis*	Indian gooseberry/Emblic myrobalan
Amlavetasa	*Garcinia pedunculata*	Garcinia
Apamarga	*Achyranthes aspera*	Rough chaff tree
Ardak	*Zingiber officinales*	Ginger
Ashwagandha	*Withania somnifera*	Winter cherry
Atasi	*Linum usitatissimum*	Linseed
Ativisha	*Aconitum heterophyllum*	Aconite/Atis
Bacopa/Brahmi	*Bacopa monniera*	Thyme-leaved gratiola
Badara	*Zizyphus jujube*	Jujube tree/plum
Bakuchi	*Psoralia corylifolia*	Bacuchi/Purple flea bane seeds
Bala	*Sida cordifolia*	Indian country mallow
Bharngi	*Clerondendron serratum*	
Bringaraj/Bhringaraj	*Eclipta alba*	Trailing eclipta
Bibithaki	*Terminalia belerica*	Beleric myrobalan
Bilva	*Aegle marmelos*	Bengal quince/Bael root
Brahmi	*Centella asiatica*	Gotu kola/Indian pennywort
Chandan/Candana	*Santalum album*	Sandalwood
Chirata/Chirayata/Chiretta	*Swertia chireta*	Chiretta
Citrak/Chitrak	*Plumbago zeylanica*	White leadwort
Dadima	*Punica granatum*	Pomegranate
Dalchini	*Cinnamomum zeylanicum*	Cinnamon
Daruharida	*Berberis vulgaris*	Barberry root
Devadaru	*Cedrus deodara*	Himalayan cedar
Dhanya	*Coriandrum sativum*	Coriander
Dhataki	*Woodfordia fructicosa/floribunda*	Downy grislea
Draksha	*Vitis vinifera*	Grape
Dugdhapheni	*Taraxacum officinale*	Dandelion
Ela	*Eletteria cardamomum*	Cardamom
Erand	*Ricinus communis*	Castor plant

(Continued)

Ayurvedic name	Latin name	English name
Gokshura	*Tribulis terrestris*	Small caltrops/Goats head/ Puncture vine
Guduchi	*Tinospora cordifolia*	Amrit
Guggulu	*Commiphora/mukul*	Indian bedellium/Myrrh
Haldi	*Curcuma longa*	Turmeric
Hapusha	*Juniperus communis*	Juniper
	Alchemilla vulgaris	Ladies mantle
	Lavendula spp.	Lavender
	Melissa officinalis	Lemon balm
Haritaki	*Terminalia chebula*	Indian gall nut
Hing	*Ferrula asafoetida*	Asafoetida
Jatamansi	*Nardostachys jatamansi*	Muskroot/Indian spikenard
Jathiphala	*Myristica fragrans*	Nutmeg
Jati	*Jasminium grandiflorum*	Jasmine
Jeera	*Cuminum cyminum*	Cumin
Jupha	*Hyssopus officinalis*	Hyssop
	Cetraria islandica	Iceland moss
Kalijeera	*Nigella sativa*	Black cumin seeds
Kankolam	*Piper cubeba*	Cubebs
Kantkari	*Solanum xanthocarpum*	Wild egg plant
Kapikacchu	*Mucuna pruriens*	Cowhage plant
Karanja	*Pongamia glabra/pinnata*	Indian beech
Katuveera	*Capsicum minimum*	Cayenne
	Houttuynai cordata	Chameleon plant
	Chamomilla recutita	Chamomile (German)
	Anthemis nobilis	Chamomile (Roman)
	Stellaria media	Chickweed
	Galium aparine	Cleavers
Khadira	*Acacia catechu*	Black catech/Cutch tree
Katikaranja	*Caesalpinia bonducella*	Bonduc nut/Fever nut
Kumari	*Aloe vera*	Aloe vera
	Angelica archangelic	Angelica
	Astragalus membranaceus	Astragalus
	Chelone glabra	Balmony
	Petasites hybridus	Butterbur
Kumkum	*Crocus sativus*	Saffron
	Salvia officinalis	Sage
	Smilax utilis/officinalis	Sasparilla
	Prunella vulgaris	Self-heal
Kushta	*Saussurea lappa*	Costrus root
Kutaki/Katuka/Kutki	*Picrorrhiza kurroa*	Yellow gentian
Lasuna	*Allium sativum*	Garlic
Lavang	*Syzygium aromaticum*	Clove
Lavang	*Eugenia caryophyllus*	Clove
	Tussilago farfara	Coltsfoot
	Symphytum officinale	Comfrey

Ayurvedic name	Latin name	English name
	Zea mays	Corn silk
	Primula veris	Cowslip
	Geranium maculatum	Cranesbill, American
Madhuka	*Madhuka indica*	Indian butter tree/Mahwa tree
Markandika	*Cassia angustifolia*	Senna
	Capsella bursa-pastoris	Shepherd's purse
	Scutellaria laterifolia	Skullcap
	Ulmus fulva	Slippery elm
		Soap nut
	Artemisia abrotanum	Southernwood
		Spearmint
	Urginea maritima	Squills
	Hypericum perforatum	St John's wort
	Drosera rotundifolia	Sundew
	Asperula odorata	Sweet woodruff
	Melaleuca alternifolia	Tea tree
	Thuja occidentalis	Thuja
	Thymus vulgaris	Thyme
	Potentilla tormentilla	Tormentil
	Actostaphylos uva-ursi	Uva ursi
	Verbena officinalis	Vervain
	Viola odorata	Violet flowers
	Prunus serotina	Wild cherry
	Baptisia tinctoria	Wild indigo
	Lactuca virosa	Wild lettuce
	Avena sativa	Wild oats
	Viola tricolor	Wild pansy
	Dioscorea villosa	Wild yam
	Hamamelis virginiana	Witch hazel
	Artemisia absinthium	Wormwood
	Achillea millefolium	Yarrow
	Rumex crispus	Yellow dock
	Tylophora asthmatica	Indian lobelia
	Tylophora indica	Indian ipecac/Anthrapachaka leaf
Mandukaparni/Brahmi	*Centella/Hydrocotyl asiatica*	Gotu kola
Manjista	*Rubia cordifolia*	Indian madder
Methi	*Trigonella foenum-graecum*	Fenugreek
Mishreya	*Anethum graveolens*	Dill
	Echinacea angustifolia/purpurea	Echinacea
	Sambucus nigra	Elder
	Inula helenium	Elecampane
	Ephedra sinica	Ephedra
	Euphorbia hirta/pilulifera	Euphorbia
	Euphrasia officinalis	Eyebright
Murva	*Clematis tribola*	Bowstring hemp
Musali	*Asparagus adscendens/officinalis*	

(Continued)

Ayurvedic name	Latin name	English name
Musta	*Cyperus rotundus*	Musta
Nagakesaka	*Messua ferra*	Cobra's saffron
Neem/nimba	*Azadirachta indica*	Margosa tree
Padmaka	*Prunus cirasoidus*	Bird cherry
Parpataka	*Fumaria indica/parviflora*	Fumitory
Patha	*Cissempelus pareira*	Velvet leaf
Patola	*Trichosanthes kirilowii*	Serpent gourd
Pippali	*Piper longum*	Long pepper
Punarnava	*Boerhavia diffusa*	Indian hogweed
Raktachandana	*Petrocarpus santalinus*	Red sandalwood
Rohisham	*Cymbopogon citratus*	Lemon grass
	Tilea europea	Limeflowers
Sahadeva	*Vernonia cineria*	Fleabane
Sariva	*Hemidesmus indicus*	Indian sarsparilla
Sarsapa	*Brassica alba or nigra*	Mustard
Shankapushpi	*Convolvulus pluricaulis*	Shankapushpi
Shata pushpa	*Foeniculum vulgare*	Fennel
Shatavari	*Asparagus racemosus*	Wild asparagus
Shilajit	*Asphaltum*	Mineral pitch
Sallaki	*Boswellia carteri/serrata*	Frankincense
	Gentiana lutea	Gentian
	Ginkgo biloba	Gingko
	Panax ginseng	Ginseng
	Solidago virgaurea	Golden rod
	Hydrastis canadensis	Golden seal
	Chelidonium majus	Greater celandine
	Grindelia camporum	Grindelia
	Nepeta hederacea	Ground ivy
	Viola tricolor	Heartsease
	Eupatorium cannabinum	Hemp
	Geranium robertianum	Herb Robert
	Lonicera spp.	Honeysuckle
	Humulus lupulus	Hops
		Horehound
	Equisetum arvense	Horsetail
Tagara	*Valeriana wallichi*	Indian valerian, tagar
Tailparna	*Eucalyptus globulus*	Eucalyptus
Talisa/Talisha/Talispatra	*Abies webbiana*	Silver fir
Tamalapatra	*Cinnamomum tamal/zeylanicum*	Cinnamon
Taruni	*Rosa* spp.	Rose
	Rosmarinus officinalis	Rosemary
Tulsi	*Ocimum sanctum*	Sacred/holy basil
Tulsi	*Ocimum basilicum*	Basil
	Laurus nobilis	Bay tree
	Sanguinaria canadensis	Blood root
	Iris versicolor	Blue flag
	Eupatorium perfoliatum	Boneset

Ayurvedic name	Latin name	English name
	Borago officinalis	Borage
	Bupleurum chinense	Bupleurum root
	Arctium lappa	Burdock
	Juglans cinera	Butternut
	Melaleuca leucadendron	Cajeput
	Nepeta cataria	Catnip
		Cat's claw bark
Udumbara	*Ficus racemosa*	Cluster fig
Vacha	*Acorus calamus*	Sweet flag
Vamsha	*Bambosa arundinacea*	Bamboo
Vamsha lochana	*Bambosa bambos*	Bamboo manna
Varuna	*Crateava nurvala*	Three leaved caper
Vasa/vasak	*Adhatoda vasica*	Malabar nut
Vidanga	*Embelia ribes*	Vidanga
	Pimpinella anisum	
	Agrimonia eupatoria	Agrimony
Yashti madhu	*Glycyrrhiza glabra*	Liquorice
	Lobelia inflata	Lobelia
		Lotus seeds
	Pulmonaria officinalis	Lungwort
	Calendula officinalis	Marigold
	Origanum marjorana	Marjoram
	Althea officinalis	Marshmallow
	Filipendula ulmaria	Meadowsweet
	Viscum album	Mistletoe
	Verbascum thapsus	Mullein
	Urtica dioica/urens	Nettle, stinging
	Quercus robur	Oak bark
	Citrus vulgaris/aurantium	Orange blossom/Neroli
	Origanum vulgare	Oregano
	Petroselinum crispum	Parsley
	Passiflora incarnata	Passionflower
	Mentha pulegium	Pennyroyal
	Mentha piperita	Peppermint
	Perilla frutescens	Perilla leaf
	Pinus sylvestris	Pine
	Plantago major	Plantain
	Asclepias tuberosa	Pleurisy root
	Portulaca oleracea	Purslane
	Pricasma excelsa	Quassia
	Rubus idaeus	Raspberry
	Trifolium pratense	Red clover
	Rheum palmatum	Rhubarb

Appendix 2

The Ayurvedic questionnaire for assessing your basic constitution: Prakruti

Characteristic	*Vata* attribute	*Pitta* attribute	*Kapha* attribute	If none specify
Weight	☐ low	☐ medium	☐ heavy	☐
Body frame	☐ small	☐ medium	☐ large	☐
Muscles	☐ not muscular	☐ muscular	☐ soft, flabby	☐
Height	☐ unusually short ☐ unusually tall	☐ medium height	☐ small and stout ☐ large and stout	☐
Hips	☐ narrow	☐ medium	☐ wide	☐
Shoulders	☐ narrow	☐ medium	☐ wide	☐
Chest	☐ small	☐ normal	☐ large	☐
Hair	☐ dry, brittle ☐ curled ☐ thin ☐ dark	☐ straight ☐ oily ☐ blond, red ☐ shiny ☐ greasy	☐ thick ☐ oily ☐ curly ☐ lustrous	☐ ☐
Body hair	☐ scanty	☐ moderate	☐ thick	☐
Face	☐ irregular features	☐ prominent features	☐ rounded	☐
Eyes	☐ small ☐ dry	☐ medium ☐ red	☐ large ☐ moist	☐
Nose	☐ small ☐ long, bent	☐ medium ☐ straight, pointed	☐ large ☐ wide	☐
Lips	☐ small ☐ dark	☐ medium ☐ soft, red	☐ large ☐ velvety	☐
Teeth	☐ not straight	☐ medium, straight	☐ large, straight	☐

Characteristic	*Vata* attribute	*Pitta* attribute	*Kapha* attribute	If none specify
Skin	☐ rough, dry ☐ cold ☐ thin ☐ tans easily	☐ oily ☐ warm, moist ☐ burns easily, freckled	☐ soft and smooth ☐ cool and oily ☐ tends to burn, pale	☐ ☐ ☐
Veins	☐ easily visible	☐ moderately visible	☐ not visible	☐
Nails	☐ brittle ☐ dry, ridged	☐ well formed ☐ soft	☐ strong, thick ☐ smooth	☐
Fingers	☐ small, long	☐ regular	☐ wide, plump	☐
Hands and feet	☐ cold, dry	☐ warm, pink	☐ cool, damp	☐
Body fat	☐ around the waist	☐ evenly distributed	☐ around thighs and buttocks	☐
Energy level	☐ very active	☐ normally active	☐ lethargic	☐
Movement	☐ rather fast	☐ medium speed	☐ slow and steady	☐
Lifestyle	☐ erratic	☐ busy, regular	☐ steady, slow	☐
Memory	☐ good short term ☐ quick to grasp ☐ quick to forget	☐ medium ☐ sharp ☐ clear	☐ good long term ☐ slow to grasp ☐ never forgets	☐
Mood	☐ changes quickly	☐ intense, changes quickly	☐ steady, non- changing	☐
Speech	☐ fast, chaotic ☐ interrupted	☐ sharp ☐ clear and precise	☐ slow, monotonous ☐ melodious	☐
Creativity	☐ rich in ideas	☐ inventive, technical	☐ methodical	☐
Sleep	☐ light, easily interrupted ☐ 5–6 hours	☐ short and even ☐ 6–8 hours	☐ long and deep ☐ over 8 hours	☐
Eating habits	☐ irregular	☐ regular	☐ snack between meals	☐
Appetite	☐ variable	☐ strong, cannot miss meals	☐ mild, can miss meals	☐

Glossary 1

Ayurvedic herbs and formulae

CHURNAS/POWDERS

Dhartree churna

- Ingredients: Triphala, liquorice, senna
- Properties: Laxative, *ama pachana*, clears toxins from the gut
- Uses: To clear *ama* from the gut in *Pitta* and *Kapha* problems. Avoid in *Vata* conditions and in small children
- Dose: $\frac{1}{2}$ tsp at night in a little warm water.

Hingwastaka churna: Asafoetida 8 compound

- Ingredients: Asafoetida, ginger, black pepper, long pepper, rock salt, cumin, black cumin, ajwan
- Properties: Carminative, stimulant, antispasmodic. Decreases *Vata* and *Kapha*, increases *Pitta*
- Uses: Abdominal distension, gas, colic, indigestion, poor appetite
- Dose: 1–4 g or 2–8 tablets, 2–3 times daily in warm water.

Lavanbhashkar churna: five salts compound

- Ingredients: 5 salts, fennel, long pepper, long pepper root, black cumin, cinnamon leaf, nagakeshar, talisha, rhubarb root, pomegranate seeds, cinnamon, cardamom
- Properties: Stimulant, carminative, laxative. Decreases *Vata*, increases *agni* and *Pitta*
- Uses: Loss of appetite, malabsorption, constipation, abdominal pain
- Dose: 1–4 g or 2–8 tablets, 2–3 times daily in warm water or buttermilk.

Rasayana churna: rejuvenation powder

- Ingredients: Guduchi, gokshura, amalaki
- Properties: Bitter tonic, demulcent, alterative, diuretic, antacid
- Uses: General debility, skin rashes, allergies, chronic fevers or infections. Good rejuvenative tonic for *Pitta*, particularly after febrile diseases
- Dose: 1–4 g or 2–8 tablets, 2–3 times daily in raw sugar and ghee, or in milk.

Sitopaladi churna: rock candy compound powder

- Ingredients: Rock candy, bamboo manna, long pepper, cardamom, cinnamon
- Properties: Expectorant, antitussive, decongestant
- Uses: Colds, coughs, lack of appetite, fever, debility, burning sensation in extremities. Major anti-*Kapha* formula, reduces *Vata*
- Dose: 1–4 g or 2–8 tablets, 2–4 times daily in honey or ghee.

Talisadi churna

- Ingredients: Talisha, trikatu, bamboo manna, cardamom, cinnamon, raw sugar
- Properties: Expectorant, antitussive, stimulant
- Uses: Colds, flu, bronchitis, asthma, loss of appetite, indigestion, chronic fever. Mainly anti-*Kapha*
- Dose: 1–4 g or 2–8 tablets, twice daily in honey.

Trikatu powder

- Ingredients: Black pepper, long pepper, ginger
- Properties: Stimulant, expectorant
- Uses: Lack of appetite, indigestion, cough, congestion. Specific for low *Agni* and high *Ama*, (weak digestive fire and accumulations of toxins). Reduces *Kapha* and *Vata*, increases *Pitta*
- Dose: 1–3 g or 2–6 tablets, 2–3 times daily in honey or warm water.

Trikulu churna

- Ingredients: Clove, cinnamon, cardomum.

Triphala churna

- Ingredients: The most famous Ayurvedic compound, Triphala, or the "three fruits" consists of fruits of three tropical trees, called "myrobalan plums", haritaki, amalaki and bibhitaki
- Properties: Laxative, tonic, rejuvenative, astringent
- Uses: Chronic constipation, abdominal gas and distension, eye diseases, chronic diarrhoea. Good for all three *doshas*
- Triphala is considered the best and safest bowel cleanser as well as a tonic and rejuvenative

(*rasayana*). It improves digestive fire, enhancing appetite and digestion and has a reputation for nourishing the nervous system. It is good for constipation in any of the *doshas,* although it is not always effective in acute constipation. As a metabolic regulator, it helps to reduce weight while having a strengthening and nutritive effect upon deeper tissues including blood, muscle and nerve tissue in those who are underweight.

- Triphala can be taken with digestive spices such as trikatu, thus combining a bowel cleanser (*ama pachana*) with remedies to raise the digestive fire (*agni deepana*). Triphala is useful not only in *ama* conditions but also part of a regular diet for preventing the accumulation of *ama.*
- Dose: 5–10 g once daily in warm water, ghee or honey before sleep.

GUGGULS

Gugguls are pills made with the purified resin of guggul, *Commipoha mukul,* a relative of myrrh. Guggul is purified by boiling it with various herbal decoctions such as Triphala and straining out the purified resin. A variety of different herbal powders or extracts are added to the purified guggul resin, often with ghee. They are mainly used for treating arthritis, nervous system disorders, skin problems, (high cholesterol and triglycerides in adults) and obesity.

Gokshuradi guggul: tribulis compound guggul

- Ingredients: Guggul, gokshura, Trikatu, musta
- Properties: Diuretic, alterative, demulcent
- Uses: Difficult urination, arthritis, urinary infections
- Dose: 2–5 pills, 2–3 times daily in cyperus tea, vetivert tea.

Triphala guggul

- Ingredients: Guggul, triphala, long pepper
- Properties: Alterative, anti-inflammatory, antibiotic, antiseptic

- Uses: Boils, abscesses, haemorrhoids, nasal polyps, oedema, arthritis. Cleansing and detoxifying for *Vata,* particularly in *Sama* conditions or when *Vata* has entered the lymph or blood
- Dose: 2–5 pills, 2–3 times daily in warm water.

HERBAL WINES

There are two types of herbal wines, *asavas* and *arishtas.* They are herbal fermentations, made in a similar way to grape wine, in large wooden vats and are considered easier on the digestion than other herbal preparations. Many contain spices which not only improve their taste but also their assimilation. They are particularly good for *Vata.*

Asavas are made with fresh herbal juices and *arishtas* are made with decoctions of herbs, i.e. they have been boiled first. Dhataki flowers are added and they are left to self-ferment.

Kumariasava: aloe herbal wine

- Ingredients: Aloe gel, jaggery, honey, trikatu, triphala and other spices
- Properties: Alterative, tonic, blood tonic
- Uses: Anaemia, poor endocrine function, cough, asthma, constipation, liver problems
- Dose: 10–25 ml with equal amount of water twice daily after meals.

Balarishta: bala herbal wine

- Ingredients: Bala, ashwagandha, jaggery, dhataki, ela, erand
- Properties: Restorative tonic
- Uses: For all symptoms associated with *Vata* derangement
- Dose: 10–25 ml with equal quantity of water twice daily after meals.

Ashwagandharishta: ashwagandha herbal wine

- Ingredients: Ashwagandha, white musali, manjishta, liquorice, turmeric, Trikatu, sandalwood, calamus, dhataki, jaggery
- Properties: Nerve tonic, sedative
- Uses: Nervous debility, convalescence, insomnia, anxiety and tension
- Dose: 10–25 ml with equal amount of water twice daily after meals.

Draksharishta: grape herbal wine

- Ingredients: Mainly raisins, honey, sugar, dhataki, and various spices
- Properties: Stimulant, carminative, diuretic
- Uses: Loss of appetite, indigestion, general debility, insomnia, cough. Good for *Vata* type weak digestion, poor absorption
- Dose: 10–25 ml with equal amount of water twice daily after meals.

Dasmularishta

- Ingredients: *Desmodium gangeticum* – shalaparni, *Ureria picta* – prusnaparni, *Solanum indicum* – vruhati, *Solanum xanthocerpum* – kantakari, *Tribulus terrestris* – Gokshura, *Aegle marmelos* – bilva, *Oroxylum indicum* – syonaka, *Smelina arborea* – gambari, *Premna integrifolia* – ganikarica
- Properties: Balances VPK, rejuvenative tonic, nervine
- Uses: Respiratory disease, skin problems, poor appetite, anaemia, urinary problems, convalescence, nourishing for all *Vata* problems
- Dose: 10–25 ml with equal amount of water twice daily after meals.

HERBAL JELLIES

These are herbal jams/jellies prepared with raw sugar, i.e. jaggery or with honey, which are considered excellent tonics. The sugar acts as a preservative, improves the taste of the preparation and enhances their tonic properties.

Chyawan prash

The most famous of all herbal jellies chyawan prash is good for almost any weakness condition or as an energy supplement for all three *doshas*. The main ingredient is amalaki, the highest natural source of vitamin C.

- Ingredients: Amalaki, long pepper, bamboo manna, cloves, bilva, cinnamon, cardamom, cubebs, ghee, raw sugar
- Properties: Nutritive tonic, rejuvenative
- Uses: General debility, convalescence, nervous exhaustion, loss of weight, poor immunity, anaemia, chronic cough, tendency to chest problems, asthma
- Dose: 1–2 tsp, 2–3 times daily in milk.

TAILAS: MEDICATED OILS

These are a speciality of Ayurveda. They are combinations of many tonic herbs and sometimes analgesic herbs, prepared mainly with sesame oil. They are used in massage and oleation therapy for external nourishment and are considered not as supplements to treatment but as a treatment in themselves.

Bringaraj taila: eclipta oil

- Ingredients: Bringaraj juice, sesame oil
- Properties: Antiseptic, hair tonic, nervine
- Uses: An excellent hair and scalp conditioner. Also calms the mind.

Brahmi taila: gotu kola oil

- Ingredients: Gotu kola and other nervine herbs in coconut oil
- Properties: Nervine, sedative, antipyretic
- Uses: Insomnia, mental agitation, headache, eye-ache, ADD + ADHD, general brain tonic.

Mahanaryan taila

- Ingredients: Contains 58 herbals including shatavari, cow's milk, ashwagandha, castor root, gokshura, neem, bilva, bala, sesame oil
- Properties: Demulcent, emollient, analgesic
- Uses: muscle + joint pain. Most commonly used oil for pain.

Ann taila

- Ingredients: Contains 32 ingredients including devadaru, cinnamon, sariva, daruharidra liquorice, musta, ela, sandalwood, Triphala, bilva
- Properties: Decongestant, antiseptic
- Uses: For colds, catarrh, rhinitis, sinusitis
- Dose: 2 drops in each nostril morning and night.

Glossary 2

Sanskrit terms

Abhyanga	massage
Agni	digestive enzymes/digestive "fire"
Ajirna/ajeerna	indigestion
Akasha	space, one of the five elements
Alochak Pitta	one of the five subtypes of *Pitta*, the form of fire governing vision
Ama	toxins, the undigested food mass
Amla	sour
Annavaha srota	digestive system channels of transport
Anupana	food medium or vehicle that transports herbs to the tissue levels (e.g., honey)
Ap	water element
Apana Vayu	one of the five *Vata* subdoshas; downward moving air
Arishta	herbal wine made with decoctions
Arogya	health
Asava	herbal wine made with juice of herbs
Asthi	bone tissue
Astivaha srota	bone channels
Atisara	diarrhoea
Avalambak Kapha	one of the five subtypes of *Kapha*, the form of water giving support
Basti	medicated enema – one of the five *pancha karma* therapies
Bhrajak Pitta	one of the five subtypes of *Pitta*, the form of fire governing complexion
Bhutagnis	five digestive enzymes/fires that metabolize the five elements
Bodhak Kapha	one of the five subtypes of *Kapha*, the form of water governing taste
Brahma	Reality; the Absolute
Chikitsa	Ayurvedic treatment
Churna	herbal powder
Chyawan prash	herbal rejuvenative jam with amalaki and ghee as its main ingredients
Dhanvantari	Divine father of Ayurveda
Dhara drava	medicated oil for the head
Dharma	life purpose or life path; God-given talent
Dhatuagnis	seven digestive enzymes that metabolize the seven tissue layers
Dhatu	tissue

Dosha	a principal humour which governs biological and psychological functions of the mind/body
Draksha	herbal wine made from grapes and other spices
Ghee	clarified butter
Ghrita	another word for ghee
Grahani	digestive disorders affecting the intestine, e.g. IBS
Guda	(jaggery) a form of pure cane sugar
Guna	prime quality of nature (prakriti)
Gunas	three qualities or the fundamental laws of nature (sattva: creation, rajas: maintenance, tamas: dissolution)
Guru	heavy (one of the gunas); that which is digested slowly and increases *Kapha*
Guti	herbal pills
Hima	cold infusions
Jaggery	(guda) a form of pure cane sugar
Jatharagni	digestive enzymes in the GI tract, digestive "fire"
Jwara	fever
Kama	healthy and spiritual use of the senses
Kapha	biological water – humour – one of the doshas
Karma	action
Kasa	cough
Kasaya	astringent (one of the six tastes/*rasas*); Increases *Vata*
Katu	pungent (one of the six tastes/*rasas*); Increases *Pitta* and *Vata*
Kaumara bhritya	paediatrics; one of the eight branches of Ayurvedic medicine
Kayachikitsa	internal medicine; one of the eight branches of Ayurvedic medicine
Khara	rough quality of food
Kichari	grain/legume meal; usually basmati rice and mungdal
Kledaka Kapha	one of the five forms of *Kapha*, the form of water governing digestion
Krimi	parasites
Kushtha	obstinate skin diseases
Kwatha	herbal decoction
Laghu	light (one of the gunas); easy to digest. Increases *Vata* and *Pitta*, decreases *Kapha*
Langhana	reduction or lightening therapy
Lavana	salty (one of the six tastes/*rasas*); Increases *Pitta* and *Kapha*
Lepa	herbal paste or poultice
Madhur	sweet (one of the six tastes/*rasas*); Increases *Kapha*, decreases *Pitta*
Majja	marrow and nerve tissue
Majjavaha srota	marrow/joint lubrication channels
Mala	waste produce (i.e., urine, sweat, faeces)
Mamsa	muscle tissue
Mamasvaha srota	muscle channels
Manas	mind
Manda	slow quality of e.g. digestion
Mandagni	low digestive "fire"
Marma	energy points on the body
Medas	fat tissue
Medovaha srota	srota adipose/fat channels
Moksha	Self-realization
Mridu	soft quality of food

Mutra	urine
Mutravaha srota	urinary channels
Nadi	nerve channels
Nasya	nasal application of herbs and oils
Neti	small vessel that looks like a miniature watering can; used for nasal washing
Netra basti	medicated eye bath
Nidana	diagnosis, aetiology, cause of disease
Nirama	conditions without Ama
Niruha basti	oily enema
Ojas	prime energy of the body
Pachaka Pitta	one of the five types of *Pitta*, the form of fire governing digestion
Pancha Karma	the five purification practices of Ayurveda
Peya	thin soup taken after *pancha karma* therapies
Phanta	hot infusions
Pinda sveda	*abhyanga* therapy using a heated bolus
Pitta	biological fire – humour, one of the doshas
Prabhava	special effects of herbs, foods
Prakriti	one's basic constitution or nature
Prana	life-force; inward-moving air
Pranayama	breathing exercises
Prana Vayu/Vata	one of the five *Vata* subdoshas, outward moving air
Pranavaha srota	channel through which *prana* flows
Pritivi	earth, one of the five elements
Purisha	faeces, waste products
Purusha	eternal, unmanifest Consciousness
Purva karma	preliminary *pancha karma* therapies (oleation and sudation)
Purvarupa	hidden or incubatory signs of disease
Pushti	nourishing
Rajas/rajasic	law of nature that maintains life; one of the three gunas
Rakta	blood tissue
Ranjaka Pitta	one of the five types of *Pitta*, the form of fire colouring the blood
Rajas	quality of energy, turbulence and distraction, one of the three gunas
Rasa	the initial taste of a substance; sweet, sour, salt, pungent, bitter or astringent and the 1st tissue/abatu
Rasayana	rejuvenative
Ruksha	unctuous (one of the gunas)
Sadhaka Pitta	one of the five types of *Pitta*, the form of fire governing intelligence
Sama Kapha	ama condition of *Kapha*
Sama Pitta	ama condition of *Pitta*
Sama Vata	ama condition of *Vata*
Samana Vayu/ Vata	one of the five types of *Vata*, equalizing air, governs digestion
Sattva	quality of clarity and harmony, the mind in its natural state, one of the three gunas
Shamana	palliation therapy
Shita	cold (one of the gunas)
Shodhana	purification therapy
Shukra	reproductive tissue
Sleshak Kapha	one of the five types of *Kapha*, the form of water lubricating joints

Snehana	oil application
Snigdha	oily (one of the gunas)
Srotas	channel systems of the body
Stanyavahasrotas	channels carrying the breast milk
Sveda	sweat
Svedana	therapeutic sweating, steam therapy
Taila	medicated oil, mainly made with sesame oil
Tarpak Kapha	one of the five types of *Kapha*, the form of water governing emotion
Tikshna	hot, fast acting, sharp (one of the gunas)
Tikta	bitter (one of the six tastes/*rasas*); Increases *Vata* and *Pitta*
Tridosha	three basic forces of the universe. The combination of the five elements gives the three doshas; which influence all mental and physical processes
Udana Vayu/Vata	one of the five types of *Vata*, upward moving air
Ushna	hot
Vamana	emesis; therapeutic vomiting
Vata	biological air-humour. One of the doshas
Vedas	ancient scriptures of India
Veerya	the potency of the drug, either heating or cooling
Vikriti	disease nature. The present constitutional balance of *Vata/Pitta/Kapha* in an individual
Vipaka	post digestive effect of a herb or food related to its taste: sweet, sour or pungent
Virechana	purgation therapy
Vyana Vayu/Vata	one of the five types of *Vata*, diffusive or outward moving air

Glossary 3

Western terms

Alterative	producing beneficial effects through detoxification
Amoebicidal	kills amoebae
Anabolic	helps in constructive metabolic processes
Analgesia	alleviation of pain
Anodyne	relieves pain
Anthelmintic	destroys worms
Antibacterial	destroys bacteria or suppresses their growth/reproduction
Anticonvulsant	prevention or relief of convulsions
Antifungal	destroys fungi or suppresses their growth/reproduction
Antihistamine	counteracts the effects of histamine in an allergic response
Anti-inflammatory	helping to counter/resolve the inflammatory process
Antimalarial	used in the treatment of malaria
Antimicrobial	kills micro-organisms or suppresses their multiplication/growth
Antineoplastic	inhibits the development and proliferation of malignant cells/tumours
Antioxidant	significantly delays or prevents oxidation by destroying free radicals
Antipyretic	reduces fever
Antiseptic	inhibits the growth and development of pathogenic micro-organisms
Antispasmodic	relieves spasm, usually of smooth muscle
Antiviral	destroys viruses or suppresses their replication
Appetizer	increases the desire for food
Astringent	causing contraction, drying
Bactericide	destroys bacteria or suppresses their reproduction
Cardiotonic	has a tonic effect on the heart, improving strength of beat
Carminative	relieves flatulence
Choleretic	stimulates the flow of bile
Counterirritant	causes a superficial irritation, intended to relieve pain in a deeper part of the body
Decoction	herbal formulation prepared by boiling the plant parts in water
Decongestant	reduces congestion
Demulcent	soothing, mucilaginous or oily formulation which allays irritation of inflamed surfaces
Dentifrice	preparation used with a toothbrush for cleaning the teeth

Deobstruent	prevents obstruction
Depurative	purifying or cleansing
Detoxification	removal of toxins and wastes
Diaphoretic	promotion of perspiration
Diuretic	promotes the excretion of urine
Emetic	causes vomiting
Emmenagogue	induces menstruation
Emollient	softens or soothes irritated skin or mucous membranes
Expectorant	promotes the expulsion of mucus from the respiratory tract
Febrifuge	reduces body temperature in fever
Free radical	highly reactive molecule with an unpaired electron that causes damage to tissues
Galactagogue	promotes the flow of milk
Haemostat	checks bleeding; styptic
Hypocholesterolaemic	reduces levels of blood cholesterol
Hypoglycaemic	lowers the level of glucose in the blood
Hypolipidaemic	reduces serum lipid concentrations
Hypotensive	lowers blood pressure
Immunomodulator	augments or diminishes immune responses
Infusion	tea made from steeping a herb in water to extract its medicinal properties
Insecticide	substance selectively poisonous to insects
Laxative	promotion of evacuation of the bowel
Refrigerant	reduces bodily heat or fever
Restorative	capable of restoring health or strength
Rubefacient	reddens the skin by increasing the blood flow
Sedative	reduces nervousness and anxiety, promotes sleep
Stimulant	produces stimulation of the central nervous system
Stomachic	enhances the functional activity of the stomach
Thermogenic	producing heat
Tonic	term used for medicinal preparations intended to restore normal tone or function to tissues
Unctuous	greasy or oily; oleaginous
Vermifuge	expels worms or intestinal parasites; anthelmintic

Index

(All major references are in **bold**)

Printed and bound by CPI Group (UK) Ltd, Croydon, CR0 4YY

03/10/2024

01040345-0010